Pharmacology

PHARMACOLOGY

A Review with Questions and Explanations

Manuchair Ebadi, Ph.D.

Professor and Chairman
Department of Pharmacology
University of Nebraska College of Medicine
Omaha

Little, Brown and Company   Boston/Toronto

Library of Congress Catalog Card No. 84-52688

ISBN 0-316-20416-1

Printed in the United States of America

MV

It is with affection and gratitude that I dedicate this book to my teachers for inspiring me to learn and to my students for encouraging me to teach

Contents

Preface

Diagnosing and treating a disease, whether by a physician, by a nurse, or by other members of the health care delivery team, is a complex undertaking that requires the acquisition of extensive knowledge in basic and clinical sciences including pharmacology and toxicology.

This review book, *Pharmacology*, is intended to give special consideration to mechanisms of action of drugs and the problems of drug-drug interactions. It does not profess to enumerate and discuss all drugs but only the agents most often used. Special care has been taken to emphasize pharmacologic concepts and their involvement in reverting pathologic states into physiologic states. Every attempt is made to discuss the potential and most often occurring side effects of drugs and how they can be avoided or minimized. This review does not offer an encyclopedic account of all reported side effects or drug interactions. This philosophy of education is consistent with the 1984 report of the Association of American Medical Colleges' panel on the General Professional Education of the Physician that "medical faculties must limit the amount of factual information that students are expected to memorize."

It is expected and hoped that the pharmacologic concepts to be learned here will then guide students of medicine to seek and gather additional extensive knowledge in pharmacology, in therapeutics, and in toxicology from the various references cited at the end of each chapter. By doing so, the physicians, the dentists, the nurses, the pharmacists, and other members of the health care delivery team will be able to fulfill their obligations to society in alleviating the physical and mental sufferings of human beings.

This review may be used in conjunction with a more extensive textbook while completing a required course in pharmacology. However, since the materials are presented in a fashion to integrate basic knowledge and clinical information, the book will be especially useful to medical, nursing, dental, pharmacy, and graduate students, and house officers when preparing for MSKP, Flex, ECFMG, VQE, national boards, specialty boards, or comprehensive examinations. In addition, the concepts outlined in the 365 questions appearing in this review book are fundamental principles often emphasized by pharmacologists or toxicologists.

I extend my appreciation to Margaret McCall and Janet Roche Johnson for their expert secretarial and artistic assistance. The interest of Dr. Reba Benschoter, Director of the Biomedical Communication Education Program, is acknowledged.

Finally, the support of the members of the faculty of the Department of Pharmacology at the University of Nebraska College of Medicine, especially that of Dr. Carl F. Gessert, is recognized and admired. Their dedication to teaching exemplifies the notion of Martin H. Fischer that knowledge is the accumulation of science, and wisdom lies in its simplification.

M. E.

Introduction

Appropriate drug therapy improves the quality of life, whereas injudicious drug therapy may result in drug-induced diseases. Physicians and dentists administer medications for diagnostic, prophylactic, or therapeutic purposes. The prescribed medications bring about the desired effects in most patients but may prove to be inert and ineffective in some or may result in totally unexpected responses and precipitate harmful reactions in others.

Iatrogenic diseases and medication-induced problems could probably be reduced substantially if physicians or other members of the health care delivery team were fully acquainted with the principles of pharmacokinetics and remained constantly cognizant of possible unexpected interactions between drugs and ailing human bodies. One way to avoid overdosage and at the same time enhance the efficacy and safety of drug therapy is to prescribe drugs, not on the basis of body weight but according to the achieved plasma concentrations of drugs in their active forms. This practice is often essential in pediatric and geriatric patients and in patients with genetic abnormalities in whom the rate of absorption, distribution, biotransformation, and excretion of drugs is developing, is declining, or is altered. Similarly, this practice is useful in chronically medicated individuals such as patients with epilepsy, Parkinson's disease, and endocrine and metabolic disorders, in whom the treatment may have to be continued during their lifetime [2].

Pharmacology may be defined as "the study of the selective biologic activity of chemical substances on living matter" [1]. Often, but not always, selective biologic activities are caused by very small amounts of drugs. For example, in hypothyroidism, one gives a daily dose of 50 μg of thyroxine for 1 to 2 weeks, a daily dose of 100 μg for 3 to 4 weeks, and then a permanent daily dose of approximately 150 ug. Similarly, the recommended daily allowance of vitamin B_{12} is small, being 0.5 μg in infants and 3.0 μg in adults. Dactinomycin is used in doses of 15 μg/kg/day for 5 days in the treatment of hospitalized patients with Wilms's tumor.

The effects of a drug should be selective, and the responses should occur in some but not all cells. Acetylcholine, which produces widespread cholinergic actions with a short duration of action, is not useful as a drug. Methacholine, carbachol, and bethanechol, the synthetic derivatives of acetylcholine, are resistant to hydrolysis and are more specific in their actions. The recognition of adrenergic receptor subtypes as $alpha_1$, $alpha_2$, and $beta_1$, $beta_2$ has resulted in the synthesis of highly specific agonists and antagonists for adrenergic receptor sites. For example, stimulation of $beta_1$ receptors causes cardiac stimula-

tion and lipolysis, whereas stimulation of $beta_2$ is responsible for bronchodilation and vasodepression. $Beta_2$ agonists are especially useful in the treatment of asthma because they produce bronchodilation without much cardiac acceleration.

The use of drugs in the treatment of a disease is termed *pharmacotherapeutics*. In managing a disease, however, the use of drugs is not always necessary. For example, adult-onset diabetes may be managed by diet and exercise alone. Although in some feverish individuals an antipyretic such as acetylsalicylic acid (aspirin) is used to reduce fever, there are infections such as neurosyphilis, some gonococcal infections, and chronic brucellosis in which pyrexia seems to be beneficial to the host.

A drug may be used substitutively, supportively, prophylactically, symptomatically, diagnostically, or correctively. In juvenile-onset diabetes mellitus and in Addison's syndrome, insulin and cortisone acetate are used respectively as substitutes or supplements for substances whose production never existed, or initially existed but now has ceased. In adult-onset diabetes mellitus, oral antidiabetic agents are used to support the physiologic function of the body by stimulating the synthesis and release of insulin.

Oral contraceptive tablets are used to prevent pregnancy. Isoniazid may be used to prevent the development of active tuberculosis (1) in individuals who have been exposed to tuberculosis but have no evidence of infection, (2) in those with a positive test for tuberculosis and no apparent disease, and (3) in individuals with a history of tuberculosis in whom the disease is currently inactive.

Drugs may eliminate or reduce the symptoms of a disease without influencing the pathology. Fever may be associated with respiratory tract infection, bacterial endocarditis, biliary tract disorders, tuberculosis, carcinoma, cirrhosis of the liver, collagen diseases, encephalitis, glomerulonephritis, Hodgkin's disease, hysteria, malaria, leukemia, measles, mumps, and plague, to name a few. Aspirin reduces fever in these cases without altering the disease processes themselves.

A drug may also be used to diagnose a disease. Histamine has been used to assess the ability of the stomach to secrete acid and to determine parietal cell mass. Anacidity or hyposecretion in response to histamine may reflect pernicious anemia, atrophic gastritis, or gastric carcinoma, whereas a hypersecretory response may be found in patients with duodenal ulcer or with the Zollinger-Ellison syndrome.

In the majority of cases, drugs do not *cure* diseases but do correct the symptoms associated with them. For example, antidiarrheal agents check diarrhea, and laxatives correct constipation. No drugs exist that cure essential hypertension, although there are some that lower blood pressure. No drugs have been synthesized that cure arthritis, although a number of them reduce the pain and immobility associated with it.

In correcting symptoms, drugs never create new functions. They stimulate or depress the functions already inherent in the cells. Oral antidiabetic agents stimulate the pancreas and not the kidney to release insulin.

In correcting symptoms, drugs may produce adverse effects, which may or may not be acceptable to the patients. Numerous agents with anticholinergic properties cause dry mouth, which is easily correctable and hence is acceptable. Conversely, some antihypertensive medications cause impotence in male patients, a condition they find unacceptable, and thus this side effect leads to lack of compliance with the prescribed medication.

It is clear that drugs resembling the proverbial double-edged sword are able to help or hurt the patients further. By comprehension of pharmacokinetics and pharmacodynamic principles, and the full understanding of drug-drug interactions, one is able to reduce unwanted side effects drastically and to enhance the therapeutic efficacy and usefulness of drugs in modern medicine.

REFERENCES

1. Bevan, J. A. *Essentials of Pharmacology*. New York: Harper & Row, 1969.
2. Ebadi, M. The pharmacokinetic basis of therapeutics with special reference to drugs used in neurology. *Adv. Neurol.* 13:333, 1975.

I. Principles of Pharmacology

1. The Pharmacokinetic Basis of Therapeutics

Poisons and medicine are oftentimes the same substance given with different intents.

Peter Mere Latham

The primary therapeutic objectives should be to prevent and to cure diseases. If these goals are not achievable, the secondary therapeutic objectives should be to mitigate and to mollify by drugs the progressive, devastating, or disabling nature of diseases. The amount of drug or drugs to be given and the duration of therapy to be instituted depend on the nature of the disease to be treated. For example, an uncomplicated urinary tract infection may be cured with 10 days' treatment with a sulfonamide, whereas a patient with grand mal epilepsy may have to be treated for life with phenytoin or phenobarbital or both.

The successful prevention, cure, or treatment of diseases will depend on using drugs in sufficient amount to obtain the desirable effects and to avoid the harmful side effects. In the past, the therapeutic regimens of numerous drugs, including morphine and cardiac glycosides, were established by empiric observations and by trial and error. Dealing often with naturally occurring drugs, physicians chose the drugs, decided on doses and frequency of administration, noted and recorded the beneficial effects, and adjusted the regimen if toxic reactions had occurred [9].

Today, advances in pharmacology and in therapeutics have broadened our appreciation of (1) the mechanisms involved in disposition of drugs by the body, (2) the inherent ability of drugs to modify the physiologic integrity of the host, and (3) the interactions between drugs when present simultaneously in the body and the competition between them for each to influence or to be influenced by the organism. By being cognizant of these pharmacologic principles, by applying them fully, and by remaining vigilant to countless interactions between drug and ailing body, one can substantially reduce the side effects of numerous drugs.

In the first three chapters, this triad of therapeutics is discussed by elaborating on the pharmacokinetics, the pharmacodynamics, and the drug-drug interactions.

PHARMACOKINETICS IN MEDICINE. Pharmacokinetic principles, which deal with the fate of drugs, discuss the absorption, distribution, binding, biotransformation, and excretion of drugs and their metabolites in the body (Fig. 1-1).

ADMINISTRATION OF DRUGS. Drugs are administered as a solid in the form of capsules, tablets, and pills (e.g., clonidine), as a volatile liquid (e.g., halothane, enflurane), as a solution (e.g., chlorpromazine), as an aerosol (e.g., beclomethasone), as a gas (e.g., oxygen, nitrous oxide), and as a crystalline suspension (e.g., insulin). The chosen route of administration is determined by the desired onset of action and duration of action of drugs, by the nature of the drugs, by special circumstances, and by the bioavailability of drugs.

In life-threatening conditions, or in circumstances wherein an immediate onset of action is required, drugs must be administered directly into the general circulation. In diabetic ketoacidosis, a large dose of insulin (2 U/kg initially, divided intravenously and subcutaneously, followed by 1 U/kg every 2 hours) is given until the concentration of glucose in the blood approaches normal values. In hypocalcemic tetany, calcium gluconate is administered as a 10% solution delivering 0.45 mEq Ca^{2+} per milliliter. Epinephrine or isoproterenol may be administered intracordally in cardiac arrest and heart block with syncopal seizures.

DURATION OF ACTION. If a long duration of action is desirable, one may administer a drug continuously or administer a drug in a long-acting form. For example, in pneumococcal meningitis, 20 to 40 million U of penicillin G are given daily by constant infusion drip or divided in doses given by intravenous bolus at 2- to 3-hour intervals. Penicillin G procaine suspension (e.g., Crysticillin, Duracillin), soluble in water only to the extent of 0.4 percent, is designed for deep intramuscular injection and slow absorption from the site of injection.

NATURE OF THE DRUGS. Proteinaceous drugs (insulin for diabetes mellitus, growth hormone for hypopituitary dwarfism, and oxytocin in dysfunctional labor) are destroyed in the stomach and naturally are not given orally. Actinomycin D (Cosmegen) used in Wilms's tumor, rhabdomyosarcoma, carcinomas of the testis and uterus, Ewing's sarcoma in adults, and choriocarcinoma, is designed for intravenous injection only. Severe necrosis has occurred when it was inadvertently deposited in tissues.

Fig. 1-1. *The pharmacokinetic principles.*

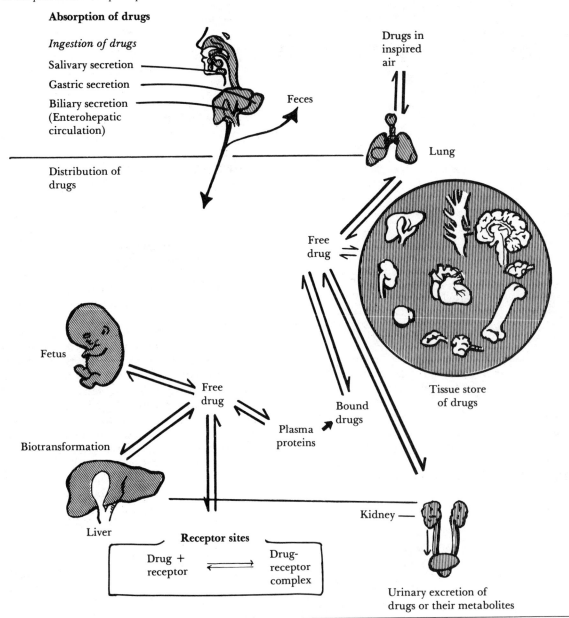

Absorption of drugs

Ingestion of drugs

Salivary secretion

Gastric secretion

Biliary secretion (Enterohepatic circulation)

Feces

Drugs in inspired air

Lung

Distribution of drugs

Free drug

Free drug

Fetus

Biotransformation

Plasma proteins

Bound drugs

Tissue store of drugs

Liver

Receptor sites

Drug + receptor ⇌ Drug-receptor complex

Kidney —

Urinary excretion of drugs or their metabolites

SPECIAL CIRCUMSTANCE. Drugs are applied to the mucous membranes of the conjunctiva, nasopharynx, and vagina for their local effects. Antidiuretic hormone (lypressin) is given by nasal spray, but the intention is to produce systemic effects. In meningeal leukemia, cytosine arabinoside (ara-C, Cytosar in a dose of 20–30 mg/m²) is injected directly into the spinal subarachnoid space. In osteoarthritis, corticosteroids are given by intraarticular injection.

BIOAVAILABILITY. The physiochemical nature of certain drugs may exclude the oral route of administration, and hence these drugs are said to have sub-

normal oral bioavailability. For example, nitroglycerin is given sublingually in angina pectoris because it is catabolized very rapidly in the liver if it is given orally. Spectinomycin in a single intramuscular injection of 2 gm is recommended in the treatment of acute genital and rectal gonorrhea in patients who are either allergic to penicillin or infected with a penicillinase-producing microorganism. Spectinomycin is not bound to plasma proteins and is excreted unchanged in active form in the urine.

ABSORPTION OF DRUGS. Although different mammalian cells vary greatly in shape, size, chemical composition, and function, they share certain basic similarities in their fine structures (e.g., plasma membrane, nucleus, mitochondria, Golgi apparatus, endoplasmic reticulum, ribosomes, lysosomes, microtubules, filaments, and centrioles). The thickness of the plasma membrane varies from cell to cell and even in the same cell at different times and with the nutritional status of the organism.

Membranes, whether belonging to a single-cell organism, such as an ameba, or to a highly complex being, such as a mammalian organism, have evolved to be functionally protective in nature. For example, the various lipoid barriers of the gastrointestinal tract, of kidney tubules, and of the central nervous system allow the absorption of essential nutrients, guard against uncontrollable disposal of electrolytes and other substances, and prevent the entrance of potentially toxic materials.

In order to reach its site of action (receptor site), a drug may have to traverse a succession of membranes. For example, phenytoin, when administered orally, must pass across the gastrointestinal epithelium, the blood-brain barrier, the plasma membrane, and finally the membranes of subcellular organelles of neurons. An understanding of how drugs traverse their various cellular and subcellular membranes is not only of academic interest, in terms of defining the nature of living membranes, but also of clinical significance, in terms of attaining the desired therapeutic level of an administered agent.

Electron microscopic studies suggest that all tissues have a fundamental structure called the unit membrane or plasma membrane. The membranes are composed of lipids and proteins in a ratio of 70:1. The current concept is that the lipid-soluble substances are able to traverse the membrane by dissolving in the lipoid phase, and the lipid-insoluble substances penetrate only when they are sufficiently small to pass through the pore. In addition, the absorption of large lipid-insoluble substances such as sugars and amino acids is accomplished by specialized transport processes.

Drug Particle Size and Drug Absorption. The rate of dissolution of a drug increases significantly as the size of drug particle decreases [8]. For example, the reduction in particle size of digoxin from 3 to 1 mm^3 increases the surface area of drug particles exposed to solution to the extent of 300 percent. The more soluble drugs are absorbed faster and more completely than the relatively insoluble ones. The oral bioavailability of numerous drugs has been increased by a reduction in particle size. On the other hand, decreasing particle size is not advantageous with compounds such as penicillin G and erythromycin that tend to decompose in the gastrointestinal tract. Similarly, it should be recalled that not all solubilized drugs are absorbed. For example, neomycin is soluble but is not absorbed from the gastrointestinal tract and is eliminated to the extent of 97 percent in the feces. Consequently, neomycin has been used orally as an intestinal antiseptic to prepare the bowel for surgery.

Passive Diffusion. Passive diffusion takes place when a drug molecule moves from a region of relatively high to one of low concentration without requiring energy. Diffusion and movement of drugs continue until an equilibrium has been achieved on both sides of the membrane. The equilibrium is achieved faster with highly permeable and hence lipid-soluble drugs and when there is a large surface area of membrane.

Carrier-Mediated Transport. The concept of "carrier-mediated" transport of drugs, although started as an armchair theory and assumption, has now been accepted. However, it is still ill defined and remains in a rudimentary stage of development. Essentially, the carrier concept assumes that the substance to be carried forms a complex with a component of the membrane on one side, the complex is carried through the membrane, the drug or the substance is released, and the carrier then returns to the original surface and state to repeat the process (Fig. 1-2A). The carrier shows specificity, since L-dopa but not D-dopa is transported [8].

Facilitated Transport. Facilitated transport is essentially the same as carrier-mediated transport, with the exception that, in addition to a carrier molecule, another transport facilitator is essential. For example, vitamin B_{12} attaches to intrinsic factor, and vitamin B_{12}–intrinsic factor complex in turn attaches to carrier molecule and is transported [8]. The transport process does not require energy and does not proceed against a concentration gradient (Fig. 1-2B).

Ion Pair Transport. Organic anions combine with organic cations to form a neutral complex, which is then transported through membrane by passive diffusion (Fig. 1-2C).

Pinocytosis. Water-insoluble substances such as vitamins A, D, E, and K are transported by being engulfed by the membranes, being dissolved in them, and then being released unchanged in the inside compartment (Fig. 1-2D).

Other Factors Controlling the Rate of Absorption of Drugs. In addition to the lipid-water partition coefficient, the factors controlling the rate of absorption of drugs are degree of ionization, surface area, blood flow through the region, and gastric emptying time.

DEGREE OF IONIZATION AND DRUG ABSORPTION. The degree of dissociation of drugs and the pH of the internal medium play important roles in the transfer of drugs across biologic membranes. Most drugs are either weak acids or bases. Therefore, in solution they exist in nonionized and ionized forms. The nonionized forms of various compounds are more lipid soluble and are able to penetrate the cellular membranes. It is interesting that the rate of passage of many drugs across various membranes becomes a function of the pK_a of the drug and the pH of the internal medium. This concept is derived from the Henderson-Hasselbalch equation as follows:

Fig. 1-2. *Various mechanisms transporting drugs. (From W. A. Ritschel,* Handbook of Basic Pharmacokinetics. *Hamilton, Ill.: Drug Intelligence Publications, Inc., 1976.)*

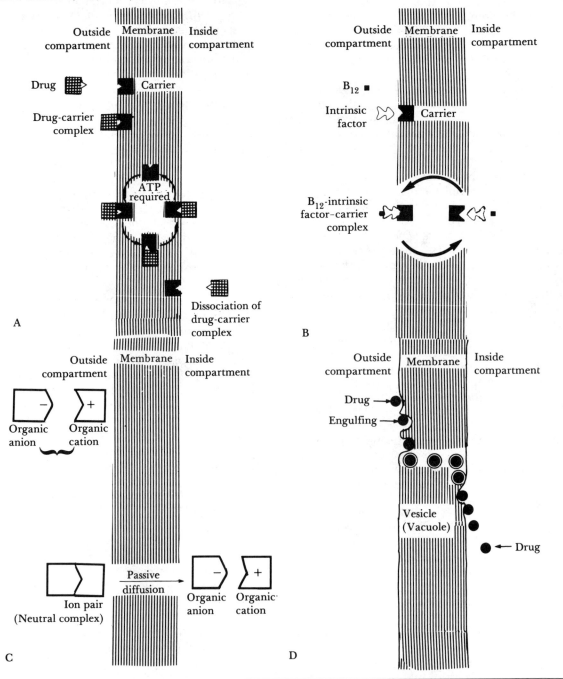

For an acid:

$$pK_a = pH + \log \frac{\text{Molecular concentration of nonionized acid}}{\text{Molecular concentration of ionized acid}}$$

For a base:

$$pK_a = pH + \log \frac{\text{Molecular concentration of ionized base}}{\text{Molecular concentration of nonionized base}}$$

For example, phenytoin is absorbed primarily from the upper intestinal tract. An acid with a pK_a of 8.3 to 9.2, phenytoin is insoluble at the pH of the gastric juice (pH = 2.0) and therefore cannot be absorbed significantly from the stomach. On passage into the small intestine, where the pH is less acidic (7.0 to 7.5), phenytoin becomes absorbed in a nonionized form. By using the Henderson-Hasselbalch equation for an acidic compound like phenytoin with a pK_a of 8.5, the degree of its ionization may be calculated as follows:

pH	% Nonionized	% Ionized
6	99.7	0.3
7	96.9	3.1
8	76.4	23.6
8.5	50.0	50.0
9	23.6	76.4
10	3.06	96.94

It is clear that at the pH 7.0 of duodenum, 96.9 percent of phenytoin is in the nonionized form, which favors its absorption. The absorption of phenytoin is greatest from the duodenum and decreases as one descends toward lower parts of the small intestine. The absorption from the cecum and the large intestine is several fold lower than that seen in the duodenum. By using the Henderson-Hasselbalch equation, one realizes that salicylic acid (pK_a 3) is 99 and 91 percent nonionized at pH 1 and pH 2 respectively. Therefore, according to this model, acetylsalicylic acid is best absorbed when the pH of the stomach is highly acidic. The high acidity, however, limits the aqueous solubility of the aspirin.

SURFACE AREA AND DRUG ABSORPTION. The influence of ionization on drug absorption is important only in circumstances in which biologic pH's vary dramatically, such as those seen in the stomach (variation from 1.5 to 7.0) and in the urine (variation from 4.5 to 7.5). The changes in pH in other biologic fluids are considerably smaller. Since both ionized and nonionized drugs are absorbed from subcutaneous and intramuscular sites of injection, the concept of ionization does not appear to play so important a role in passage of drugs across the capillary wall [10]. Finally, although drugs such as acetylsalicylic acid are best absorbed from an acidic medium (as seen, e.g., in stomach), the major portion of aspirin is nevertheless absorbed in the upper small intestine, which has considerably greater absorptive surface. The total absorptive area of the small intestine and its microvilli has been estimated to be greater than 200 m^2 for intestine versus 1 m^2 for stomach. Similarly, the perfusion rate of intestine is considerably higher than that of stomach. As a matter of fact, most drugs, whether nonionized or ionized, whether acidic, basic, or neutral in character, are absorbed mainly from the small intestine [10]. Consistent with this view is the observation that buffered acetylsalicylic acid preparations are dissolved faster and absorbed better chiefly in the intestine. Similarly, patients with achlorhydria or those who have undergone gastrectomy have little difficulty absorbing orally ingested drugs.

BLOOD FLOW AND DRUG ABSORPTION. Absorption of drugs in solution from intramuscular and subcutaneous sites of injection is perfusion rate limited [9]. Failure to recognize this important concept has resulted in fatality. For example, morphine sulfate is often administered subcutaneously in a dose of 10 mg for a 70-kg person. This dose is sufficient to produce analgesia in 70 percent of patients having moderate to severe pain. In circulatory collapse and shock (e.g., septic shock in bacteremia due to release of endotoxin) where the peripheral circulation may be impaired, morphine is not absorbed. In some cases

reported in the literature, lack of analgesia prompted additional injection of morphine, all of which remained at the injection sites and in subcutaneous capillary beds. Upon improvement of peripheral circulation, the massive amount of morphine given by repeated injection became absorbed, causing death primarily from respiratory depression.

Increasing blood flow enhances the absorption of drugs whereas decreasing blood flow has the opposite effect. Massaging the site where a drug has been administered increases the rate of absorption of drug whereas placing an ice pack on it retards it. On the other hand, one may take advantage of this concept and deliberately retard the absorption of drugs by reducing the peripheral circulation. Local anesthetics are often combined with a vasoconstricting substance such as epinephrine and injected as a mixture. Epinephrine causes vasoconstriction, hence producing a bloodless field of operation. It also prevents the rapid absorption of local anesthetics and hence enhances its duration of action. By retarding the absorption of the local anesthetic, epinephrine prevents systemic toxicity by local anesthetics.

GASTRIC EMPTYING TIME. Since drugs are mostly absorbed from the upper part of the small intestine, the rate of gastric emptying plays a crucial role in drug absorption. If rapid absorption is desired, drugs should be taken on an empty stomach. Meals, especially those with high fat content, retard the absorption of drugs. The desire for rapid absorption necessitates that the interactions between food and drugs be monitored carefully [8, 9].

Drugs such as clindamycin and lincomycin should be taken on an empty stomach. These agents are effective against streptococci, pneumococci, and susceptible staphylococci (as is penicillin) and are used for treating patients who are allergic to penicillin. Clindamycin and lincomycin are absorbed only to the extent of 20 to 35 percent from the gastrointestinal tract. Taking these agents with a meal will further hinder their absorption and produce plasma concentration of antibiotics that are ineffective.

The tetracyclines should be taken orally 1 hour before or 2 hours after meals. These agents are useful in rickettsial and bacterial diseases, in infections produced by *Mycoplasma* organisms, and in disorders caused by *Chlamydia* organisms. In an empty stomach, the amount of an oral dose that is absorbed is 30 percent for chlortetracycline, 60 to 80 percent for oxytetracycline, demeclocycline, and tetracycline, 95 percent for doxycycline, and 100 percent for minocycline. Absorption of these agents is impaired by milk and milk products and by concomitant administration of aluminum hydroxide gels, sodium bicarbonate, calcium and magnesium salts, or iron preparations, because of the chelation of divalent and trivalent cations by tetracyclines.

Anticholinergic drugs such as propantheline should be taken 1 hour before meals. Anticholinergic drugs are able to inhibit the secretion of gastric juice that is ordinarily stimulated by food. In the past, in the management of acid-pepsin disease, antacids were given 1 hour after meals and anticholinergic drugs were administered 1 hour before the meals. Initially, the presence of food neutralizes excess acid in the stomach. In the absence of food, antacids given 1 hour after meals neutralizes excess acid. Since the onset of action of anticholinergic drugs is between 1½ and 2 hours, giving them before meals allows them to exert their peak effects at a time when antacids remain in the stomach.

HEPATIC FIRST-PASS EFFECT. There are several possible mechanisms by which the oral administration of a drug may result in an inadequate plasma concentration of the drug or its active metabolite(s) [8, 9]. A drug such as penicillin G or erythromycin may be destroyed by acid hydrolysis. Drug compounds such as tetracyclines may form insoluble complexes with polyvalent ions such as Ca^{2+}. A drug such as neomycin will not be absorbed when given orally and will appear in the feces unchanged. However, by far the most important reason an orally or a parenterally administered drug may not develop an adequate plasma concentration is the "first-pass effect," which may be defined as the loss of drug as it passes through the liver for the first time. For example, nitroglycerin for the management of patients with angina pectoris is given sublingually. Given orally, nitroglycerin will be rapidly inactivated in the liver, producing inadequate concentration to be of immediate value to the patient. Sublingually administered nitroglycerin bypasses the liver and enters the superior vena cava and, in turn, perfuses the coronary circulation. Other examples of drugs showing extensive first-pass hepatic elimination and hence very low oral bioavailability are desipramine (antidepressant), morphine (analgesic), propranolol (beta-adrenergic receptor blocker), lidocaine (antiarrhythmic agent, local anesthetic), and verapamil (a Ca^{2+} channel blocking agent).

The first-pass effect can at times be overcome by raising the dosage; this is done with desipramine and propranolol. Occasionally, raising the dosage creates secondary problems such as severe hypotension, seen with larger doses of nitrites. Therefore, nitroglycerin and other nitrites are not given orally in the management of angina pectoris. The nitrites may, however, be used parenterally as vasodilators in congestive heart failure and in myocardial infarction. If the metabolite(s) of a drug resulting from first passage through the liver is (are) pharmacologically less active, the oral dose should be much larger than the parenteral dose. For example, in the management of cardiac arrhythmia, propranolol may be given in the dose range of 40 to 80 mg per day orally. For emergency use, propranolol is administered intravenously in a dose of 0.5 to 1.0 mg every 3 to 5 minutes, provided the patient may be monitored carefully with ECG.

DISTRIBUTION OF DRUGS IN THE BODY. Administered drugs, whether given orally or parenterally, become distributed nonuniformly throughout the body. Factors regulating this distribution are the lipophilic characteristic of drugs, the blood supply to the tissues, and the chemical composition of various organs and tissues. The distribution of drugs not only influences their onset of actions but also at times determines their duration of actions. For example, thiopental, an intravenous anesthetic, causes unconsciousness after 10 to 20 seconds following its administration. Consciousness returns in 20 to 30 minutes. The rapid onset of action is due to the rapid transport of thiopental to the brain. The short duration of action is due to the subsequent redistribution to other tissues, such as muscle and fat.

BINDING OF VARIOUS DRUGS TO PLASMA PROTEINS. In an ideal therapeutic regimen a sufficient amount of the drug should reach the locus of action (receptor site) to bring about the desired effect but not so much as to produce toxicity. Furthermore, the drug should not disappear too rapidly from the locus of action or the therapeutic effects will be transient and hence of limited value. The binding of drugs to plasma proteins and various subcellular components tends to accomplish the above-mentioned objectives. Various techniques (e.g., gel filtration, nuclear magnetic resonance spectroscopy, and fluorescence quenching) have facilitated the detection of active centers and binding sites and the estimation of the rate of drug-protein interaction. It has been shown that a number of plasma proteins, especially albumin, have a high affinity for binding drugs, so that at a given total plasma concentration only a portion of the total amount of drug is free in the plasma water. The remainder is bound to plasma proteins and in this form does not exert any pharmacologic effects. The interaction between drug and protein is not a chemical one but a reversible attachment (by various forces including electrostatic, London–van der Waals, hydrogen binding, and some combination of these). This drug-protein complex is readily reversible, and there is a continuous shift of bound to unbound drugs (see Fig. 1-1). The binding site of endogenously occurring acidic substances (e.g., bilirubin, vitamin C, and bile acids) and acid drugs (e.g., phenylbutazone, penicillins, and sulfonamides) is the *N*-terminal amino acid. The basic drugs (e.g., diphenhydramine, streptomycin, chloramphenicol, and coumarin anticoagulants) bind nonspecifically [8].

The response to a drug is determined by the unbound fraction that is in the plasma water. This is the fluid through which the drug is transported to sites of action, metabolism, and excretion. The concentration of unbound drug, rather than the concentration of total drug, is often a better index of the effective therapeutic level of the drug. The clinical laboratory assessment of the plasma level of a drug involves, in most cases, the measurement of bound plus unbound amounts of the agent. The greater the amount of bound drug, the less rapidly will the plasma level of unbound drug decline, as it is continuously being replenished through dissociation of the complex. The binding of drug to plasma protein is not usually a disadvantage; in fact, without such binding most drugs would elicit too transient an effect to be of much value. They would have to be administered so frequently that the plasma concentration would oscillate between toxic and ineffective levels. Therapy is easier to control when a drug is stable in the body and the plasma concentration does not fluctuate widely. In addition to enhancing the absorption rates of drugs, and serving as a storage site (silent sites or acceptor sites) for them, hormones and vitamins are also bound and maintained throughout the body [8].

The percent protein binding of drugs at therapeutic levels varies dramatically. Some drugs such as allopurinol, heparin, and isoniazid do not become bound. Other drugs such as antipyrine, ethambutol, and theophylline become bound to the extent of only 4 to 15 percent. Several drugs such as ampicillin (25%) and digoxin (23%) show low protein binding, some drugs such as atropine (50%) and meperidine (40%) show moderate protein binding, and some drugs such as carbamazepine (72%), furosemide (75%), nitrofurantoin (70%), and rifampin (85%) show high degrees of protein binding. Some drugs such as bishydroxycoumarin (97%), diazepam (96%), phenylbutazone (98%), and diazoxide (96%) bind to plasma proteins extensively [8]. The binding sites of the protein are not unlimited and are subject to saturation. When this occurs, toxicity may develop with further drug administration, since the later portion of the drug remains free. Consistent with this statement is the observation that in individuals suffering from hypoalbuminemia or altered plasma and tissue proteins toxic manifestations of drugs are quite frequent and considerably higher.

Drugs may alter the protein binding of other agents. For instance, aspirin decreases the binding of thyroxine, and the binding of bilirubin is hindered by many pharmacologic agents. The more tightly bound drugs can displace the less firmly bound agents. The intensity of the effect of displaced drug on the patient will simply depend on the blood level of free drug and its nature. At times the effect may be highly undesirable and even fatal. Only a slight displacement of a highly bound drug like bishydroxycoumarin (an oral anticoagulant) by phenylbutazone, which has greater affinity for binding sites, can cause serious hemorrhage. Because only 3 percent of the anticoagulant is free, an additional displacement of 3 percent increases its effects by 100 percent.

TISSUE LOCALIZATION OF DRUGS. After a drug has been absorbed, the initial phase of its distribution into the tissues is based on cardiac output and regional blood flow. Highly perfused organs such as the brain, heart, liver, and kidney receive most of the drug. Diffusion into the interstitial component occurs rapidly. Lipid-soluble and lipid-insoluble drugs have different patterns of distribution, and thiopental, a highly lipid-soluble substance, distributes into

the brain rapidly [9]. In addition to having their distribution affected by regional blood flow and the degree of lipid-solubility, some drugs have a propensity to accumulate in select tissues. For example, steroids, digitalis, iodine, quinacrine, organic mercurials, and tetracyclines are concentrated in the fat, heart, thyroid gland, liver, kidney, and bone respectively. Since the perfusion of the bone with blood is not extensive, local blood flow may not play a role in accumulation of tetracycline in the bone. Active transport (e.g., accumulation of lithium in the bone) and the presence of specific binding proteins (e.g., thyroglobulin in the thyroid gland) are responsible for accumulation of lithium and thyroid hormones in the bone and the thyroid gland respectively. The accumulation of antimalarial agent chloroquine in the liver is due to its interaction with hepatic DNA involving intercalations between adjacent pairs of the double helix.

APPARENT VOLUME OF DISTRIBUTION OF DRUGS. Volume of distribution (V_D) is defined as the amount of drug in the body in relation to the concentration of drug in the plasma.

$$V_D = \frac{\text{Amount of the drug in the body}}{\text{Concentration of the drug in the plasma}}$$

Assume you have given 300 mg of phenytoin to an epileptic patient. When equilibrium has been reached, the plasma concentration of phenytoin is 10 μg per milliliter, and the apparent volume of distribution of phenytoin would be 30 liters. The "one-compartment model" of distribution assumes that administered drug is homogeneously distributed throughout the tissue fluids of the body. Ethyl alcohol will distribute uniformly throughout the body, and any body fluid may be used to assess its concentration. The "two-compartment model" of distribution envisions two or multiple central or peripheral compartments. The central compartment involves blood volume and the extracellular fluid volume of the highly perfused organs (brain, heart, liver, and kidney, which receive three-quarters of the cardiac output); and the peripheral component consists of relatively less perfused tissues such as muscle, skin, and fat depots. When distributive equilibrium has occurred completely, the concentration of drug in the body will be uniform [13].

The rate of distribution of a drug from blood to a tissue depends on the extent of binding of that drug to plasma proteins (only free drug is able to distribute), on the ability of that drug to diffuse through tissue membrane (in general, lipophilic drugs are able to diffuse), on the degree of perfusion of that tissue (unit of blood/minute/volume of tissue), and on the properties of tissue membrane. All other factors remaining equal, the higher the tissue perfusion, the higher the amount of drug to be diffused. For example, the perfusion rate of lung, kidney, heart, brain, muscle, and fat is 10.0, 4.0, 0.6, 0.5, 0.025, and 0.03 respectively. Naturally, it takes much longer for a drug in blood to achieve equilibrium with fat than with the lungs [9].

In comparing thiopental and penicillin, one learns that thiopental enters the brain more rapidly than muscle whereas the reverse is the case with penicillin. Thiopental is a lipophilic substance that diffuses easily into both muscle and brain. Since the perfusion of brain is higher than that of muscle, thiopental diffuses into the brain more quickly. Penicillin is a polar substance that does not enter brain at all. However, since the muscle capillaries are porous in nature, they allow many drugs including penicillin to diffuse across the membrane rapidly. Drugs that show extensive tissue binding are said to have an apparent volume of distribution many times the total body size. For example, digoxin, which binds to plasma protein to the extent of 23 percent, has an apparent volume of distribution of 8 liters/kg. The apparent volume of distribution of quinacrine with its extensive tissue binding is greater than 500 liters/kg. The volume of distribution of drugs that do not bind to plasma or tissue proteins varies between the extracellular fluid volume (16 liters) and the total body water (42 liters). Inulin, Na^+, Br^-, and I^- are confined to extracellular water whereas antipyrine, caffeine, and ethanol are distributed in total body water [9].

THE BLOOD-BRAIN BARRIER. The brain capillaries are tightly joined together and covered by a footlike sheath that arises from astrocytes. Thus, a drug leaving the capillaries in the brain has to traverse not only the nonporous capillary cell wall itself but also the membranes of the astrocyte in order to reach the neurons. Such a structure, frequently described as the blood-brain barrier, tends therefore to limit the entry of many drugs into the brain.

Five areas of brain—the pituitary gland, the pineal gland, the area postrema, the median eminence, and the choroid plexus—have capillaries that are relatively permeable.

THE PLACENTAL BARRIER. The membrane separating fetal blood from maternal blood in the intervillous space, the so-called placental barrier, resembles other membranes. Lipid-soluble substances diffuse readily, while water-soluble substances do not diffuse, or diffuse poorly. Anesthetics and analgesics readily cross both the blood-brain and the placental barriers. Morphine-induced respiratory depression and miosis may occur both in the mother and in her newborn infant. The children of narcotic-addicted mothers will be born addicted to narcotics.

SITES OF ACTION OF DRUGS (RECEPTOR SITES). It is generally accepted that most but not all drugs (e.g., anesthetics, antiseptics) exert their potent and specific effects by forming a bond, generally reversible, with a cellular component called a receptor site. Receptor sites should be differentiated from acceptor sites or "silent sites," which are the locations where drugs are stored. Drugs that interact with a receptor and elicit a response are called agonists. Drugs that interact with receptors preventing the action of agonists are referred to as antagonists. For example, acetylcholine, causing bradycardia, is an agonist whereas atropine, blocking the action of acetylcholine and preventing bradycardia, is an antagonist. Discussion of the effects of two drugs often refers to potency, which is a measure of the dosage required to bring about a response, and to efficacy, which is a measure of the inherent ability to exert an effect.

In a comparison of the pharmacologic properties of two compounds, one may be more potent and efficacious than the other. As an analgesic, morphine is more potent and efficacious than acetylsalicylic acid. Two compounds may be equally efficacious but one could be more potent. Haloperidol and chlorpromazine are both efficacious neuroleptics in the management of schizophrenic symptomatology, but haloperidol is more potent than chlorpromazine.

Differentiation should also be made between affinity and intrinsic activity, which implies that drug binds to the receptor and results in pharmacologic actions. Affinity is a measure of the degree to which a drug binds to the receptor—whether it exerts a pharmacologic action (as an agonist) or simply blocks the receptor (as an antagonist).

NATURE AND TYPE OF PHARMACOLOGIC RECEPTOR SITES. Receptors may be located on the plasma membrane of a cell. For example, muscarinic cholinergic receptors are located on parasympathetic effector cells such as smooth muscle, cardiac muscle, exocrine glands, and brain [3]. Acetylcholine-induced vasodilation, negative chronotropic effect, and negative inotropic effect are mediated by interaction of acetylcholine directly with its membrane-bound receptor (Fig. 1-3A).

Numerous hormones and peptides combine with receptors in the plasma membranes, triggering the activation of adenylate cyclase and catalyzing the formation of cyclic AMP—"second messenger"—from ATP [1]. For example, epinephrine or glucagon binds with its membrane receptor, triggering the guanosine triphosphate (GTP)–dependent activation of adenylate cyclase (Ac) by a membrane-bound coupling protein. The activation of adenylate cyclase catalyzes the conversion of ATP to cyclic AMP, which in turn activates cyclic AMP–dependent protein kinase, which mediates the conversion of inactive phosphorylase to active phosphorylase in the liver, which subsequently results in conversion of stored glycogen to glucose (Fig. 1-3B).

Numerous steroids, including testosterone, exert their effects by binding initially with a cytoplasmic receptor (R), which becomes translocated to the nucleus in its activated state [4]. The testosterone-receptor complex binds to nuclear chromatin, initiating the synthesis of specific messenger RNA (mRNA) and specific RNA. The newly synthesized RNA traverses the nucleus and is translated on cytoplasmic ribosomes, causing testosterone-directed induction of

Fig. 1-3. *A. Cholinergic receptors—the muscarinic cholinergic receptor. (Modified from A. Goth, Medical Pharmacology [11th ed.]. St. Louis: Mosby, 1984.) B. Catecholamine receptor—the receptor for epinephrine or glucagon and cyclic AMP–mediated conversion of glycogen to glucose. (Concepts from R. W. Butcher, Role of cyclic AMP in hormone functions. N. Engl. J. Med. 279:1378, 1968.) C. Steroid receptor—the receptor for testosterone. (Modified from M. M. Grumbach and F. A. Conte, Disorders of Sex Differentiation. In R. H. Williams [ed.], Textbook of Endocrinology [6th ed.]. Philadelphia: Saunders, 1981.) D. GABA-benzodiazepine receptors—the GABA, benzodiazepine, and chloride ionophore complex. (Modified from W. Haefely et al., Neuropharmacology of Benzodiazepines: Synaptic Mechanisms and Neural Basis of Action. In E. Costa [ed.], The Benzodiazepines: From Molecular Biology to Clinical Practice. New York: Raven Press, 1983.)*

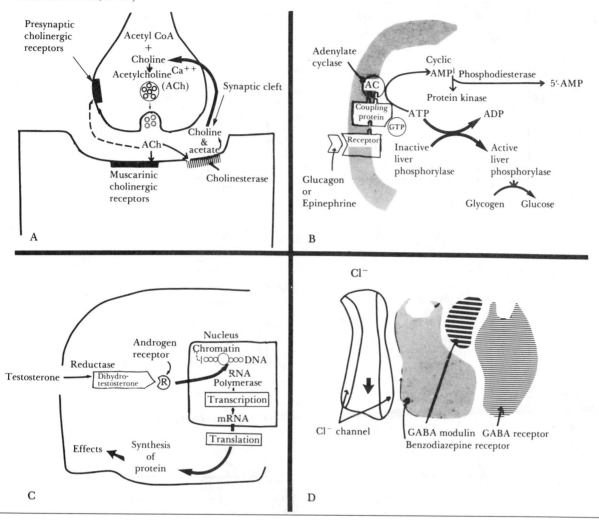

specific proteins, creating the actions of testosterone (Fig. 1-3C).

Numerous neuropharmacologic agents including anticonvulsants exert their effects by interacting with a GABA receptor–chloride ionophore complex [5]. This complex consists of GABA recognition site, benzodiazepine receptor site, picrotoxin-barbiturate binding site, the chloride channel, and various proteins modulating these actions and interactions. (Fig. 1-3D).

DOSE-RESPONSE RELATION. The relation between the amount of drug administered (e.g., morphine) or the concentration of the administered drug in the plasma and the magnitude of desired response obtained (e.g., analgesia) is referred to as a dose-response relation [11]. Naturally, when no morphine is present at the receptor site, no analgesia is obtained (Fig. 1-4A). When all the available receptor sites are occupied, one may hypothesize that maximum response will be obtained (Clark's hypothesis). This linear dose-response relationship, depicted in Figure 1-4A, may be expressed in a logarithmic scale (Fig. 1-4B).

POTENCY AND EFFICACY. *Potency* refers to the lowest dose that produces maximum effect. Morphine in a dose of 10 mg given subcutaneously pro-

Fig. 1-4. *Dose-response relationship (A and B), of unequal potency of two compounds with equal efficacy (C), and of a competitive antagonism between an agonist and an antagonist (D). (Modified from R. J. Tallarida and L. S. Jacob,* The Dose-Response Relation in Pharmacology. *New York: Springer-Verlag, 1979.)*

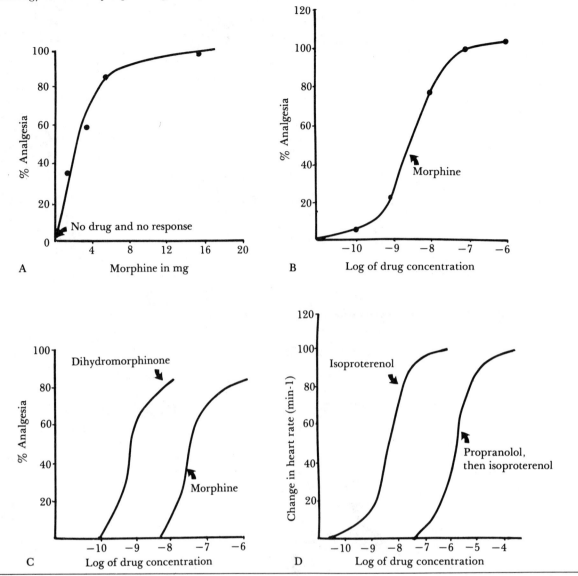

duces analgesia. Dihydromorphinone (Dilaudid) is able to accomplish the same degree of analgesia in a dose of 2 mg. Therefore, morphine and dihydromorphinone are equally efficacious whereas dihydromorphinone is more potent than morphine (Fig. 1-4C).

The interaction between a drug and a receptor site is similar to a reversible interaction between a substrate and an enzyme. An agonist is a pharmacologic substance that interacts with a receptor site and elicits a response. Drugs that interact with the receptor site preventing the binding and hence the actions of agonists are referred to as antagonists. The antagonism is called competitive or surmountable antagonism if the inhibition is overcome by increasing the concentration of the agonist (Figs. 1-4D and 1-5A). Propran-

olol (a beta-adrenergic receptor antagonist) is a competitive antagonist to isoproterenol (a beta-adrenergic receptor agonist). Atropine is a competitive antagonist of acetylcholine at the muscarinic cholinergic receptor site. Naloxone is a competitive antagonist of morphine at its receptor site. Diphenhydramine is a competitive antagonist of histamine at (H_1) receptor sites. In examining the kinetic nature of competitive antagonists, one realizes that parallel dose-response curves having the same maximum effect (Figs. 1-4D and 1-5A) are produced for the agonists in the presence and absence of a fixed amount of antagonist [11].

In contrast to competitive antagonism, when the antagonist binds irreversibly to the receptor site producing permanent chemical changes or inactivation

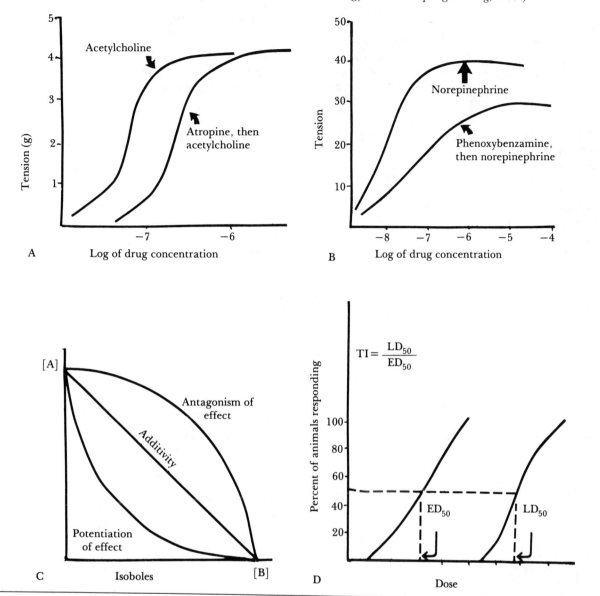

Fig. 1-5. *Competitive antagonism (A). Noncompetitive antagonism (B). Isobole (C). Concept of a therapeutic index (D). (Modified from R. J. Tallarida and L. S. Jacob,* The Dose-Response Relation in Pharmacology. *New York: Springer-Verlag, 1979.)*

of the receptor site, one speaks of a noncompetitive antagonism or of nonequilibrium blockade. Phenoxybenzamine, an alpha-adrenergic receptor blocking agent, noncompetitively and irreversibly blocks the alpha-adrenergic receptor site, preventing norepinephrine from exerting its full action (Fig. 1-5B) [11].

PHYSIOLOGIC AND PHARMACOLOGIC ANTAGONISM. If two drugs, one an agonist and another an antagonist, bind to the same receptor site, either producing or preventing an effect, this association is called pharmacologic antagonism. Naloxone, atropine, and diphenhydramine are pharmacologic

and specific antagonists of morphine, acetylcholine, and histamine at their respective receptor sites. In physiologic antagonism, the drugs do not bind to the same receptor sites but produce functionally opposite results. For example, histamine produces vasodilation whereas epinephrine produces vasoconstriction, but they interact with two separate receptor sites. Physiologic antagonism is utilized extensively in medicine, especially in overcoming the toxicity of pharmacologic agents. For instance, diazepam (Valium) may be used to overcome the CNS excitation produced by physostigmine, an acetylcholinesterase inhibitor that results in enhancement of the concentration of acetylcholine. Diazepam overcomes the acetylcholine-mediated CNS excitation by enhancing the activity of gamma-aminobutyric acid (GABA), an inhibitory neurotransmitter.

ENHANCEMENT OF DRUG ACTION. Numerous agents acting at two or more receptor sites may magnify each other's effects, producing responses greater than the one produced by each drug alone. For example, angiotensin II enhances the vasoconstricting effects of norepinephrine; histamine augments the hypotensive effects of acetylcholine. If the quantitative summation of the effects produced by two drugs is greater than the algebraic sum of the effects produced by each drug alone, the result is called potentiation of effects. For example, diazepam, chlorpromazine, and alcohol, taken individually, will all cause sedation. However, when alcohol is ingested either with diazepam or with chlorpromazine, pronounced CNS depression may ensue, and fatalities have occurred with injudicious combined uses of these CNS depressants. In this case alcohol potentiates the CNS depression induced by diazepam or chlorpromazine. In depicting the potentiation of two drugs, an isobole plotting the effects of drugs A and B is used (Fig. 1-5C).

THERAPEUTIC INDEX. The therapeutic index (Fig. 1-5D), which is obtained from animal experimentation, deals with the ratio of lethal doses to 50 percent of the population (LD_{50}) over the median effective dose (ED_{50}).

$$\text{Therapeutic index} = \frac{LD_{50}}{ED_{50}}$$

The higher the therapeutic index, the safer the drug, and the lower the therapeutic index, the greater the possibility of causing toxicity. The therapeutic index for barbiturates as a class is 10 whereas the therapeutic index for cardiac glycosides as a class is 3. Since the usual therapeutic doses of cardiac glycoside is 1 mg, fatality may result if only 3 mg has been administered to a patient.

BIOTRANSFORMATION OF DRUGS. Biotransformation may be defined as enzyme-catalyzed alteration of drugs by the living organism. Although few drugs are eliminated unchanged, urinary excretion is a negligible means of terminating the action of most drugs or poisons in the body. As a matter of fact, the urinary excretion of a highly lipid-soluble substance such as pentobarbital is so slow that it would take the body a century to rid itself of the effect of a single dose of the agent. Therefore, through evolutionary adaptation, the mammalian and terrestrial animals have developed systems that enable them to convert most lipid-soluble substances into water-soluble ones, so that they may be easily excreted by the kidney.

SITES OF DRUG BIOTRANSFORMATION— NONHEPATIC METABOLISM. In general, biotransformation may be divided into hepatic and nonhepatic metabolism. Among the nonhepatic drug–metabolizing systems, those found in the intestinal epithelium, lung, and plasma have been studied. Some of the drugs metabolized in the blood are the following.

Plasma. Succinylcholine, a muscle relaxant, is hydrolyzed by the pseudocholinesterase of liver and plasma to succinylmonocholine. The short duration of action of succinylcholine (5 minutes) is due to its rapid hydrolysis in the plasma. Patients with atypical cholinesterase who cannot metabolize succinylcholine develop pronounced apnea. Procaine, a local anesthetic, is also hydrolyzed by pseudocholinesterase.

Lung. Lung is involved in activation as well as inactivation of numerous physiologic and pharmacologic substances. For example, in the lung angiotensin I becomes converted to angiotensin II. Serotonin, norepinephrine, histamine, prostaglandins, and steroids are examples of agents metabolized and inactivated by the lung.

Intestinal Epithelium. The intestinal epithelium is capable of removing numerous agents [6].

HEPATIC DRUG METABOLISM. By far the major portion of biotransformation is carried out in the liver by a group of highly nonspecific enzymes located in the "smooth surface" microsomes of the endoplasmic reticulum [2]. The biotransformations in the liver are commonly grouped into two phases (Table 1-1).

During phase I, most drugs are inactivated pharmacologically, some drugs remain unaltered, and some become more active and toxic in nature. For example, phenytoin in the liver is first hydroxylated to hydroxyphenytoin (phase I) and then conjugated with glucuronic acid (phase II) and excreted by the kidney as phenytoin glucuronide conjugate. During phase I, in addition to the introduction of a polar group such as OH group, a potential polar group may also be unmasked from the drug to be metabolized. For example, compound $R-OCH_3$ is converted to compound $R-OH$ by demethylation. Codeine becomes demethylated to morphine. The free or the unmasked polar group is then conjugated with glucuronate, sulfate, glycine, or acetate.

SCHEME OF MIXED-FUNCTION OXIDATION REACTION PATHWAY. The hepatic endoplasmic reticulum possesses oxidative enzymes called mixed-function oxidases or monooxygenase with specific requirement for both molecular oxygen and reduced nicotinamide adenine dinucleotide phosphate (NADPH). Essential in the mixed-function oxidase system is a hemoprotein designated as cytochrome

Table 1-1. *General Pathways of Drug Metabolism by Nonspecific Enzymes in the Liver*

Reactions	Localization of Enzymes	Enzymes
Phase I		
Oxidations		
Hydroxylations	Microsomes	Cytochrome P450 (oxidases)
Dealkylations	Microsomes	
Oxide formation	Microsomes	
Desulfuration	Microsomes	
Dehalogenation	Soluble, microsomes (minor)	
Aldehyde oxidation	Soluble	
Reductions		
Aldehyde reduction	Soluble	Flavin enzymes
Azoreduction	Microsomes	
Nitroreduction	Microsomes, soluble	
Hydrolyses		
Deesterification	Microsomes, soluble	Esterases
Deamidation	Microsomes, soluble	
Phase II		
Glucuronide conjugation	Microsomes	Transferases
Acylation	Mitochondria, soluble	
Methylation	Soluble	
Mercapturic acid formation	Soluble	
Sulfate conjugation	Soluble	
Glycine conjugation	Soluble	

Modified from J. R. Gillete, Factors affecting drug metabolism. *Ann. N.Y. Acad. Sci.* 179:43, 1971.

P450 (absorbs light at 450 nm when exposed to carbon monoxide). The primary electron donor is NADPH whereas the electron transfer involves cytochrome P450, a flavoprotein. The presence of a heat-stable fraction is necessary for the operation of the system.

A drug substrate to be metabolized binds to oxidized cytochrome P450, which in turn is reduced by cytochrome P450 reductase. Drug-reduced cytochrome P450 complex then combines with molecular oxygen. A second electron and two hydrogen ions are acquired from the donor system, and the subsequent products are oxidized drug and water with regeneration of the oxidized cytochrome P450 (Fig. 1-6). This process is summarized as follows:

1. NADPH + oxidized cytochrome P450 + H$^+$ →
reduced cytochrome P450 + NADP$^+$

2. Reduced cytochrome P450 + O$_2$ →
"active oxygen complex"

3. "Active oxygen complex" + drug substrate →
oxidized drug + oxidized cytochrome P450 + H$_2$O

NADPH + O$_2$ + drug substrate + H$^+$ →
NADP$^+$ + oxidized drug + H$_2$O

CONSEQUENCE OF BIOTRANSFORMATION REACTIONS.

The process of biotransformation usually inactivates or detoxifies (or both) the administered drugs or the ingested poisons, but other reactions may also take place.

Precursor Activation. Occasionally, an inactive precursor such as levodopa is converted to an active metabolite such as dopamine.

Metabolic Activation of Drugs. Often an active drug becomes converted to another pharmacologically active substance. The following are a few examples:

Drug		Active Metabolite
Trimethadione	becomes demethylated to	dimethadione
Mephobarbital	becomes demethylated to	phenobarbital
Primidone	becomes oxidized to	phenobarbital
Codeine	becomes demethylated to	morphine
Imipramine	becomes demethylated to	desmethylimipramine
Acetophenetidin	becomes deethylated to	*p*-acetaminophen
Chloral hydrate	becomes reduced to	trichloroethanol
Prednisone	becomes reduced to	prednisolone

Conversion to Metabolites with Dissimilar Actions. In certain instances, the body converts a drug to several active metabolites with dissimilar pharmacologic properties. For example, phenylbutazone undergoes aromatic hydroxylation to produce a metabolite that has sodium-retaining and antirheumatic activities, and an alkyl-chain oxidation to produce a metabolite with strong uricosuric property. Phenylbutazone itself has both uricosuric and antirheumatic effects.

Fig. 1-6. *Oxidation of a drug by the enzyme cytochrome P450 visualized here as a sequential process. The enzyme (1) is a complex of a protein and the oxygen-binding compound heme, which contains an iron atom that is initially in the ferric (Fe^{3+}) form (open circle). The cytochrome binds the drug (2). Then (3) the enzyme cytochrome P450 reductase, utilizing the coenzyme NADPH, reduces the iron of the heme to the ferrous (Fe^{2+}) form (black dot), in which it can bind a molecule of oxygen (4). It supplies one atom of oxygen to oxidize the drug and one generally to form water, in the process reverting to its oxidized form (5). The drug, oxidized and in most cases inactive, is thereupon released (6). (Reprinted with permission from A. Kappas and A. P. Alvares, Sci. Am. 232:30, 1975.)*

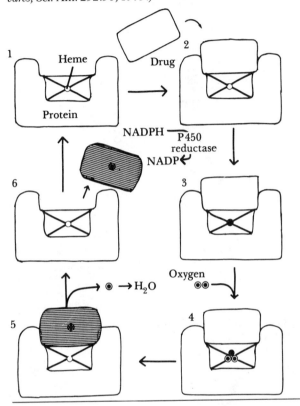

LETHAL SYNTHESIS. The metabolism of drugs and agents does not always lead to detoxification, because occasionally the metabolites are toxicologically more potent. Some examples are [7, 12]:

Drug	Metabolite
Sulfamethazine	N_4-Acetylsulfamethazine
Aminopyrine	4-Aminoantipyrine
Parathione	Paraoxon

DRUG METABOLITE KINETICS. In the majority of cases, drugs are converted to metabolites, which, in the more polar and water-soluble forms, are readily excreted. Often the concentration of metabolite far exceeds the concentration of drug. For example, an orally administered propranolol becomes rapidly converted to 4-hydroxypropranolol, whose concentration is several hundredfold higher than that of propranolol [9]. Sometimes the metabolites are able to inhibit the further metabolism of the parent drug.

For example, phenytoin becomes metabolized to hydroxyphenytoin. When given in higher than recommended individualized doses, hydroxyphenytoin inhibits the hydroxylase system that metabolizes phenytoin, increasing its concentration in free form and its potential to produce toxicity.

Enterohepatic circulation may sometimes prolong the half-life of a drug. A drug that is absorbed from the gastrointestinal tract, excreted in the bile, and resorbed from the intestine is said to have undergone "enterohepatic cycling." Drugs are delivered to the liver by means of both portal vein and hepatic artery and returned to the rest of the body by the hepatic vein. The difference between the concentration of drug taken to and removed from the liver accounts for the amount of drug metabolized or excreted in the bile. Let us assume that the liver has conjugated a drug with glucuronic acid to its metabolite. The conjugated product may appear in the bile and finally be excreted in the small intestine. The possibility exists that in the intestine the beta-glucuronidase originating from the resident flora may hydrolyze the glucuronide-drug conjugate back to the parent drug, allowing the parent drug to be resorbed. The continuous enterohepatic cycling will increase the half-life of this agent in the body [9].

FACTORS THAT MODIFY THE METABOLISM OF DRUGS. Many environmental factors and pathophysiologic conditions inhibit or stimulate the activity of drug-metabolizing enzymes and hence may alter the outcome of a therapeutic regimen. Pharmacogenetics, immaturity of drug-metabolizing enzyme systems, and drug-drug interactions are a few of the factors that have been shown to alter drug metabolism.

PHARMACOGENETICS. Pharmacogenetics may be defined as the study of the hereditary variation in the handling of drugs. Pharmacogenetic abnormalities may be entirely innocuous unless the particular individual is challenged with drugs. The alterations in handling of a drug may be attributed to abnormalities at anatomic or at molecular levels. For example, in inherited subaortic stenosis, digitalis may cause an adverse drug reaction. Molecular abnormalities may be due to alteration in the receptor sites or result from absence or deficiency of a particular enzyme. The hyposensitivity and resistance of certain individuals to coumarin anticoagulants and the hypersensitivity of patients with Down's syndrome to atropine are probably caused by abnormalities in their respective receptor sites. Acatalasia and the decrease in the activities of pseudocholinesterase, acetylase, and glucose 6-phosphate dehydrogenase are examples of enzymatic deficiencies that may produce mild to very severe adverse reactions.

INFLUENCE OF AGE ON DRUG METABOLISM. Drug metabolism is very deficient qualitatively and quantitatively in the newborn. For example, chloramphenicol, when used injudiciously, may cause gray syndrome, characterized by vomiting, refusal to suck, irregular and rapid respiration, abdominal distention, periods of cyanosis, passage of loose green stools, cardiovascular collapse, and death. The mechanism of chloramphenicol toxicity is apparently failure of the newborn to conjugate chloramphenicol with glucuronic acid due to inadequate activity of hepatic glucuronyl transferase. This, in combination with inadequate renal excretion of drug in the newborn, results in a higher than expected level of chloramphenicol in the plasma. Therefore, the newborn should receive chloramphenicol in doses not greater than 25 to 50 mg per kilogram of body weight. Similarly, the elderly are prone to toxicity of numerous drugs, including cardiac glycosides. A dose of digitoxin which was totally "therapeutic" and innocuous at age 60 may produce severe toxicity and even death at age 70. The abilities of the liver to metabolize drugs and of the kidney to excrete drug metabolites decline with the aging process.

ENZYME INDUCTION AND INHIBITION.

The activities of microsomal drug-metabolizing enzymes in laboratory animals and humans can be enhanced by an alteration in the level of endogenous hormonal concentrations, such as androgens, estrogens, progestational steroids, glucocorticoids, anabolic steroids, norepinephrine, insulin, and thyroxine. This effect can also be brought about by the administration of exogenous substances, such as drugs, food preservatives, coloring agents, insecticides, volatile oils, urea herbicides, and polycyclic aromatic hydrocarbons. The increase in the activities of drug-metabolizing enzymes appears to be due to an elevation in the rate of synthesis of the enzyme protein; hence it is truly an "enzyme induction" phenomenon. The rise in the activities of drug-metabolizing enzymes is blocked by substances such as ethionine, puromycin, or actinomycin D, the known inhibitors of de novo protein synthesis.

Liver microsomal enzyme inducers that are lipid soluble at physiologic pH may be characterized and classified into two general groups. Some, like phenobarbital, tend to stimulate all enzymes whereas others, such as 3-methylcholanthrene, tend to be selective. It is generally agreed that there is no relation between the dosage, the structure of the inducers, and the intensity and degree of microsomal enzyme induction. In addition, agents such as steroids, phenobarbital, and carcinogenic substances bring about their effects through varied mechanisms. For example, maximum elevation in the activity of drug-metabolizing enzymes following phenobarbital administration is not reached for at least 3 days whereas the polycyclic hydrocarbons seem to exert this effect in a few hours. Furthermore, the administration of phenobarbital increases the amounts of NADPH–cytochrome c reductase and cytochrome P450, and the rate of cytochrome P450 reduction. In contrast, the administration of 3-methylcholanthrene increases the amount of cytochrome P450 but not the activity

of NADPH–cytochrome c reductase; nor does it increase the rate of cytochrome P450 reduction.

Clinical Implication of Enzyme Induction and Inhibition. Patients are often given several drugs at the same time. The possibility that one drug may accelerate or inhibit the metabolism of another drug should always be kept in mind. In cases in which the phenomenon has occurred, the removal of an enzyme inducer could be hazardous. The following examples may reveal the consequence of enzyme induction.

Phenylbutazone is an analgesic, antipyretic, uricosuric, and antiinflammatory agent. Among its side effects are activation of peptic ulcer and gastrointestinal hemorrhage. If one treats a dog with large amounts of phenylbutazone, side effects such as vomiting and diarrhea with bloody stool ensue. However, as the administration of phenylbutazone continues for several days, these side effects disappear. In this case, phenylbutazone "induces" its own hydroxylation, which results in a lower plasma level of the drug and the absence of the side effects. Chronic treatment with phenylbutazone and many other drugs—chlorpromazine, pentobarbital, phenobarbital, chlordiazepoxide, and the like—that stimulate their own metabolism should be expected to result in decreased effectiveness and toxicity.

Patients who are on anticoagulant therapy may develop severe hemorrhage several days after discharge from the hospital. Often the hospitalized patients are sedated with barbiturates, which tend to stimulate the enzymes that metabolize bishydroxycoumarin. Abrupt withdrawal from barbiturates after discharge is likely to revert the activity of the drug-metabolizing enzymes to their prebarbiturate stage, which consequently raises the free circulating level of the anticoagulant, resulting in hemorrhage. Naturally, treatment with phenobarbital should be expected to alter the maintenance dosage of anticoagulants.

RENAL EXCRETION OF DRUGS.

An orally administered drug will gradually begin to become absorbed. As the amount of drug in the body increases by 50 percent, the amount of the drug at the absorption site should decrease by the same amount. The absorbed drug will gradually become metabolized or excreted mostly by the kidneys. In addition to their elimination by the kidneys, drugs and their metabolites are eliminated in the bile, in the milk, in the sweat, and by the lungs. The excretion of drugs into milk may become significant to a breast-fed child, and the excretion of drugs, especially gaseous anesthetics, from the lungs becomes important in specialized circumstances [9].

Rate of Excretion of Drugs by Kidneys. The amount of a drug (and its metabolites) to appear in the urine depends on the amount of drug undergoing glomerular filtration, tubular secretion, and tubular resorption. This simple concept may be elaborated. Metabolism plays a major role in drug excretion, since the metabolites are more water-soluble substances, which are excreted. Drugs are excreted in free forms, and the plasma protein–bound drugs and tissue-stored drugs naturally are not excreted.

The excretion of drugs from the kidneys, like the absorption of drugs from the gastrointestinal tract, depends on lipid-solubility and on the degree of ionization of drugs and the pH of the urine. Nonionized lipid-soluble drugs are resorbed and not eliminated. Generally, drugs that are bases are excreted when the urine is acid whereas acidic compounds are excreted more favorably if the urine is alkaline. For example, in phenobarbital (weak acid pK_a of 7.3) poisoning, alkalinization of urine with sodium bicarbonate will be helpful in eliminating phenobarbital. In amphetamine toxicity, acidification of urine with ammonium chloride will be required.

Drugs that undergo glomerular filtration as well as active tubular secretion have a very short half-life. Penicillin is one such compound. Its half-life is prolonged by coadministration of probenecid, a uricosuric drug that inhibits the tubular secretion of penicillin. Most drugs, however, have relatively longer half-lives than penicillin because they undergo glomerular filtration, partial tubular resorption, and no active tubular secretion [9].

Significance of Blood Flow on Clearance of Drugs. In general, the rate of extraction of drug from blood and the rate of clearance by the kidney depends on blood flow and the ability of the kidney to extract the drug (extraction ratio). If all of the drug is removed from the blood as it traverses the kidneys, the extraction ratio will be 1. The higher the blood flow, the higher will be the rate of excretion of that drug, and the clearance is said to be perfusion rate limited. For example, the extraction ratio of one of the cardiac glycosides, digoxin, is low, and toxicity is likely to occur in renal failure. Similarly, the hepatic extraction ratio of digitoxin is low, and toxicity is likely to occur in hepatic failure. Consequently, cardiologists have long recognized that digitoxin and digoxin should be avoided in liver and in renal failure respectively [9].

HALF-LIFE OF A DRUG. The half-life of a drug or its elimination half-life is the time required to reduce its concentration in the blood by one-half. For penicillin G, the half-life is 20 minutes; that is, after its intravenous administration, only 50 percent of it will remain in the blood after 20 minutes. The intravenously administered drug and the orally administered identical drug, once it has reached the general circulation, have identical half-lives. When given at a regular interval, a drug or its metabolite reaches a plateau concentration after approximately four to five half-lives. This plateau will change only if the dose or frequency of administration has been altered.

QUESTIONS ON PHARMACOKINETICS

Select one answer or explanation that best answers the question or completes the statement.

_____ 1. Drugs interact with their receptor sites by forming:
   A. Ionic bonds.
   B. Hydrogen bonds.
   C. Van der Waals forces.
   D. All of the above.

_____ 2. The hepatic mixed-function oxidase system:
   A. Requires both NADPH and O^2.
   B. Must bind reversibly with its substrate.
   C. Requires cytochrome P450 as a component.
   D. All of the above.

_____ 3. A drug is being metabolized by zero-order kinetics. This indicates that:
   A. A constant amount of drug is being catabolized each hour.
   B. A constant fraction of the drug is being catabolized each hour.
   C. The drug is a water-soluble substance.
   D. The time required to catabolize half of the drug is independent of the initial concentration of the drug.

_____ 4. A drug is being metabolized by first-order kinetics. If 50 percent of this drug is metabolized in 12 minutes, then 75 percent would be metabolized in:
   A. 18 minutes.
   B. 24 minutes.
   C. 30 minutes.
   D. 36 minutes.

_____ 5. In advanced cirrhosis of the liver, the dosage of which of the following drugs should be altered?
   A. Penicillin.
   B. Morphine.
   C. Sulfisoxazole.
   D. Succinylcholine.
   E. All of the above.

_____ 6. Which of the following two drugs are poorly excreted by the kidney?
   A. Neostigmine and succinylcholine.
   B. Penicillin and chloramphenicol.
   C. Aspirin and indomethacin.
   D. Diazepam and chlorpromazine.

_____ 7. A weak base with a pK_a of 5 is now at equilibrium in the body. What would be the stomach-plasma ratio of this base when the stomach pH is 2 and that of plasma is 7?
   A. $10^{-3}:1$.
   B. $10^{-1}:1$.
   C. $10^1:1$.
   D. $10^3:1$.

_____ 8. A weak base with a pK_a of 5 is now at equilibrium in the body. What would be the urine-plasma ratio of this base when the pH of urine is 3 and that of plasma is 7?
   A. 1,000:1.
   B. 100:1.
   C. 10:1.
   D. 1:1.

_____ 9. At equilibrium, a drug is distributed uniformly in the extracellular fluid, is excreted unchanged by glomerular filtrates, and is not resorbed. What would be the approximate half-life of this drug?
   A. 15 minutes.
   B. 30 minutes.

C. 60 minutes.

D. 120 minutes.

____ 10. A drug undergoes glomerular filtration and now is found in renal tubular fluid. This finding probably indicates that:

A. The drug was free and not bound to plasma protein.

B. The drug does not require catabolism.

C. The drug has a quaternary N^+

D. The drug has a volume of distribution of 50,000 liters.

____ 11. When a drug has a low therapeutic index, that drug should be:

A. Used mostly orally.

B. Used only intravenously.

C. Considered a potentially toxic substance.

D. Given only in submilligram doses.

____ 12. The urinary elimination of a weak base (e.g., amphetamine) is enhanced when:

A. The urine is more acidic.

B. The urine is more basic.

C. The pH of the urine approximates the pK_a of the drug.

D. The pH of the plasma approximates the pK_a of the drug.

____ 13. Probenecid is sometimes administered with penicillin:

A. To enhance the urinary excretion of penicillin and hence reduce hypersensitivity reaction.

B. To make the pH of the urine more basic.

C. To convert penicillin from ionized to nonionized form.

D. To interfere with active tubular secretion.

____ 14. The apparent volume of distribution of ethyl alcohol in a 70-kg person is:

A. 12 liters.

B. 40 liters.

C. 4 liters.

D. Cannot be estimated.

____ 15. The duration of action of a drug is dependent on its:

A. Plasma and tissue binding.

B. Metabolism.

C. Tubular filtration and secretion.

D. All of the above.

ANSWERS AND EXPLANATIONS ON PHARMACOKINETICS

1. D.

Explanation: The interaction between drugs and receptors is not a chemical one and is reversible in nature. Only a few drugs, such as irreversible cholinesterase inhibitor, form a covalent bond with their receptors.

2. D.

3. A.

4. B.

5. E.

Explanation: Penicillin, methicillin, ampicillin, and nafcillin are stored in liver. Morphine is metabolized in part by glucuronic acid conjugation. Sulfisoxazole is metabolized by acetylation. Succinylcholine is metabolized by pseudocholinesterase of liver and plasma, a factor responsible for its short duration of action.

6. A.

Explanation: Drugs containing quaternary nitrogen usually do not cross the placental barrier or the blood-brain barrier, nor are they readily excreted by the kidneys.

7. D.

Explanation: Calculation of the equilibrium distribution ratio of total drug concentration in two compartments at different pH's.

$$R_{1:2} = \frac{1 + 10^{pK_a - pH_1}}{1 + 10^{pK_a - pH_2}} \text{ (for a base)}$$

$$R_{1:2} = \frac{1 + 10^{5-2}}{1 + 10^{5-7}} = \frac{1 + 10^3}{1 + 10^{-2}} = \frac{1001}{1.01} = 10^3 : 1$$

8. B.

9. C.

Explanation: Assume that the extracellular fluid is 12 liters and the GFR is 135 ml/min; then

$$t\, 1/2 = 0.69 \times V_D/c$$
$$t\, 1/2 = 0.69 \times 12,000/135$$
$$t\, 1/2 = 61.6$$

10. A.

Explanation: Only protein-unbound "free" drugs are able to be metabolized or excreted.

11. C.

12. A.

13. D.

14. B.

15. D.

REFERENCES

1. Butcher, R. W. Role of cyclic AMP in hormone functions. *N. Engl. J. Med.* 279:1378, 1968.

2. Gillette, J. R. Factors affecting drug metabolism. In E. S. Vesell, (ed.), Drug metabolism in man. *Ann. N.Y. Acad. Sci.* 179:43, 1971.

3. Goth, A. *Medical Pharmacology* (11th ed.). St. Louis: Mosby, 1984. P. 118.

4. Grumbach, M. M., and Conte, F. A. Disorders of Sex Differentiation. In R. H. Williams (ed.), *Textbook of Endocrinology* (6th ed.). Philadelphia: Saunders, 1981. P. 445.

5. Haefely, W., et al. Neuropharmacology of Benzodiazepines: Synaptic Mechanisms and Neural Basis of Action. In E. Costa (ed.), *The Benzodiazepines: From Molecular Biology to Clinical Practice.* New York: Raven Press, 1983. P. 23.

6. Kalant, H., and MacLeod, S. M. Drug Biotransformation. In P. Seeman, E. M. Sellers, and W. H. E. Roschlau (eds.), *Principles of Medical Pharmacology* (3rd ed.). Toronto: University of Toronto Press, 1979. Pp. 45–56.

7. LaDu, B. N., Mandel, H. G., and Way, E. L. *Fundamentals of Drug Metabolism and Drug Deposition.* Baltimore: Williams & Wilkins, 1971.

8. Niazi, S. *Textbook of Biopharmaceutics and Clinical Pharmacokinetics.* New York: Appleton-Century-Crofts, 1979.

9. Rowland, M., and Tozer, T. N. *Clinical Pharmacokinetics. Concepts and Application.* Philadelphia: Lea & Febiger, 1980.

10. Seeman, P. Drug Absorption. In P. Seeman, E. M. Sellers, and W. H. E. Roschlau (eds.), *Principles of Medical Pharmacology* (3rd ed.). Toronto: University of Toronto Press, 1979. Pp. 21–33.

11. Tallarida, R. J., and Jacob, L. S. *The Dose-Response Relation in Pharmacology*. New York: Springer-Verlag, 1979.

12. Vesell, E. S. (ed.). *Ann. Acad. Sci.* 179 (whole issue), 1971.

13. Wartak, J. *Clinical Pharmacokinetics. A Modern Approach to Individualized Drug Therapy*. New York: Praeger, 1983.

2. Pharmacodynamics

The desire to take medicine is perhaps the greatest feature which distinguishes man from the animals.

Sir William Osler

Pharmacodynamics may be defined as the study of the actions and effects of drugs on organs and tissues at cellular and subcellular levels. Therefore, pharmacodynamics provides information on how drugs bring about their beneficial effects and how they cause their side effects. By understanding and applying the knowledge gained in studying pharmacodynamics, physicians and other members of the health care delivery team are able to render effective and safe therapeutic care to their patients.

Chapter 1, on pharmacokinetics, discussed the processes of absorption, binding, distribution, biotransformation, and excretion of drugs. These processes are efficiently designed to provide sufficient quantity of drugs to their receptor sites to bring forth the desired therapeutic effects.

Pharmacodynamics discusses the sites of action, the modes of action, and the mechanisms of action of drugs. For example, when 10 to 15 mg of morphine sulfate is administered subcutaneously to a patient with multiple fractures, analgesia, sedation, respiratory depression, emesis, miosis, suppression of the activity of gastrointestinal tract, and oliguria may occur. These diversified effects are caused at multiple peripheral and central sites and by numerous modes and mechanisms of actions.

SITE OF ACTION. The receptor site where a drug acts to initiate a group of functions is the site of action of that drug. The central sites of actions of morphine include the cerebral cortex, hypothalamus, and medullary center.

MODE OF ACTION. The character of an effect produced by a drug is called the mode of action of that drug. Morphine, by depressing cerebral cortex, hypothalamus, and medullary center, is responsible for decreasing pain perception (analgesia), inducing narcosis (heavy sedation), depressing the cough center, stimulating initially and then depressing the vomiting center, and depressing respiration.

MECHANISM OF ACTION. The identification of molecular and biochemical events leading to an effect is called the mechanism of action of that drug. Morphine causes respiratory depression by depressing the responsiveness of the respiratory center to CO_2.

STRUCTURE-ACTIVITY RELATIONSHIP. A definite and strong relationship seems to exist be-

tween the structure of most pharmacologic compounds and their inherent pharmacologic properties. For example, modification of the structure of acetylcholine alters its pharmacologic properties dramatically. Acetylcholine mediates cholinergic function at various anatomic sites. In fact, with the exception of the sensory fibers and postganglionic sympathetic neurons, all the nerves of the mammalian peripheral nervous system are probably cholinergic. Examination of the structure of acetylcholine reveals quaternary nitrogen in one end of the molecule and an ester at the other end, separated by two-carbon linkage. Substituting a keto group for the ester group diminishes the cholinergic properties of acetylcholine according to the following scale [2]:

Compound		Activity Relative to Acetylcholine
Acetylcholine	$(CH_3)_2N^+ - CH_2 - CH_2O - \overset{\displaystyle O}{\overset{\|}{C}} - CH_3$	1
4-Ketoamyl-trimethyl-ammonium ion	$(CH_3)_2N^+ - CH_2 - CH_2 - CH_2 - \overset{\displaystyle O}{\overset{\|}{C}} - CH_3$	1/12
3-Ketoamyl-trimethyl-ammonium ion	$(CH_3)_2N^+ - CH_2 - CH_2 - \overset{\displaystyle O}{\overset{\|}{C}} - CH_2 - CH_3$	1/160
2-Ketoamyl-trimethyl-ammonium ion	$(CH_3)_2N^+ - CH_2 - \overset{\displaystyle O}{\overset{\|}{C}} - CH_2 - CH_2 - CH_3$	1/620

Therefore, one recognizes that the maintenance of the structure of acetylcholine is essential for its cholinergic activity. Acetylcholine, an important physiologic agent, is not useful as a drug, since its short-lived actions are massive and nonspecific in character. The various synthetic derivatives of acetylcholine differ from acetylcholine in being more resistant to hydrolysis by cholinesterase (longer duration of action) and having relatively organ-specific action(s). For example, bethanechol chloride

$$(CH_2)_3N^+ - CH_2 - \overset{\overset{\displaystyle H}{\|}}{\underset{\underset{\displaystyle CH_3}{|}}{C}} - O - \overset{\overset{\displaystyle O}{\|}}{C} - NH_2 \cdot Cl^-$$

is useful in treating urinary retention, megacolon, and delayed gastric emptying that one sees following vagotomy for amelioration of the symptoms of severe peptic ulceration.

DRUG ACTIONS UNRELATED TO STRUCTURES. Where drugs exert their effects by interacting with specific receptors, structural modification does dramatically alter the expected effects. However, it should be understood that not all drugs produce their effects by interacting with specific receptors. For example, general anesthetics such as thiopental, halothane, cyclopropane, and nitrous oxide have vastly dissimilar structures. Antacids, such as sodium bicarbonate, and aluminum hydroxide are similar in functions but not in structures. Diuretics such as triamterene, chlorothiazide, and furosemide do not share any specific structure-activity relationships. Phenol, hydrogen peroxide, ethyl alcohol, hexachlorophene, and benzalkonium chloride are excellent antiseptics with dissimilar structures.

DRUG RECEPTOR–SPECIFIC INTERACTION.
Contemporary ideas of drug action and drug specificity are based on the assumption that the initial process in drug action is the formation of a reversible complex between the drug and a cell component generally known as the "drug receptor." The interaction of a drug with a specific receptor site is characterized by at least three factors.

Chemical and Structural Specificity. Alteration in structure of compounds does alter their pharmacologic properties. For example, nalorphine, a narcotic antagonist, varies from morphine, a narcotic agonist, by replacement of the CH_3 group on the morphine's nitrogen by the allyl radical $-CH_2CH=CH_2$.

Stereoisomeric Specificity. Only the $(-)$ enantiomorph of morphine and certain other opioids can interact with ("enter") the receptor site. For example, levorphanol, a synthetic narcotic, is 5 to 10 times more potent than morphine, and its L $(+)$ enantiomorph dextrorphan is devoid of analgesic activity.

Potency. Drugs that interact with receptor sites may exert their effects in extremely small doses. For example, etorphine is 10,000 times more potent than morphine.

RECEPTOR-RELATED DISEASES. Numerous diseases are related to alteration in or loss of integrity of pharmacologic receptors. For example, myasthenia gravis is a remitting and relapsing neuromuscular disease of humans characterized by muscular fatigability that is thought to result initially from breakdown of immunologic tolerance, inflammatory responses at the neuromuscular junction, alteration of morphology of neuromuscular junction, and reduction in acetylcholine receptors. The beneficial effects of steroids may be attributed to their antiinflammatory and immunosuppressive properties. The usefulness of neostigmine during the acute attack may be due to its ability to inhibit acetylcholinesterase and increase the concentration of acetylcholine at the cholinergic receptors to compensate for reduction in these receptors. Insulin-resistant diabetes mellitus and testicular feminization are also examples of diseases brought on by resistance of receptors to their agonists (i.e., insulin and androgen respectively) [1, 3, 4].

DRUG-RELATED RECEPTOR ALTERATION.
Numerous drugs when taken in large doses and chronically may alter receptor functions, involving a decrease in receptor number, an increase in receptor number, or a decrease in the adaptability of receptors to physiologic events. Neuroleptic-induced tardive dyskinesia is an example of the alteration of striatal dopaminergic receptor sites.

RECEPTOR DOWN REGULATION. Receptor down regulation, also referred to as desensitization or tachyphylaxis, is an alteration in receptor number occurring upon continuous presence of a drug. Alpha-adrenergic receptors and insulin receptors are examples of receptors that manifest down regulation [4].

CELLULAR SITES OF ACTIONS OF DRUGS.
Being very reactive in nature, many drugs bring about their effects or side effects by interacting with coenzymes, enzymes, or nucleic acids, as well as other macromolecules and physiologic processes such as transport mechanisms. An appreciation of the complex interactions between drugs and physiologic parameters may be gained by noting some examples.

Drug-Coenzyme Interactions. ISONIAZID AND PYRIDOXAL PHOSPHATE: AN INDICATION FOR PYRIDOXINE. The primary drugs in the treatment of tuberculosis are isoniazid, ethambutol, and rifampin. Isoniazid is prescribed orally in doses of 4 to 5 mg per kilogram of body weight. If pyridoxine is not given concurrently with isoniazid, peripheral neuritis is the most common side effect. Toxic doses may cause optic neuritis, muscular twitching, dizziness, ataxia, paresthesias, and convulsions, especially in malnourished patients. These neuropathies are thought to result from chemical interaction between isoniazid and pyridoxal phosphate and reduction in the level of this important coenzyme in the body. The coadministration of pyridoxine averts these side effects.

PYRIDOXAL PHOSPHATE NULLIFICATION OF LEVODOPA EFFECTS: A CONTRAINDICATION FOR PYRIDOXINE. Levodopa, given orally on a chronic basis, is effective in combating the pathophysiology of parkinsonism characterized by tremor, rigidity, postural abnormalities, and akinesia, which are thought to result in part from deficiency of dopamine in the striatum. The administration of pyridoxine to a parkinsonian patient benefiting from levodopa will nullify the therapeutic beneficial effects of levodopa. The mechanism of nullification is thought to be due to pyridoxal phosphate–stimulated dopa decarboxylase and the conversion of a higher than ordinary proportion of levodopa to dopamine in the periphery, resulting in reduction in the formation of dopamine in the striatum. At the present time, most patients are treated concurrently with levodopa and a dopa decarboxylase inhibitor, such as carbidopa, which circumvents this problem.

FOLIC ACID AND TRIMETHOPRIM-SULFAMETHOXAZOLE. In acute and chronic urinary tract infection, the combination of trimethoprim-sulfamethoxazole (Bactrim, Septra) exerts a truly synergistic effect on bacteria. The sulfonamide inhibits the utilization of *p*-aminobenzoic acid in the synthesis of folic acid, while trimethoprim, by inhibiting dihydrofolic acid reductase, blocks the conversion of dihydrofolic acid to tetrahydrofolic acid, which is essential to bacteria in the de novo synthesis of purines, pyrimidines, and certain amino acids. Since mammalian organisms do not synthesize folic acid but require it as a vitamin in their daily diets, the trimethoprim-sulfamethoxazole combination does not interfere with the metabolism of mammalian cells.

DICUMAROL AND VITAMIN K. Phytonadione is identical to naturally occurring vitamin K_1, which is required for the synthesis of blood coagulation factors such as prothrombin (II), proconvertin (VII), Christmas factor or plasma thromboplastin component (IX), and Stuart-Power factor (X) in the liver. Dicumarol and ethyl biscoumacetate act as competitive antagonists of vitamin K and interfere with the synthesis of these factors in the liver. Similarly, the bleeding induced by hypoprothrombinemia can be rectified by the administration of vitamin K.

The examples cited indicate clearly that drugs may produce their actions or side effects by interacting with coenzymes, such as pyridoxal phosphate, folic acid, and vitamin K.

Drug-Enzyme Interactions. Numerous drugs exert their effects or side effects by interacting with enzymes.

ALLOPURINOL, XANTHINE OXIDASE, AND HYPERURICEMIC STATES. Allopurinol is used to lower uric acid levels in primary gout, prophylactically in myeloproliferative neoplastic disease, investigationally in Lesch-Nyhan Syndrome, and adjunctively with thiazide diuretics or with ethambutol. The mechanism of action of allopurinol is to inhibit the enzyme xanthine oxidase, which converts hypoxanthine into xanthine, which in turn becomes oxidized into uric acid.

$$\text{Hypoxanthine} \xrightarrow[\text{oxidase}]{\text{Xanthine}} \text{xanthine} \xrightarrow[\text{oxidase}]{\text{Xanthine}} \text{uric acid}$$

When xanthine oxidase is inhibited by allopurinol, there is a fall in the plasma level of uric acid and a decrease in the size of the urate pool in the body.

DRUGS AND BRONCHIAL ASTHMA. Bronchial asthma is characterized by respiratory distress, apnea, wheezing, flushing, and cyanosis. Since bronchoconstriction seems to be the common denominator of pathogenesis of asthma, bronchodilation is usually considered an effective pharmacologic intervention. Theophylline given intravenously is used in status asthmaticus patients who are refractory to epineph-

rine. In addition, in severe acute asthma attacks, epinephrine is administered subcutaneously and is considered the sympathomimetic drug of choice. Epinephrine may also be given along with theophylline. It is thought that bronchodilation in part is associated with enhanced concentration of cyclic AMP, which is metabolized according to the following scheme:

$$\text{ATP} \xrightarrow[\text{cyclase}]{\text{Adenylate}} \text{cyclic AMP} \xrightarrow{\text{Phosphodiesterase}} 5' \text{ AMP}$$

Epinephrine stimulates the beta-adrenergic receptors in the bronchioles, which in turn activate the membrane-bound adenylate cyclase to synthesize more cyclic AMP, whereas theophylline inhibits the activity of phosphodiesterase, conserving the previously synthesized cyclic AMP. Corticosteroids, also effective in the symptomatic treatment of certain types of asthma, exert their beneficial effects in part by enhancing the catecholamine effects, and by antagonizing the cholinergic actions, one of which is bronchoconstriction.

TRANYLCYPROMINE AND ENDOGENOUS DEPRESSION. Tranylcypromine, a monoamine oxidase inhibitor, is effective in the symptomatic treatment of endogenous depression. Monoamine oxidase, an enzyme found primarily in neurons, in liver, and in lungs, catalyzes the oxidative deamination of serotonin, epinephrine, and norepinephrine.

$$\text{Norepinephrine} \xrightarrow{\text{Monoamine oxidase}}$$
3-methoxy-4-hydroxyphenylethylene glycol (MHPG)

As a monoamine oxidase inhibitor, tranylcypromine increases the concentrations of monoamines in the body. The simultaneous administration of tranylcypromine and ingestion of food substances containing biogenic amines, such as cheese and wines containing high tyramine, may produce a hypertensive crisis, characterized by marked hypertension, occipital headache, palpitation, dilated pupils, and, in some cases, intracranial and fatal hemorrhage. These side effects are caused by accumulation of catecholamine released by tyramine from, for example, cheese and by inhibition of its catabolism imposed by tranylcypromine.

The examples cited indicate that drugs may bring forth their effects or side effects by interacting with enzymes, such as xanthine oxidase, adenylate cyclase, phosphodiesterase, and monoamine oxidase.

Drug–Nucleic Acid Interactions. Chemotherapeutic agents useful in neoplastic diseases exert their therapeutic effects by modifying the synthesis or the functions of nucleic acids. For example, 6-mercaptopurine inhibits purine ring biosynthesis, cytarabine inhibits DNA polymerase, alkylating agents cross-link DNA, and hydroxyurea inhibits the conversion of ribonucleotides into deoxyribonucleotides. However, other pharmacologic agents such as chlorpromazine, a neuroleptic, also modify nucleic acid synthesis. One of the side effects of chlorpromazine is mild to severe agranulocytosis. Chlorpromazine reduces the synthesis of DNA by inhibiting the activity of thymidine kinase according to the following scheme:

$$\text{Thymidine} + \text{ATP} \xrightarrow[\text{kinase}]{\text{Thymidine}} \text{thymidine 5'} \text{ phosphate} + \text{ADP}$$

In addition to chlorpromazine, phenylbutazone (analgesic and antiinflammatory agent), sulfonamides (chemotherapeutic agents), chlorothiazide (diuretic), thiouracil and methimazole (antithyroid drugs), phenytoin (antiepileptic drug), pyribenzamine (antihistaminic), and chloramphenicol (antimicrobial agent) may cause agranulocytosis in susceptible individuals. The incidence of this side effect is highest among persons with lower than normal proliferative capacity of the bone marrow.

INTERACTIONS OF DRUGS WITH NEURONAL ELEMENTS.

Neuropharmacology may be defined as the study of drugs that affect the nervous system and its neuronal components. The functions of the nervous system are intimately linked with the synthesis, storage, release, and uptake of many transmitters and their modulators. An extensive number of drugs bring about their beneficial effects or side effects by interacting with these neurotransmitter-neuromodulator systems. A few examples will be cited, limiting the discussion to the effects of selected drugs on the synthesis, storage, and release of norepinephrine.

Reserpine and Hypertension. Reserpine may be used in conjunction with a diuretic in the treatment of mild to moderate hypertension. It is thought that reserpine brings about its antihypertensive effect by preventing the storage and hence reducing the pool of norepinephrine in the body. This amine-depleting action of reserpine not only has beneficial effects but also causes side effects. For instance, reserpine may tranquilize and lead to depression (depletes catecholamine from brain); may cause bradycardia, increase the motility of the gastrointestinal tract, and cause miosis (enhanced cholinergic activity secondary to decreased sympathetic activity); and may increase atrioventricular conduction time resulting from an increase in the refractory period of the AV conduction system (depletion of myocardial norepinephrine).

Alpha-Methyldopa and Hypertension. Alpha-methyldopa is used in the treatment of mild to moderate hypertension. The proposed mechanism of action is suppression of renin release, stimulation of central alpha inhibitory adrenergic receptor, and possibly formation of false transmitter, such as alpha-methylnorepinephrine. Substances activating beta-adrenergic receptor sites, such as angiotensin II, increase the release of norepinephrine whereas substances activating alpha-adrenergic receptor sites, such as dopamine, acetylcholine, and prostaglandins (PGE_1 and PGE_2 but not $PGF_{2\alpha}$), reduce the release of norepinephrine. In addition to reducing the blood pressure, alpha-methyldopa causes sedation (interference with function of norepinephrine), parkinsonism (interference with function of dopamine), psychosis (interference with function of serotonin), and decreased libido and impotence (interference with function of norepinephrine).

INTERACTION OF DRUGS WITH THE ENDOCRINE SYSTEM.

The nervous system and the endocrine system are linked and interrelated functionally and demonstrate pharmacologic cross reactivities. The endocrine system, which is an effector arm of the nervous system, is adrenergic in character. A few examples will be cited showing the interactions of drugs with the endocrine system.

Alpha-Methyldopa and Renin. Hypotension and decreased renal perfusion pressure promote the release of renin from the juxtaglomerular apparatus of the kidney. Renin converts angiotensin I to angiotensin II, a potent endogenously occurring vasoconstrictor in the body. Catecholamine can also release renin, and this effect is blocked by propranolol, a beta-adrenergic receptor blocking agent. Drugs altering the renin level are able to alter blood pressure. Alpha-methyldopa suppresses renin release whereas the oral contraceptive medications have the opposite effect. In addition, promising new antihypertensive medications such as captopril specifically inhibit angiotensin-converting enzyme, hence preventing the formation of angiotensin II.

Drugs and Prolactin. The release of prolactin from the adenohypophysis is a centrally mediated event involving dopaminergic neurons. Stimulation of dopaminergic neurons blocks prolactin production whereas blockade of dopaminergic function causes lactation. Chlorpromazine (which blocks dopamine receptor), reserpine (which depletes dopamine), and alpha-methyldopa (which forms a false transmitter such as alpha-methyldopamine) are all able to cause inappropriate lactation in a woman.

Diabetes Mellitus and Insulin Release. A sulfonylurea such as tolazamide may be used in patients with maturity-onset diabetes mellitus in whom the disease cannot be controlled by diet or exercise alone, and in diabetes patients without complicating factors such as infections, ketosis, and acidosis where crystalline zinc insulin may be required. The hypoglycemic effects of tolazamide appear to be caused by stimulation of insulin secretion from the beta cells of the pancreatic islets, which is mediated via beta-adrenergic receptor sites. Pharmacologic agents such as isoproterenol, which stimulates beta receptors, or phentolamine, which blocks alpha receptor sites, promote the release of insulin. Examples of agents that may cause hyperglycemia in certain circumstances are aldosterone, caffeine, catecholamines, chlorpromazine, corticosteroids, ethacrynic acid, furosemide, glucagon, indomethacin, nicotine, oral contraceptives, and thiazide diuretics. Examples of drugs causing hypoglycemia are alcohol, isoniazid, methimazole, propranolol, and salicylate.

This discussion clearly points to the fact that drugs do not create functions but merely stimulate or inhibit functions already inherent in the cells. Pharmacodynamics-related interactions take place at various levels of cellular activities, including ion transport, and involve enzymes, coenzymes, nucleic acids, and numerous other biochemical modalities yet to be delineated.

QUESTIONS ON PHARMACODYNAMICS

Select one answer or explanation that best answers the question or completes the statement.

16. All of the following drugs exert their effects by interacting with one or more receptor site(s) except which one?
    A. Neostigmine.
    B. Diazepam.
    C. Echothiophate.
    D. Halothane.

17. In general, all drugs that exert their effects by interacting with receptor sites show the following specific properties:
    A. Structural specificity and stereoisomeric specificity.
    B. Supersensitivity and tachyphylaxis.
    C. Up regulation but not down regulation.
    D. Covalent bonding, and act as suicide inhibitor.

18. A desired clinical response may be delayed, altered, or blocked by:
    A. A drug that does not go into solution.
    B. A drug that does not get to its site of action.
    C. Abnormal pharmacogenetics.
    D. Lack of absorption from the site of administration.
    E. All of the above.

19. Alpha-methyldopa is thought to exert its antihypertensive effect by:
    A. Forming a false transmitter.
    B. Stimulating alpha inhibitory adrenergic receptors in the CNS.
    C. Inhibiting renin function.
    D. All of the above.

20. Aspirin is thought to exert its effects by altering the synthesis of:
    A. Vitamin A.
    B. Cyclic AMP.
    C. ATP.
    D. Prostaglandin.

21. Dihydrofolic acid reductase is inhibited by:
    A. Acetylsalicylic acid.
    B. Dicumarol.
    C. Methotrexate and trimethoprim.
    D. Chlorpromazine.

22. In angina pectoris, nitroglycerin is given sublingually because:

    A. It is not absorbed orally.
    B. It causes severe hypotension and bradycardia.
    C. It is hepatotoxic.
    D. None of the above.

23. The isoniazid-induced convulsions in a patient with tuberculosis may result from:
    A. Depletion of pyridoxal phosphate from neurons.
    B. Stimulation of glutamic acid decarboxylase.
    C. Reduction in norepinephrine concentration.
    D. Depletion of ascorbic acid from adrenal gland.

24. In the management of a urinary tract infection, trimethoprim-sulfamethoxazole preparation exerts a truly synergistic effect because the combination:
    A. Blocks two consecutive steps in bacterial metabolism.
    B. Facilitates the synthesis of folic acid in humans.
    C. Facilitates the synthesis of purine and pyrimidine in bacteria.
    D. Eliminates the hypersensitivity reaction in patients sensitive to sulfamethoxazole.

25. Allopurinol is useful in preventing or alleviating hyperuricemia by:
    A. Enhancing the excretion of uric acid.
    B. Converting the uric acid into a more soluble metabolite.
    C. Inhibiting the synthesis of uric acid.
    D. Correcting the state(s) causing hyperuricemia.

26. The beneficial effects of epinephrine and theophylline are mediated by altering the activities of which two enzymes?
    A. Acetylcholinesterase and choline acetylase.
    B. Monoamine oxidase and carboxypeptidase.
    C. Dihydrofolate reductase and pyridoxal kinase.
    D. Adenylate cyclase and phosphodiesterase.

27. The chlorpromazine-induced agranulocytosis is in part due to inhibition of:
    A. Adenine phosphoribosyltransferase.
    B. Thymidine kinase.
    C. 5-Phosphoribosyl-1-pyrophosphate synthetase.
    D. Glutamine PRPP aminotransferase.

28. Levorphanol is an analgesic drug and dextrorphan is not. In terms of drug receptor interaction, this is an example of:
    A. Stereoisomeric specificity.
    B. Tachyphylaxis at the receptor site.
    C. Irreversible receptor occupancy.
    D. The Huckel electron approximation.

29. The depression by morphine of the respiratory center is an example of:
    A. Drug-nullified physiologic process.
    B. Drug-stimulated physiologic process.
    C. Drug-inhibited physiologic process.
    D. Drug-potentiated physiologic process.

30. Receptor down regulation results in which of the following events?
    A. Reduction in the number of receptor sites and attenuation of inherent pharmacologic activity.
    B. Increase in the number of receptor sites and potentiation of inherent pharmacologic activity.

C. Increase in the number of receptor sites and creation of novel pharmacologic activity.
D. Constancy in the number of receptor sites with loss of inherent activity.

ANSWERS ON PHARMACODYNAMICS

16. D.
17. A.
18. E.
19. D.
20. D.
21. C.
22. D.
23. A.
24. A.
25. C.
26. D.
27. B.
28. A.
29. C.
30. A.

REFERENCES

1. Essman, W. B. *Neurotransmitters, Receptors and Drug Actions.* Jamaica, N.Y.: SP Medical and Scientific Books, 1980.
2. Goldstein, A., Aronow, L., and Kalman, S. M. *Principles of Drug Action. The Basis of Pharmacology* (2nd ed.). New York: Wiley, 1974.
3. Lamble, J. W. *Toward Understanding Receptors.* Amsterdam: Elsevier North-Holland, 1981.
4. Lefkowitz, R. J. *Receptor Regulation.* London: Chapman & Hall, 1981.

3. Adverse Reactions and Drug–Drug Interactions

> Imperative drugging—the ordering in any and every malady—is no longer regarded as the chief function of the doctor.
>
> *Sir William Osler*

It is commonplace for patients to receive two or more drugs concomitantly. Furthermore, it is becoming increasingly obvious to physicians and other members of the health care delivery team that many drug combinations, when used inappropriately and injudiciously, have the inherent potential to interact adversely and to cause side effects and even fatal toxicity [1, 3, 4].

Whether drugs are given individually or in combination, some adverse reactions are inevitable and may not be eliminated. For example, patients undergoing treatment with antineoplastic drugs will develop expected side effects such as hair loss. While arresting the rapidly multiplying cancerous cells, antineoplastic agents also arrest or retard the multiplication and growth of normal but rapidly dividing host cells. Nevertheless, many adverse effects of drugs or drug-drug interactions either are avoidable or may be minimized substantially.

The varied and complex mechanisms may be broadly classified as pharmacokinetic interactions or pharmacodynamic interactions [2]. In pharmacokinetic interactions, some drugs interfere with or alter the absorption, distribution, biotransformation, or excretion of other drugs. In pharmacodynamic interactions, already discussed in Chapter 2, drugs may modify the intended and expected actions of other drugs. Before discussion and further elaboration on pharmacokinetic interactions, some terms will be defined [5].

IATROGENIC REACTIONS. *Iatrogenic reactions* are, broadly, any adverse reactions produced unintentionally by physicians in their patients. For example, many antihistaminic preparations cause heavy sedation. Patients engaged in physical and mental activities requiring constant alertness—operating machinery or driving long distances, for example—should be forewarned by physicians and other health professionals about these side effects.

ALLERGIC REACTIONS. *Drug allergy* refers to reactions to a drug in a patient who was previously exposed to, was sensitized with, and developed antibodies to that drug. The underlying immunologic mechanisms may be varied and complex, involving anaphylactoid immediate reactions (e.g., to penicillin, due to formation of specific immunoglobulin E), cytotoxic reactions (e.g., drug-induced hemolytic anemias), and delayed allergic reactions (drug-induced contact dermatitis). Careful history taking prior to administration of drugs and watchful monitoring of the patients after administration of drugs will lessen the incidence and the severity of the drug-induced allergic reactions.

IDIOSYNCRATIC REACTIONS. *Idiosyncrasy* refers to an abnormal, unexpected, or peculiar reaction seen in some patients. For example, succinylcholine may cause prolonged apnea in patients with pseudocholinesterase deficiency. Hemolytic anemia may be seen following administration of an extensive number of drugs, including sulfonamides in patients with glucose 6-phosphate dehydrogenase deficiency. Malignant hyperpyrexia may occur in patients anesthetized with halothane as a general anesthetic. Paradoxic rage reaction is seen in some patients following administration of chlordiazepoxide, an antianxiety agent. Idiosyncratic reactions become manifest only in the presence of insulting drugs. Although they are inevitable when they occur unexpectedly for the first time in a patient, they may be circumvented altogether in patients who have previously shown such abnormal reactions.

TOLERANCE AND TACHYPHYLAXIS. *Tolerance* refers to decreased responses following chronic administration of drugs. For example, after repeated administration of morphine, tolerance occurs to all its effects except miosis and constipation, which continue unabated. Morphine causes respiratory depression less readily in a tolerant patient. Although it is generally accepted that tolerance may develop with many depressant drugs such as alcohol, benzodiazepine antianxiety agents, and barbiturates, it may also occur with other agents such as clonazepam (an antiepileptic agent), carbamazepine (an antiepileptic agent, and a drug of choice in trigeminal and glossopharyngeal neuralgias), and chlorpromazine (a neuroleptic).

Tachyphylaxis refers to a quickly developing tolerance brought about by rapid and repeated administration of drugs. For example, indirect-acting sympathomimetic agents such as tyramine, which exert their effects through releasing norepinephrine, are able to cause tachyphylaxis. Where no norepinephrine is present, tyramine fails to have an effect until the supply of norepinephrine in nerve terminals has been replenished.

Although tachyphylaxis is innocuous and is not regarded as a major problem in medicine, the lack of appreciation of tolerance as an entity may be devastating in character. For example, respiratory depression is not seen in a morphine-tolerant patient, and an amount much higher than normally considered therapeutic dosage is required to induce an effect. However, tolerance is lost or lessened following discontinuation of administration of morphine. In a nontolerant patient, the administration of the dose of morphine that was quite innocuous prior to loss of tolerance would prove fatal by causing severe respiratory depression.

PHARMACOKINETIC INTERACTIONS. Drugs may affect the absorption, distribution, metabolism, or excretion of other drugs. Thus gastrointestinal absorption of a drug is increased or decreased, plasma protein binding is affected, drug metabolism is stimulated or inhibited, or urinary excretion is enhanced or inhibited.

Interaction at the Site of Absorption. The rate or extent of drug absorption from the gastrointestinal tract can be influenced in a number of ways.

ALTERATION OF GASTRIC pH. Iron poisoning is characterized by vomiting, abdominal pain, gastroenteritis, and shock, and, if not properly treated, by severe metabolic acidosis, coma, and death. Deferoxamine, which binds iron, is used as a chelating agent of choice in iron poisoning. The metabolic acidosis may be appropriately treated with sodium bicarbonate. However, since deferoxamine chelates iron more effectively in an acidic medium, it should not be administered orally concomitantly with sodium bicarbonate. Ideal treatment of iron poisoning consists in gastric aspiration, followed by lavage with phosphate solution to form insoluble iron salts. Then deferoxamine should be given intravenously or intramuscularly to chelate the iron that has been absorbed. Sodium bicarbonate may be administered by the intravenous route. In order to absorb any residual iron remaining in the stomach, deferoxamine may then be instilled into the stomach.

FORMATION OF COMPLEX. Tetracyclines, as broad-spectrum antibiotics, are the drug of choice in infections with *Mycoplasma pneumoniae*. Most tetracyclines are absorbed to various degrees (30–100%) from the gastrointestinal tract, primarily from the stomach and upper part of the small intestine. The absorption of tetracyclines is hindered by milk and milk products, by numerous antacids such as aluminum hydroxide, sodium bicarbonate, and calcium carbonate, and by iron preparations such as ferrous sulfate. Naturally, these and similar substances should not be administered together orally.

ALTERATION IN GASTRIC EMPTYING TIME. Agents that reduce gastrointestinal motililty and prolong gastric emptying time will reduce the rate of absorption of drugs whose absorption takes place primarily in the duodenum. Furthermore, by keeping the poorly soluble drugs longer in the stomach, one may alter their bioavailability. Hence, compounds with strong anticholinergic properties such as propantheline (for peptic diseases), glycopyrrolate (for asthma), benztropine (for parkinsonism), and imipramine (for depression) are potentially able to alter the absorption of other drugs concomitantly administered. The absorption of digoxin and dicumarol is altered by imipramine and other tricyclic antidepressants. On the other hand, some drugs such as antacids may speed gastric emptying time.

Interactions at the Plasma Protein-Binding Sites. Drugs may compete for binding sites on the plasma or tissue protein or may displace the previously bound drugs. For example, phenylbutazone may compete with phenytoin for binding to albumin. Similarly, phenylbutazone (an antiinflammatory agent) is able to displace warfarin (an anticoagulant) from its binding site and enhance the free circulating concentration of anticoagulant. Sulfonamides (chemotherapeutic agents) are able to displace sulfonylureas (oral antidiabetic agents) and cause hypoglycemia. Estradiol, by inhibiting the hepatic metabolism of proteins, may increase the amount of binding proteins. For example, women taking estrogen-containing oral contraceptives may demonstrate elevated protein-bound iodine (PBI) while remaining euthyroid.

Interactions at the Stage of Drug Biotransformation. Drug biotransformation usually converts the nonpolar active drugs into more water-soluble but pharmacologically inactive products. Drugs may stimulate or inhibit the metabolism of other drugs. These interactions may be either innocuous or detrimental to the expected therapeutic objectives.

AGENTS STIMULATING THE BIOTRANSFORMATION OF DRUGS. The ingestion of alcohol or phenobarbital on a chronic basis induces drug biotransformation. The maximum inducing effects vary from drug to drug, usually occurring and subsiding in 7 to 10 days. The sudden withdrawal of an inducing agent has proved fatal in some circumstances. For example, hypnotic sedatives cause an increase in the rate of metabolism of coumarin anticoagulants. A physician may have to administer coumarin at increased doses in order to achieve the desired prothrombin time and therapeutic effects. Sudden withdrawal from a hypnotic-sedative agent may revert the coumarin-catabolizing enzyme to pretreatment level, and in the presence of large concentrations of free coumarin, hemorrhage may result. Since physicians anticipate that their patients may not require hypnotic-sedative agents after being discharged from the hospital, the maintenance doses of coumarin anticoagulants are gradually reduced 2 to 3 days in advance of the discharge date.

On the other hand, drugs may inhibit the metabolism of other drugs. For example, allopurinol (a xanthine oxidase inhibitor that inhibits the synthesis of uric acid) increases the effectiveness of anticoagulants by inhibiting their metabolism. Chloramphenicol (a potent inhibitor of microsomal protein synthesis) and cimetidine (an H_2 receptor blocker used in acid-pepsin disease) have similar properties. In addition, drugs may compete with each other for metabolism. In methyl alcohol (methanol) poisoning, ethyl alcohol given intravenously may be used to avert methanol-induced blindness and minimize the severe acidosis. Ethyl alcohol competes with methyl alcohol for catabolism by liver alcohol dehydrogenase. The unmetabolized and less toxic methanol is excreted unchanged in the urine.

Interactions at the Site of Excretion. Numerous drugs are able to either enhance or inhibit the excretion of other drugs. Sodium bicarbonate enhances the excretion of phenobarbital. Probenecid interferes with active secretion of penicillin and hence prolongs its half-life. Probenecid's uricosuric effects will be nullified by acetylsalicylic acid, which also possesses a uricosuric effect. When given concomitantly, both become excreted.

QUESTIONS ON ADVERSE REACTIONS AND DRUG-DRUG INTERACTIONS

Select one statement or answer that best completes the sentence or answers the question.

____ 31. No interaction of clinical significance is known to be involved between:
  A. Dicumarol and vitamin K.
  B. Levodopa and pyridoxine (B_6).
  C. Isoniazid and pyridoxine.
  D. Digoxin and vitamin A.

____ 32. Allopurinol is helpful in the gouty state through its interactions with which enzyme?
  A. Xanthine oxidase.
  B. Monoamine oxidase.
  C. Carboxypeptidase.
  D. Uric acid dehydrogenase.

____ 33. Which of the following drugs produce *opposite* functions on certain physiologic, biochemical, or pharmacologic parameters?
  A. Oral contraceptive and alpha-methyldopa.
  B. Alpha-methyldopa and reserpine.
  C. Dicumarol and acetylsalicylic acid.
  D. Thiazide diuretic and digoxin.

____ 34. Which one of the following drug combinations produces a synergistic effect?
  A. Tetracycline given with a glass of milk.
  B. Deferoxamine given with $NaHCO_3$.
  C. Norepinephrine and thyroxine.
  D. Probenecid and acetylsalicylic acid.

____ 35. Which one of the following drug combinations may increase the plasma concentration of one of the drugs?
  A. Probenecid and penicillin.
  B. Phenobarbital and $NaHCO_3$.
  C. NH_4Cl and amphetamine.
  D. Phenobarbital and dicumarol.

____ 36. Which one of the following is not an example of drug-drug interactions?
  A. An increase in metabolism of oral anticoagulants after phenobarbital.
  B. Increased CNS depression upon administration of both a barbiturate and a narcotic analgesic (e.g., meperidine).

  C. Drowsiness caused by antihistamines.
  D. Enhanced toxicity of cardiac glycosides when given with thiazide diuretics.

____ 37. In which of the following drug pairs is the second drug pharmacologically not related (a) to the same receptor sites, (b) to the same binding site, or (c) to the same related phenomenon?
  A. Reserpine and norepinephrine.
  B. Tranylcypromine and tyramine.
  C. Physostigmine and ephedrine.
  D. Metoprolol and isoproterenol.
  E. Bishydroxycoumarin and clofibrate.

____ 38. With one exception, all the following drug pairs interact in the gastrointestinal tract by one drug's interfering with the absorption or action of the other. This exception is:
  A. Tetracyclines and magnesium antacid products.
  B. Folic acid and cytarabine.
  C. Digoxin and aluminum antacid products.
  D. Tetracyclines and vitamin K.

____ 39. With one exception, all the following drug pairs interact at the transport or uptake site by one drug's interfering with the transport or uptake of the other. This exception is:
  A. Imipramine and guanethidine.
  B. Cholestyramine and digoxin.
  C. Amantadine and trihexyphenidyl.
  D. Cocaine and norepinephrine.

____ 40. With one exception in the following drug pairs, the interaction of one drug enhances the action or the toxicity of the other drug. The exception is:
  A. Phenytoin and isoniazid.
  B. Corticosteroid and epinephrine.
  C. Diazepam and ethyl alcohol.
  D. Chlorpromazine and amphetamine.

ANSWERS AND EXPLANATIONS ON ADVERSE REACTIONS AND DRUG-DRUG INTERACTIONS

31. D.
32. A.
33. A.
  Explanation: Oral contraceptives elaborate renin and may oppose the antihypertensive effects of alpha-methyldopa.
34. C.
35. A.
36. C.
37. C.
  Explanation: Reserpine releases norepinephrine, dopamine, and serotonin. Tyramine releases norepinephrine, and tranylcypromine inhibits its catabolism. Metoprolol is a beta₁-adrenergic receptor antagonist, and isoproterenol is a beta agonist. Both bishydroxycoumarin and clofibrate bind to albumin and compete with others for binding.
38. B.
  Explanation: Cytarabine (Cytosar) is used intravenously in acute granulocytic and lymphocytic leukemias. Tetracyclines decrease the intestinal bacteria flora that synthesize vitamin K.
39. C.
  Explanation: Tricyclic antidepressants including imipramine block the transport of guanethidine into ad-

renergic neurons and hence may interfere with its antihypertensive activity.

40. D.

Explanation: Isoniazid inhibits the metabolism of phenytoin and enhances its toxicity. Clorpromazine antidotes the toxicity of amphetamine, and vice versa.

REFERENCES

1. Cadwallader, D. E. *Biopharmaceutics and Drug Interactions* (3rd ed.). New York: Raven Press, 1983.

2. Hansten, P. D. *Drug Interactions* (4th ed.). Philadelphia: Lea & Febiger, 1979.

3. Levine, R. R. *Pharmacology: Drug Actions and Reactions* (3rd ed.). Boston: Little, Brown, 1983.

4. Melman, K. L., and Morrelli, H. F. *Clinical Pharmacology. Basic Principles in Therapeutics.* New York: Macmillan, 1978.

5. Meyler, L., and Peck, H. M. *Drug-Induced Diseases*, Vol. 4. Amsterdam: Excerpta Medica, 1972.

II. Autonomic Pharmacology

4. The Pharmacology of the Autonomic Nervous System

> What we learn with pleasure we never forget.
>
> *Alfred Mercier*

The nervous system and the endocrine system control an extensive number of functions in the body. The nervous system is divided into the central nervous system and the peripheral nervous system. The peripheral nervous system is further divided into the somatic nervous system (a voluntary system innervating skeletal muscles) and the autonomic nervous system (Fig. 4-1) (an involuntary system innervating smooth muscle, cardiac muscle, and glands) [10, 13]. The somatic nervous system and the autonomic nervous system differ anatomically and physiologically in the following respects [6]:

Somatic Nervous System	Autonomic Nervous System
Target tissues are skeletal muscles.	Target tissues are smooth muscle, cardiac muscle, and glands.
Cell bodies of somatic efferent neurons are found at all levels of the spinal cord.	Cell bodies are absent in cervical, lower lumbar, and coccygeal levels of the spinal cord.
The neurons have voluntary and involuntary (reflex) regulation.	The neurons have involuntary regulation only.
Target tissues (effectors) receive only one efferent neuron.	Target tissues receive two types (sympathetic and parasympathetic) of efferent neurons.
Only one myelinated neuron is interposed between the CNS and the effector organ.	The neurons between the CNS and the organ are myelinated preganglionic fibers and unmyelinated postganglionic fibers.
Acetylcholine is the transmitter.	Acetylcholine and norepinephrine are the transmitters.
Transmitter is necessary for skeletal muscle contraction, which is rapid.	Separate transmitters are necessary for contraction and relaxation of smooth muscles, which are slow in nature.
Denervation causes paralysis of skeletal muscle.	Smooth muscle shows autoregulation.
Only drugs causing skeletal muscle relaxation are used in medicine.	Both stimulants and depressants of smooth muscles are used in medicine.

Drugs influencing the autonomic nervous system are used in wide-angle glaucoma, in diagnosis of myasthenia gravis, as gastrointestinal and urinary tract stimulants in postoperative abdominal distention and urinary retention, as antidotes to poisoning from skeletal muscle relaxant such as curare, as antidotes to poisoning by tricyclic antidepressants, as preanesthetic medications, as mydriatics, as cycloplegics, in peptic acid oversecretion to diminish vagally mediated secretion of gastric juices, in slowing of gastric emptying, in vestibular disorders, in parkinsonism, in combination with local anesthetics, in hypotension and shock, in heart block to improve atrioventricular conduction and to stimulate ventricular automaticity, in bronchial asthma, as nasal decongestants, in narcolepsy, in minimal brain dysfunction, in diagnosis and treatment of pheochromocytoma, in cardiac arrhythmias, in angina pectoris, in hypertension, in thyrotoxicosis, and in tremor. In addition, numerous drugs such as neuroleptics and antidepressants bring about side effects through modifying the function of the autonomic nervous system.

The autonomic nervous system consists of (1) central connections, (2) visceral afferent fibers, and (3) visceral efferent fibers. The hypothalamus is the principal focus of integration of the entire autonomic nervous system and is concerned in the regulation of blood pressure, body temperature, water balance, metabolism of carbohydrate and lipids, sleep, emotion, and sexual reflexes. In addition to the hypothalamus, the medulla oblongata, the limbic system, and the cerebral cortex to a lesser extent integrate, coordinate, and adjust the functions of the autonomic nervous system [1, 2, 5].

Most blood vessels, sweat glands, and the spleen are innervated only by one division of the autonomic nervous system. In salivary glands, the two divisions of the autonomic nervous system supplement each other. In bladder, bronchi, gastrointestinal tract, heart, pupil, and sex organs, the two divisions of the autonomic nervous system have opposing effects (Table 4-1) [5, 10, 13].

NEUROCHEMICAL BASIS OF CHOLINERGIC TRANSMISSION. Acetylcholine, an ester of choline and acetic acid, is synthesized in cholinergic neurons according to the following scheme:

Fig. 4-1. *Divisions of the autonomic nervous system into sympathetic and parasympathetic.*

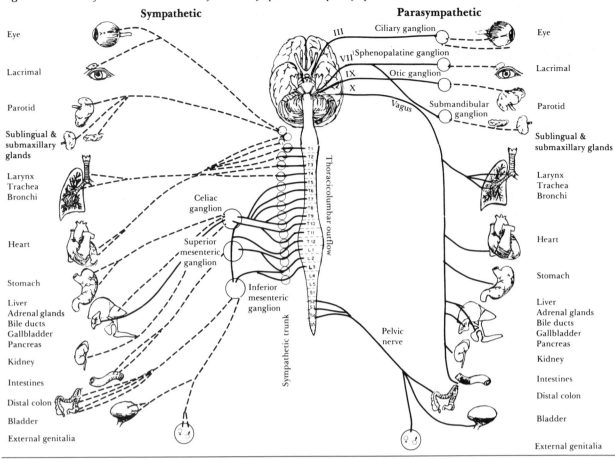

$$\text{Acetyl CoA} + \text{choline} \xrightarrow[\text{acetyltransferase}]{\text{Choline}} \text{acetylcholine}$$

Choline is actively transported into nerve terminals (synaptosomes) by a high-affinity uptake mechanism. Furthermore, the availability of choline regulates the synthesis of acetylcholine (Fig. 4-2).

Hemicholinium blocks the transport of choline into synaptosomes whereas botulinum toxin blocks the release of acetylcholine. The released acetylcholine is hydrolyzed rapidly by acetylcholinesterase to choline and acetate.

Acetylcholine receptors are classified as muscarinic and nicotinic receptors. The alkaloid muscarine mimics the effects produced by stimulation of the parasympathetic system. These effects are postganglionic and are exerted on exocrine glands, cardiac muscle, and smooth muscle. The alkaloid nicotine mimics the actions of acetylcholine that include stimulation of all autonomic ganglia, stimulation of the adrenal medulla, and contraction of skeletal muscle.

Dimethylphenylpiperazinium stimulates autonomic ganglia, tetraethylammonium and *hexamethonium* block autonomic ganglia, phenyltrimethylammonium stimulates skeletal motor muscle end plates, *decamethonium* produces neuromuscular blockade, while d-*tubocurarine* blocks both autonomic ganglia

and motor fiber end plates.

Among the agents cited, only *d*-tubocurarine is useful as a drug (skeletal muscle relaxant); and the rest are useful merely as research tools. Cholinesterase, found in liver and plasma, can hydrolyze other esters such as succinylcholine (a skeletal muscle relaxant). Cholinergic peripheral receptors are located on

1. Postganglionic parasympathetic fibers
2. Postganglionic sympathetic fibers
3. All autonomic ganglia
4. Skeletal end plate [12]

In addition, cholinergic receptors are distributed extensively in the CNS, participating in diversified functions such as audition, vision, learning and memory, ingestive behaviors (thirst, hunger), thermoregulation, locomotor activity, diurnal rhythms, sleep, and sexual activity. Alterations in cholinergic neurons have also been seen in neurologic syndromes such as catalepsy, stereotypy, and tremor and in psychiatric disorders such as schizophrenia. Furthermore, cholinergic neurons have been implicated in addiction to opiates and alcohol and in physiologic dependence and withdrawal syndromes [7].

The role of acetylcholine in schizophrenia has been widely studied. For example, anticholinergic

Table 4-1. *Responses of Effector Organs to Adrenergic and Cholinergic Impulses*

Effector Organs	Adrenergic Impulses		Cholinergic Impulses
	Receptor Type	Responses	Responses
Heart			
SA node	β_1	Increase in heart rate	Decrease in heart rate; vagal arrest
Atria	β_1	Increase in contractility and conduction velocity	Decrease in contractility and in conduction velocity
AV node and conduction system	β_1	Increase in conduction velocity	Decrease in conduction velocity: AV block
His-Purkinje system	β_1	Increase in conduction velocity	
Ventricles	β_1	Increase in contractility, conduction velocity, automaticity, and rate of idiopathic pacemakers	
Blood vessels			
Coronary	α,β_2	Constriction, dilatation	
Skin and mucosa	α_1	Constriction	
Skeletal muscle	α,β_2	Constriction, dilatation	Dilatation
Pulmonary	α,β_2	Constriction, dilatation	
Cerebral	α	Slight constriction	
Abdominal viscera	α,β_2	Constriction dilatation	
Lung			
Bronchial muscle	β_2	Relaxation	Contraction
Bronchial glands	?	Inhibition (?)	Stimulation
Stomach, intestine			
Motility and tone	α_2,β_2	Decrease (usually)	Increase (strong)
Sphincters	α_1	Contraction (usually)	Relaxation (usually)
Secretion		Inhibition	Stimulation
Intestine			
Motility and tone	α_2,β_2	Decrease	Increase (strong)
Sphincters	α	Contraction (usually)	Relaxation
Secretion		Inhibition (?)	Stimulation
Urinary bladder			
Detrusor	β	Relaxation (usually)	Contraction
Trigone and sphincter	α_1	Contraction	Relaxation
Kidney	β_2	Renin secretion	
Ureter			
Motility and tone	α	Increase (usually)	
Uterus	α,β_2	Pregnant (contraction) Nonpregnant (relaxation)	Variable
Male sex organ	α	Ejaculation	Erection
Liver	α,β_2	Glycogenolysis; gluconeogenesis	Glycogen synthesis
Pancreas			
Acini	α	Decreased secretion	Secretion
Islets (β cells)	α	Decreased secretion	
	β_2	Increased secretion	
Splenic capsule	α,β_2	Contraction	
Adrenal medulla		None	Secretion of epinephrine and norepinephrine
Salivary glands	α	Thick, viscous secretion	Profuse, watery secretion
Lacrimal glands			Secretion
Nasopharyngeal glands			Secretion
Eye			
Radial muscle iris	α_1	Contraction (mydriasis)	
Sphincter muscle iris			Contraction (miosis)
Ciliary muscle			

Adapted from S. E. Mayer, Neurohumoral Transmission and the Autonomic Nervous System. In A. G. Gilman, L. S. Goodman, and A. Gilman (eds.), *The Pharmacological Basis of Therapeutics.* New York: Macmillan, 1980.

Fig. 4-2. *Cholinergic transmission. Cholinergic nerve terminal depicting the synthesis, storage, release, and catabolism of acetylcholine.*

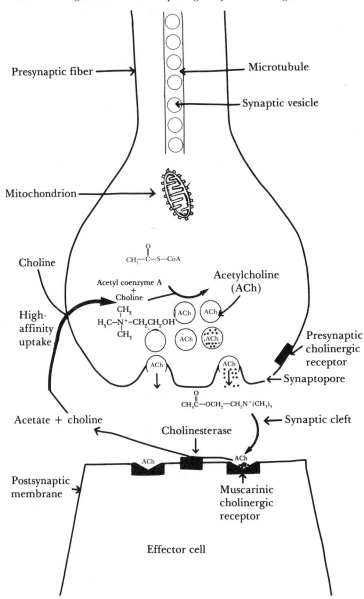

drugs such as atropine, benztropine, and trihexyphenidyl result in an acute exacerbation of schizophrenic psychosis, or they may cause toxic psychosis in nonpsychotic patients similar to paranoid schizophrenia. On the other hand, cholinomimetic agents such as physostigmine ameliorate schizophrenic symptoms [9].

CHOLINERGIC (CHOLINOMIMETIC) RECEPTOR AGONISTS. Methacholine, carbachol, and bethanechol (Fig. 4-3) are cholinomimetic agents that mimic the effects of stimulation of cholinergic nerves. The two derivatives of acetylcholine currently used are bethanechol (Urecholine Chloride) and carbachol (Miostat). Unlike acetylcholine, both agents are resistant to hydrolysis by cholinesterase. Both agents are muscarinic agonists. The nicotinic action of carbachol is greater than that of acetylcholine whereas bethanechol is devoid of nicotinic action. The cardiovascular actions of acetylcholine are vasodilation, negative chronotropic effects, and a negative inotropic effect. The cardiovascular effects of methacholine are more pronounced than those of acetylcholine, which in turn are greater than those of carbachol or bethanechol. The gastrointestinal effects (increase in tone, amplitude of contractions, and peristaltic activity) of bethanechol and carbachol are

Fig. 4-3. *Structures of cholinomimetics and of reversible and irreversible cholinesterase inhibitors.*

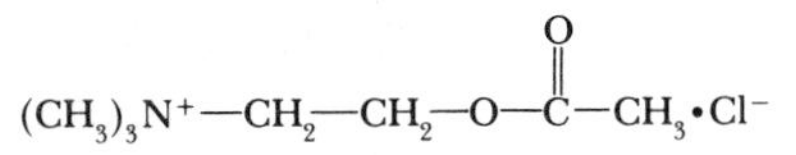

Acetylcholine chloride

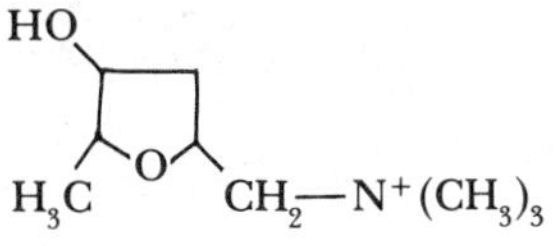

Muscarine

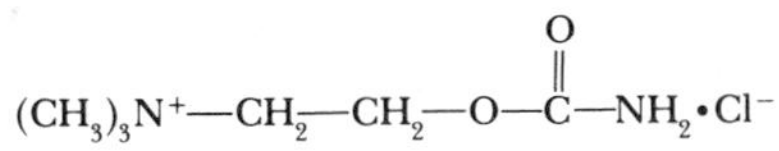

Carbachol chloride

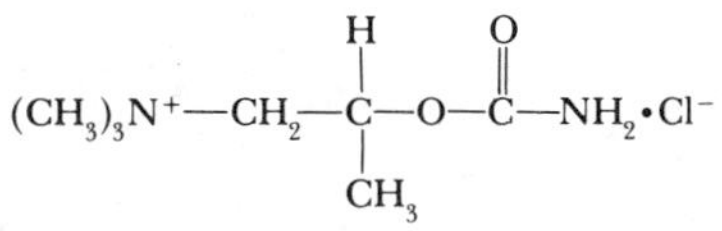

Bethanechol chloride

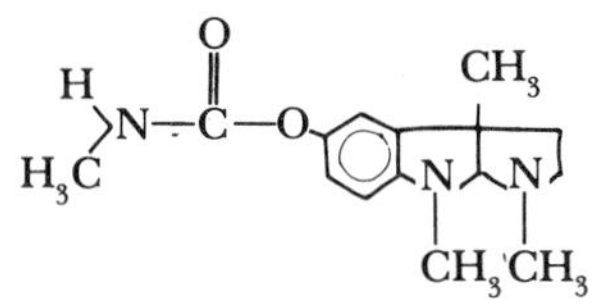

Physostigmine

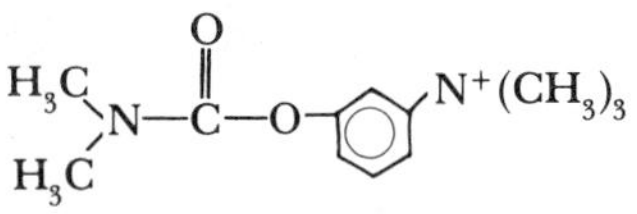

Neostigmine

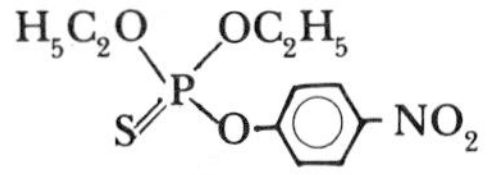

Parathion

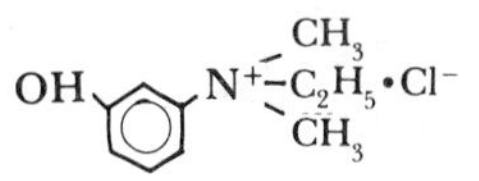

Edrophonium chloride

equal and are greater than those produced by acetylcholine. The effects of carbachol and bethanechol on the urinary tract, consisting in ureteral peristalsis, contraction of the detrusor muscle of the urinary bladder, and an increase in voluntary voiding pressure, are equal and are greater than those produced by acetylcholine.

The miotic effects of carbachol and bethanechol are greater than those produced by acetylcholine.

Atropine is able to antagonize all cholinergic (muscarinic) effects exerted by acetylcholine, methacholine, carbachol, and bethanechol. However, this antagonism is least evident with carbachol.

Bethanechol is of value in postoperative abdominal distention, gastric atony or stasis, and urinary retention. Carbachol (0.25–3.0%) may be used chronically for therapy of noncongestive, wide-angle glaucoma.

Pilocarpine is a naturally occurring (active ingredient of poisonous mushrooms, *Amanita muscaria*) cholinomimetic agent with both muscarinic and nicotinic effects (stimulates autonomic ganglia). It causes miosis, reduces intraocular pressure, and is used in wide-angle glaucoma. In addition, it may be applied topically by being placed in the eye as a drug reservoir (Ocusert).

ANTICHOLINESTERASE AGENTS. Anticholinesterases are drugs that inhibit or inactivate acetylcholinesterase, causing the accumulation of acetylcholine at the cholinergic receptors (Fig. 4-4). This produces effects similar to prolonged stimulation of cholinergic fibers. Anticholinesterases are classified as reversible and irreversible inhibitors.

The reversible inhibitors, which have a short to moderate duration of action, fall into two categories. Type one, exemplified by edrophonium, forms an ionic bond at the anionic site and a weak hydrogen bond at the esteratic site of acetylcholinesterase. Type two, exemplified by neostigmine, forms an ionic bond at the anionic site and a hydrolyzable covalent bond at the esteratic site.

Fig. 4-4. *Hydrolysis of acetylcholine by acetylcholinesterase, inhibition of acetylcholinesterase with DFP, and reactivation of the enzyme by pralidoxime. A. Acetylcholine and acetylcholinesterase. B. Acetylcholine-acetylcholinesterase complex. C. Choline and acetylated acetylcholinesterase + H_2O. D. Acetylcholinesterase phosphorylated with DFP. E. Pralidoxime. F. Acetylcholinesterase. (Concepts from S. E. Mayer, Neurohumoral Transmission and the Autonomic Nervous System. In A. G. Gilman, L. S. Goodman, and A. Gilman [eds.], The Pharmacological Basis of Therapeutics.* New York: Macmillan, 1980.)

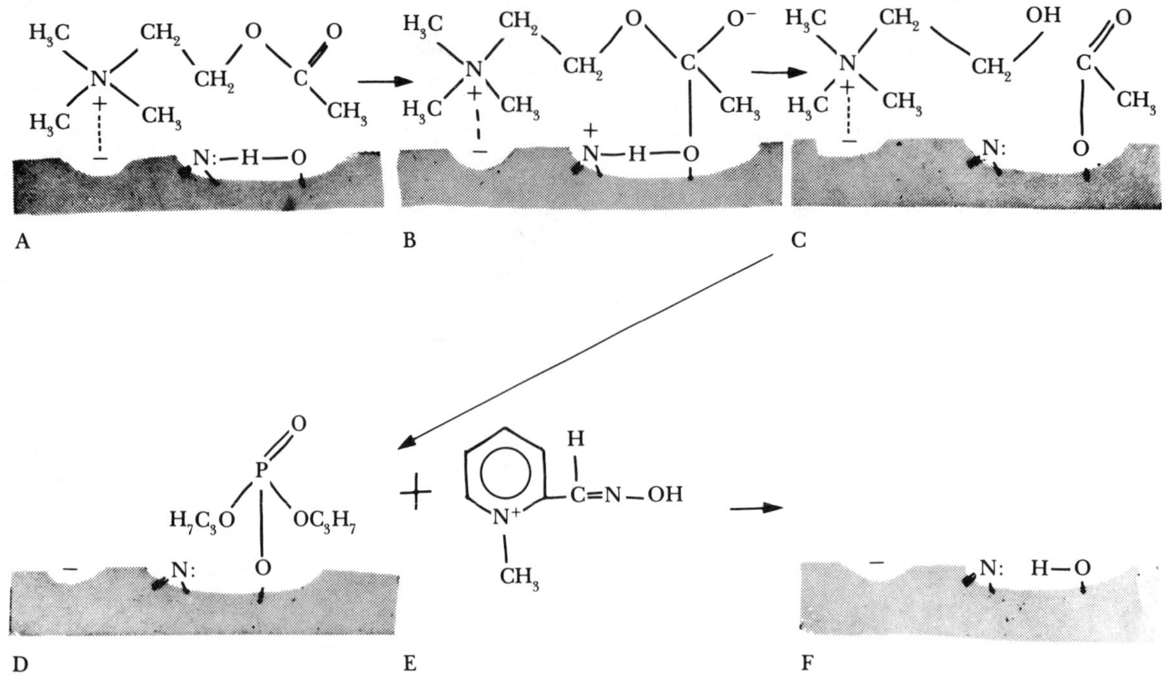

The irreversible inhibitors, exemplified by organophosphorus compounds (DFP, parathion, malathion, diazinon), have long durations of action and form a covalent bond with acetylcholinesterase that is hydrolyzed very slowly and negligibly, but the inhibition may be overcome by cholinesterase activators such as pralidoxime (2-PAM).

Cholinesterase inhibitors may also be classified as those agents possessing tertiary nitrogens (e.g., physostigmine and most organophosphorus compounds) and those containing quaternary nitrogen (e.g., neostigmine, pyridostigmine, and some organophosphorus compounds such as echothiophate). The following summarizes the comparative properties of these agents:

	Physostigmine	Neostigmine
Oral absorption	Good	Poor
Passing across blood-brain barrier	Well	No
Stimulating nicotinic receptors (skeletal muscle)	Yes	Yes
Used to combat the CNS toxicity of numerous anticholinergic drugs	Yes	No

Physostigmine (eserine sulfate) causes miosis and spasm of accommodation. It lowers intraocular pressure and hence may be used in wide-angle glaucoma. Being a lipid-soluble substance, it penetrates the brain rapidly, raises the concentration of acetylcholine, and in toxic amounts may cause cholinergic CNS toxicity, characterized by restlessness, insomnia, tremors, confusion, ataxia, convulsions, respiratory depression, and circulatory collapse. These effects are "antidoted" by atropine.

Neostigmine, unable to penetrate the blood-brain barrier, does not cause CNS toxicities. However, it may produce a dose-dependent and full range of muscarinic effects characterized by miosis, blurring of vision, lacrimation, salivation, sweating, increased bronchial secretion, bronchoconstriction, bradycardia, hypotension, and urinary incontinence. Atropine is able to oppose these muscarinic effects. Moreover, neostigmine, having a direct action as well as action through acetylcholine on end-plate nicotinic receptors, may cause muscular fasciculation, muscular cramps, weakness, and even paralysis. These effects are not countered by atropine. Furthermore, neostigmine enhances gastric contraction and secretion. Neostigmine itself is metabolized by plasma acetylcholinesterase.

The therapeutic uses of neostigmine are to combat atony of the urinary bladder and postoperative abdominal distention. In addition, it antagonizes the action of *d*-tubocurarine and curariform drugs. Edrophonium, neostigmine, or pyridostigmine may be used to diagnose myasthenia gravis. Since edrophonium has the shortest duration of action, it is most often used for this purpose.

The irreversible cholinesterase inhibitors such

as diisopropylfluorophosphate (DFP, isoflurophate, Floropryl) are used only locally in wide-angle glaucoma. Their pharmacologic effects, which are similar to those produced by physostigmine, are intense and of long duration. As organophosphorus insecticides, they are of paramount importance in accidental poisoning and in suicide and homicide attempts. They produce cholinergic crisis, which must be treated by (1) decontamination of the surroundings, (2) supporting respiration, (3) blocking the muscarinic effects by atropine, and (4) reactivating the inhibited cholinesterase by pralidoxime (2-PAM) (Fig. 4-4).

CHOLINERGIC RECEPTOR BLOCKING AGENTS.

Atropine and scopolamine, which are belladonna alkaloids, as well as other synthetic anticholinergic drugs, inhibit the actions of acetylcholine and cholinomimetic drugs at muscarinic receptors in smooth muscles, heart, and exocrine glands. In addition to these peripheral effects, anticholinergic drugs, by blocking the acetylcholine receptor sites in the CNS, produce pronounced CNS effects such as restlessness, irritability, excitement, and hallucinations. Scopolamine, on the other hand, depresses the CNS and in therapeutic doses causes fatigue, hypnosis, and amnesia. Therefore, it is used extensively in numerous medications, often in combination with antihistaminics.

The pharmacologic effects of atropine in general are dose dependent. For example, in small doses, atropine depresses sweating, elevates body temperature, decreases salivary and bronchial secretions, and relaxes bronchial smooth muscles. In somewhat larger doses (1–3 mg), it produces mydriasis (blockade of the iris sphincter muscle), cycloplegia (blockade of the ciliary muscle), and cardiovascular effects characterized by transient bradycardia (central vagal stimulation) and tachycardia (vagal blockade at the SA node). Since it has no significant effects on circulation, atropine is often used as a preanesthetic medication to depress bronchial secretion and to prevent pronounced bradycardia during abdominal surgical procedures. In still larger doses, it depresses the tone and motility of the gastrointestinal tract, the tone of the urinary bladder, and the gastric secretion. Obviously, then, the effective doses to be used in acid-pepsin diseases are preceded by numerous side effects.

Atropine is absorbed orally and crosses the placental barrier, causing fetal tachycardia. It has been used to examine the functional integrity of the placenta.

Atropine toxicity is characterized by dry mouth, burning sensation in the mouth, rapid pulse, mydriasis, blurred vision, photophobia, dry and flushed skin, restlessness, and excitement.

Physostigmine (administered intravenously) counteracts both the peripheral and the central side effects of atropine and other anticholinergic drugs such as thioridazine (neuroleptic), imipramine (antidepressant), and benztropine (antiparkinson medication). The clinical uses of atropine and related anticholinergics are as follows:

Ophthalmology
- Homatropine
  - Produces mydriasis and cycloplegia
- Eucatropine
  - Produces only mydriasis

Preoperative uses
- Atropine
  - To prevent excess salivation and bradycardia
- Scopolamine
  - In obstetrics to produce sedation and amnesia

Cardiac uses
- Atropine
  - To reduce severe bradycardia in hyperactive carotid sinus reflex
  - Diagnostically in Wolff-Parkinson-White syndrome to restore the PRS complex to normal duration

Gastrointestinal disorders
- In peptic ulcer
  - To diminish vagally mediated secretion of gastric juices and slow down gastric emptying
- In diarrhea associated with dysenteries and diverticulitis
- In excess salivation associated with heavy-metal poisoning or in parkinsonism

Neurologic diseases
- In parkinsonism (trihexyphenidyl or benztropine)
- In drug-induced pseudoparkinsonism (trihexyphenidyl or benztropine)
- In vestibular disorders such as motion sickness (scopolamine)

Contraindications to atropine and related drugs are glaucoma and prostatic hypertrophy. Methantheline and propantheline are synthetic derivatives that, in addition to possessing antimuscarinic effects, are ganglionic blocking agents and block the skeletal neuromuscular junction.

NEUROCHEMICAL BASIS OF ADRENERGIC TRANSMISSION.

Dopamine, norepinephrine, and epinephrine are classified as catecholamines and are synthesized according to the scheme depicted in Figure 4-5.

Tyrosine is converted to dopa by the rate-limiting enzyme tyrosine hydroxylase, which requires tetrahydropteridine, and is inhibited by alpha-methyltyrosine. Dopa is decarboxylated to dopamine by L-aromatic amino acid decarboxylase, which requires pyridoxal phosphate (vitamin B_6) as a coenzyme. Carbidopa, which is used with L-dopa in parkinsonism, is an inhibitor of this enzyme. Dopamine is converted to norepinephrine by dopamine beta-hydroxylase, which requires ascorbic acid (vitamin C) and is inhibited by diethyldithiocarbamate. Norepinephrine is converted to epinephrine by phenylethanolamine N-methyltransferase (PNMT), requiring S-adenosylmethionine (SAM). The activity of PNMT is stimulated by corticosteroids.

The catecholamine-synthesizing enzymes are able to synthesize dopamine and norepinephrine not only from physiologically occurring substrate such as L-dopa but also from exogenous substrates such as alpha-methyldopa, which becomes converted to alpha-methyldopamine and in turn to alpha-methylnorepinephrine. Alpha-methyldopamine and alpha-methylnorepinephrine are called false trans-

Fig. 4-5. *Adrenergic transmission. Synthesis, storage, release, and catabolism of norepinephrine.*

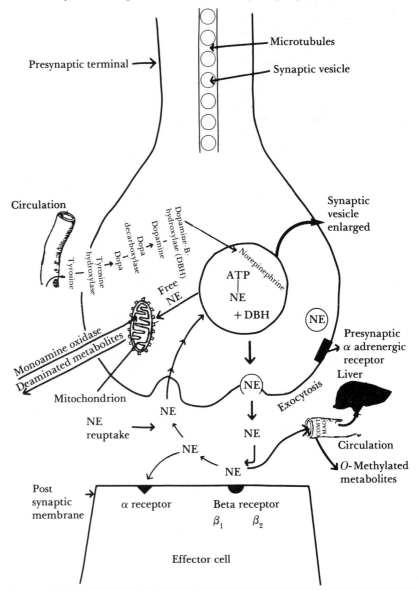

mitters, and the former is in general a weaker agonist. Alpha-methyldopa is used in hypertension.

In addition to being synthesized in the peripheral nervous system, dopamine is synthesized in corpus striatum and in the mesocortical, mesolimbic, and tuberoinfundibular systems. Norepinephrine is synthesized and stored primarily in sympathetic noradrenergic nerve terminals, in the brain, and in the adrenal medulla. Epinephrine is synthesized and stored primarily in the adrenal medulla, and to a certain extent in hypothalamic nuclei.

In sympathetic nerve terminals, in the brain, in the adrenal medulla, and in sympathetic postganglionic terminals, osmophilic granules (synaptic vesicles) are present that are capable of storing high concentrations of catecholamine (a complex with ATP and protein). The stored amines are not metabolized by intersynaptosomal mitochondrial enzyme (monoamine oxidase).

The stimulation of sympathetic neurons, in addition to releasing norepinephrine (through exocytosis), also releases ATP, storage protein, and dopamine beta-hydroxylase. The released norepinephrine interacts with receptor sites located postsynaptically (alpha$_1$) to produce the desired effects.

The action of norepinephrine is terminated by "reuptake" mechanisms. Two uptake mechanisms have been identified: *Uptake 1* is located in the presynaptic membrane, requires energy for the transport, is Na$^+$- and temperature-dependent, and is inhibited by ouabain (a cardiac glycoside), cocaine (a local anesthetic), and imipramine (an antidepressant). *Uptake 2* is located extraneuronally in various smooth muscles and glands, requires energy, and is temperature dependent. Approximately 20 percent of the amine is taken up by the uptake 2 mechanism or is metabolized.

There are two enzymes capable of metabolizing

catecholamines: *Monoamine oxidase (MAO)*, a mitochondrial enzyme, oxidatively deaminates catecholamines, tyramine, serotonin, and histamine. This enzyme is further subclassified as either monoamine oxidase A, which metabolizes norepinephrine and is inhibited by tranylcypromine, or monoamine oxidase B, which metabolizes dopamine and is inhibited by L-deprenyl. *Catechol-O-methyltransferase (COMT)*, a soluble enzyme present mainly in the liver and kidney, is also found in postsynaptic neuronal elements. About 15 percent of norepinephrine is metabolized postsynaptically by COMT.

DENERVATION SUPERSENSITIVITY.

A denervated structure, whether it be a skeletal muscle or a postganglionic nerve fiber to an autonomic effector cell such as a smooth muscle, shows enhanced sensitivity to its agonists (e.g., potassium ion, acetylcholine, histamine, and serotonin). Denervation supersensitivity becomes especially pronounced following application of norepinephrine and is thought to be caused by lack of amine uptake mechanism. The innervated skeletal muscle is sensitive to acetylcholine only at the end plates whereas the entire muscle fiber becomes sensitive following denervation. It is speculated that denervation results in creation of additional receptor sites [3]. Denervation sensitivity occurs not only following deafferentation but also following chronic administration of numerous drugs including neuroleptics.

ADRENERGIC RECEPTORS.

Adrenergic receptors are classified into alpha and beta and their subtypes.

Alpha$_1$—excitatory postsynaptic receptor
Alpha$_2$—inhibitory presynaptic receptor
Beta$_1$—excitatory postsynaptic receptor
Beta$_2$—inhibitory postsynaptic receptor

ADRENERGIC RECEPTOR AGONISTS.

Epinephrine acts on both alpha and beta receptors. Norepinephrine acts on both alpha receptors and primarily on beta$_1$ receptors. Isoproterenol is a pure beta agonist. The functions associated with alpha receptors are (1) vasoconstriction, (2) mydriasis, and (3) intestinal relaxation.

The functions associated with beta receptors are (1) vasodilatation, (2) cardioacceleration, (3) bronchial relaxation, (4) positive inotropic effect, (5) intestinal relaxation, and (6) glycogenolysis and fatty acid release.

Beta receptors are of two types: beta$_1$ and beta$_2$. Beta$_1$ is responsible for cardiac stimulation and lipolysis. Beta$_2$ is responsible for bronchodilatation and vasodepression. Beta$_2$ agonists are especially useful in the treatment of asthma because they produce bronchodilation without much cardiac acceleration.

PHARMACOLOGY OF NOREPINEPHRINE AND EPINEPHRINE. Cardiovascular Effects.

The actions of norepinephrine and epinephrine on the cardiovascular system may be quite different when both drugs are administered in small doses (0.1–0.4 μg/kg/minute slow intravenous infusion). They are essentially the same with large doses [3].

Cardiovascular Effects of Small Dose of Norepinephrine in Humans

Systolic pressure	Increased
Diastolic pressure	Increased
Mean pressure	Increased
Heart rate	Slightly decreased
Cardiac output	Slightly decreased
Peripheral resistance	Increased

Cardiovascular Effects of Small Dose of Epinephrine in Humans

Systolic pressure	Increased
Diastolic pressure	Decreased (increased by large dose)
Mean pressure	Unchanged
Cardiac output	Increased
Peripheral resistance	Decreased

Epinephrine increases (1) heart rate, (2) force of contraction, (3) irritability, and (4) coronary blood flow.

The inherent chronotropic effect of norepinephrine is opposed by reflex slowing secondary to vasoconstriction and elevated blood pressure.

Bronchodilator Effect. Epinephrine is a dilator of bronchial smooth muscle (beta$_2$ receptor) whereas norepinephrine is a weak dilator. Isoproterenol is more active than epinephrine.

Metabolic Actions. Epinephrine and isoproterenol elevate blood glucose by glycogenolysis, and by inhibiting glucose utilization. The therapeutic uses of epinephrine (or related drugs) are:

As bronchodilator (beta$_2$ receptor activation in asthma)
As mydriatic (contracts radial muscle)
In glaucoma (lowers intraocular pressure)
For allergic reactions (prevents antigen-induced histamine releases)
In hypotension (increasing mean pressure)
As nasal decongestant (mephentermine)
For local anesthesia (to produce a bloodless field of operation, to delay absorption and give longer duration of anesthetic action, and to protect brain and heart against toxic effects of local anesthetics)
As cardiac stimulant (epinephrine or isoproterenol may be injected in heart block to improve atrioventricular conduction velocity and to stimulate ventricular automaticity)

SUMMARY PHARMACOLOGY OF OTHER ADRENERGIC (SYMPATHOMIMETIC) RECEPTOR STIMULANTS.

In general, these agents may be divided into three categories: *Direct-acting agents* exert their effects directly on the receptor sites. *Indirect-act-*

ing agents such as amphetamine and tyramine exert their effects by releasing norepinephrine. *Mixed-acting agents* such as ephedrine and to a certain extent amphetamine are direct agonists and also release norepinephrine.

Ephedrine. Ephedrine is a naturally occurring sympathomimetic drug, used in the past in prevention and treatment of bronchial asthma. It acts by releasing norepinephrine and has actions similar to those of epinephrine and norepinephrine. Ephedrine is effective orally, has a long duration of action, and causes CNS stimulation.

Phenylephrine (Neo-Synephrine). Phenylephrine is a direct-acting and long-acting vasoconstrictor and has little effect on the CNS or the heart. It is used to prevent hypotension during spinal anesthesia and as a nasal decongestant.

Methoxamine (Vasoxyl). Methoxamine is a long-acting vasoconstrictor and does not cause cardiac stimulation.

Mephentermine (Wyamine). Mephentermine is a long-acting vasoconstrictor but causes cardiac stimulation. In addition, it is a nasal decongestant.

Metaraminol (Aramine). Metaraminol resembles phenylephrine in action but acts directly and indirectly.

Isoproterenol. Isoproterenol is a potent activator of beta-adrenergic receptors, possessing both bronchodilating and heart-stimulating properties. It is used in bronchial asthma, atrioventricular block, and cardiac arrest.

Amphetamine. Compared to other adrenergic agonists, dextroamphetamine has greater central and less cardiovascular effects. It produces anorexia, and in the past it was used in the treatment of obesity. Currently, it is used in narcolepsy or minimal brain dysfunction.

Sympathomimetic agents are contraindicated in hypertension and hyperthyroidism. In addition, they should not be used with anesthetics that sensitize the heart to catecholamine.

Dopamine (Intropin). Stimulation of dopamine receptors in renal and mesenteric arteries causes vasodilatation that is not blocked by propranolol (beta antagonist) but is blocked by a dopamine receptor blocking agent such as chlorpromazine. Dopamine increases renal blood flow, enhances the glomerular filtration rate, and causes sodium diuresis. Dopamine (5 μg/kg/minute) is used in the shock syndrome, myocardial infarction, trauma, endotoxin, septicemia, renal failure, or congestive heart failure.

Terbutaline (Brethine) and Metaproterenol (Alupent, Metaprel). These agents are selective beta$_2$-adrenergic receptor stimulants causing pronounced bronchodilatation with negligible cardiac stimulation in therapeutic doses.

ADRENERGIC BLOCKING (ANTIADRENERGIC) DRUGS. These agents exert their effects by blocking the access of circulating epinephrine, norepinephrine, and other sympathomimetic amines to the adrenergic receptors.

Alpha-Adrenergic Blockers. PHENOXYBENZAMINE (DIBENZYLINE). This agent is a noncompetitive alpha-adrenergic receptor blocker, and its action cannot be nullified by increasing the amount of agonist(s). It causes "epinephrine reversal." The administration of epinephrine after pretreatment with phenoxybenzamine causes vasodilation. The administration of phenoxybenzamine after epinephrine rapidly reverts epinephrine-mediated vasoconstriction to vasodilatation.

PHENTOLAMINE (REGITINE). This agent is a competitive alpha-adrenergic blocker, and its action can be nullified by increasing the amount of agonist(s). Phenoxybenzamine and phentolamine have limited therapeutic value. They are occasionally used (1) in peripheral vascular disease (Raynaud's disease), (2) diagnostically in pheochromocytoma, and (3) during surgery of pheochromocytoma.

PRAZOSIN (MINIPRESS). This agent, which is used in hypertension, causes alpha-adrenergic blockade and direct vasodilatation.

Beta-Adrenergic Blockers. These agents are competitive blockers of both beta$_1$ and beta$_2$ receptor sites.

Beta-adrenergic receptor blocking agents block sympathomimetic actions other than vasoconstriction (i.e., vasodilatation, cardiac acceleration, increased cardiac output, bronchiolar dilatation, and hyperglycemia) [8, 11]. They are used therapeutically in (1) cardiac arrhythmias, (2) digitalis-induced arrhythmias, (3) ventricular tachycardia, (4) atrial flutter or fibrillation, (5) pheochromocytoma, (6) prevention of angina pain, (7) treatment of hypertension, and (8) thyrotoxicosis.

PROPRANOLOL (INDERAL). The levorotatory (−) form of propranolol is 100 times more potent than the dextrorotatory (+) form in blocking beta$_1$- and beta$_2$-adrenergic receptor sites. However, both isomers are equally effective in their membrane-stabilizing or quinidinelike (local anestheticlike) effects. Propranolol has negative chronotropic and inotropic effects, reduces cardiac output, and is a cardiac depressant. Since it decreases atrioventricular conduction velocity and automaticity, it is employed as an antiarrhythmic substance. Propranolol is used in hypertension. It exerts its effect by decreasing cardiac output, blocking the release of renin and the formation of angiotensin II. Propranolol causes bronchoconstriction and is contraindicated in asthmatic patients. It should be used cautiously in diabetic patients because pronounced hypoglycemia may result following insulin administration. Since propranolol crosses the blood-brain barrier, it may cause behavioral disturbances, especially in elderly patients [4].

METOPROLOL (LOPRESSOR). Metoprolol is a competitive blocker of beta$_1$ receptor sites in therapeutic doses. Therefore, it causes fewer side effects such as bronchoconstriction and hypoglycemia. Furthermore, since it does not cross the blood-brain barrier, it is devoid of CNS toxicity.

The pharmacology of other beta blocking agents is hereby summarized [11]:

Drug	Beta$_1$ and Beta$_2$ Blockade	Beta$_1$ Blockade (Cardioselective)	Intrinsic Sympath-omimetic Effect	Quinidine-like Effect
Propranolol	+	–	–	+
Nadolol	+	–	–	–
Timolol	+	–	–	+
Atenolol	–	+	–	–
Metoprolol	–	+	–	+
Pindolol	+	–	+	+
Betaxolol	–	+	–	+

+ indicates that the drug possesses the assigned property.
– indicates that it does not.

Ergot Alkaloids. Ergot alkaloids block alpha-adrenergic receptors, have oxytocic properties, and are used in the treatment of migraine headache.

QUESTIONS ON AUTONOMIC PHARMACOLOGY

Select one answer that best answers the question or completes the statement.

41. Amphetamine toxicity should be treated with:
    A. Chlorpromazine.
    B. Acidification of urine.
    C. Both A and B.
    D. Propranolol.
42. The bronchoconstricting effect of propranolol is potentiated by:
    A. Morphine.
    B. Histamine.
    C. Methacholine.
    D. All of the above.
43. Which one of the following beta-adrenergic receptor blocking agents would be least detrimental in a patient with sick sinus syndrome?
    A. Propranolol.
    B. Pindolol.
    C. Metoprolol.
    D. Nadolol.
44. Which one of the following drugs is useful in the treatment of postoperative urinary retention?
    A. Bethanechol (Urecholine).
    B. Atropine.
    C. Hexamethonium.
    D. Methacholine (Mecholyl).
    E. Diisopropylfluorophosphate (Floropryl).
45. Cholinergic crisis is treated with:
    A. Physostimine.
    B. Atropine.
    C. Diisopropylfluorophosphate (Floropryl).
    D. Choline.
    E. Propranolol (Inderal).
46. The synthesis of acetylcholine depends on:
    A. The activity of acetylcholinesterase.
    B. The activity of choline acetyltransferase.
    C. The availability of choline.
    D. Acetyl coenzyme A.
    E. Acetate.
47. Dopamine (Intropin) is useful in:
    A. Oliguria.
    B. Cardiogenic and bacteremic shock.
    C. Chronic refractory congestive heart failure.
    D. All of the above.
48. Mydriasis is produced by all of the following agents except which one?
    A. Eucatropine (Euphthalmine).
    B. Phenylephrine (Neo-Synephrine).
    C. Homatropine.
    D. Cocaine.
    E. Neostigmine (Prostigmin).
49. The cardiovascular effects of tyramine are blocked by which one of the following drugs?
    A. Propranolol (Inderal).
    B. Atropine.
    C. Hexamethonium.
    D. Phentolamine (Regitine).
    E. Physostigmine.
50. Acetylcholine is characterized by all of the following actions except which one?
    A. A decrease in the rate of diastolic depolarization.
    B. A decrease in the strength of atrial muscle contraction.
    C. Bronchodilatation.
    D. A slowing of the heart rate.
51. Atropine toxicity may be characterized by the following symptoms except which one?
    A. Tachycardia.
    B. Mydriasis.
    C. Urinary retention.
    D. Profuse sweating.
52. Which one of the following statements is true about botulinus toxin?
    A. It prevents the release of acetylcholine.
    B. It prevents the uptake of dopamine.
    C. It blocks muscarinic receptor.
    D. It causes direct vasodilatation.
53. The management of myasthenia gravis may include the administration of:
    A. Neostigmine (Prostigmin).
    B. Acetylcholine (Miochol).
    C. Physostigmine.
    D. Edrophonium (Tensilon).
    E. Methantheline (Banthine).
54. Which one of the following agents has both ganglionic blocking action and muscarinic cholinergic blocking action?
    A. Atropine.
    B. Propranolol (Inderal).
    C. Methantheline (Banthine).
    D. Metoprolol (Lopressor).
    E. Neostigmine (Prostigmin).
55. The toxicity of irreversible cholinesterase inhibitors is treated with:
    A. Atropine.
    B. Physostigmine.
    C. Pralidoxime (2-PAM).
    D. Methantheline (Banthine).
    E. Atropine and pralidoxime (2-PAM).
56. Which one of the following agents antagonizes the bronchodilating and vasodilating effects of isoproterenol?
    A. Phentolamine (Regitine).

B. Phenoxybenzamine (Dibenzyline).
C. Reserpine.
D. Cocaine.
E. Propranolol (Inderal).

____ 57. All the following agents dilate the pupil except which one?
A. Morphine.
B. Ephedrine.
C. Phenylephrine.
D. Hydroxyamphetamine.

____ 58. Prazosin, a recently introduced antihypertensive agent, exerts its antihypertensive property by:
A. Blocking postsynaptic alpha$_1$ receptors.
B. Blocking muscarinic cholinergic receptors.
C. Releasing norepinephrine.
D. Blocking postsynaptic beta$_2$ receptors.

____ 59. Which one of the following statements is not true about propranolol?
A. It is metabolized in the liver to 4-hydroxy-propranolol.
B. It is not effective when given orally.
C. It is bound extensively (90%–95%) to plasma proteins.
D. It is combined with diuretic in the management of hypertension.

____ 60. Timolol (Timoptic) is characterized by the following properties except which one?
A. Reduces intraocular pressure.
B. Is a selective beta-adrenergic antagonist.
C. Is 10 times more potent than propranolol in its beta receptor blocking action.
D. Is useful in hypertension.

ANSWERS AND EXPLANATIONS ON AUTONOMIC PHARMACOLOGY

41. C.
Explanation: Acidification of urine by an agent such as ammonium chloride enhances the excretion of amphetamine whereas the administration of $NaHCO_3$ enhances the excretion of phenobarbital.

42. D.
Explanation: Histamine and methacholine cause bronchoconstriction. Morphine, besides depressing respiration directly, releases histamine.

43. B.
Explanation: Conduction delays and pacemaker cell failure of the SA and AV nodes may cause marked sinus bradycardia, called sick sinus syndrome. Pindolol has inherent sympathomimetic activity.

44. A.
45. B.
46. C.
47. D.
48. E.
49. D.
50. C.
51. D.
52. A.
53. A.
54. C.
Explanation: Methantheline contains a quaternary ammonium and differs from other anticholinergic agents such as methscopolamine, homatropine, and atropine in having both anticholinergic effects and ganglionic blocking action. Toxic doses cause neuromuscular blockade and respiratory paralysis.

55. E.

56. E.
57. A.
58. A.
59. B.
60. B.

REFERENCES

1. Appenzeller, O. *The Autonomic Nervous System: An Introduction to Basic and Clinical Concepts.* Amsterdam: Elsevier North-Holland, 1982.

2. Everett, N. B. The Autonomic Nervous System. In N. B. Everett (ed.), *Functional Neuroanatomy* (6th ed.). Philadelphia: Lea & Febiger, 1971. Pp. 242–253.

3. Goth, A. *Medical Pharmacology. Principles and Concepts* (11th ed.). St. Louis: Mosby, 1984.

4. Hornykiewicz, O., and Flattery, K. V. Drugs Acting on the Sympathetic Nervous System. In P. Seeman, E. M. Sellers, and W. H. E. Roschlau (eds.), *Principles of Medical Pharmacology* (3rd ed.). Toronto: University of Toronto Press, 1980. Pp. 153–175.

5. Ito, M., et al. *Integrative Control Functions of the Brain.* Amsterdam: Elsevier North-Holland, 1979.

6. Jenkins, T. W. *Functional Mammalian Neuroanatomy.* Philadelphia: Lea & Febiger, 1972.

7. Karczmar, A. G. Exploitable aspects of central cholinergic functions, particularly with respect to the EEG, motor, analgesic and mental functions. In D. J. Jenden (ed.), Cholinergic mechanism and psychopharmacology. *Adv. Behav. Biol.* 24:679, 1977.

8. Kielholz, P. *Beta-Blockers and the Central Nervous System.* Baltimore: University Park Press, 1976.

9. Lloyd, K. G. Observations Concerning Neurotransmitter Interaction in Schizophrenia. In K. G. Lloyd (ed.), *Cholinergic-Monoaminergic Interactions in the Brain.* New York: Academic, 1978. Pp. 363–392.

10. Mayer, S. E. Neurohumoral Transmission and the Autonomic Nervous System. In A. G. Gilman, L. S. Goodman, and A. Gilman (eds.), *The Pharmacological Basis of Therapeutics.* New York: Macmillan, 1980. Pp. 56–90.

11. Morselli, P. L., et al. *Betaxolol and Other β_1-Adrenoceptor Antagonists.* New York: Raven Press, 1983.

12. Tucek, S. *The Cholinergic Synapse. Progress in Brain Research.* Vol. 49. Amsterdam: Elsevier North-Holland, 1979.

13. Winters, P. R., Bell, R. D., and Rosenberg, R. N. Autonomic Nervous System. In R. N. Rosenberg (ed.), *Neurology.* New York: Grune & Stratton, 1980. Pp. 495–510.

III. Neuropharmacology

5. Drugs for Parkinson's Disease

He who truly knows has no occasion to shout.
Leonardo da Vinci

Four separate groups of symptoms are now described as part of the symptom complex of parkinsonism [6].

SYMPTOMS. Tremor.
The parkinsonian tremors have been referred to as "pill-rolling," "cigarette-rolling," and "to-and-fro" movements. In general, distal muscles are more commonly involved than proximal muscles. These tremors are present during rest and often disappear on purposeful movement or during sleep. During stress or anxiety-provoking situations, tremors increase, and initiation of movement "becomes increasingly difficult, extremely fatiguing, and ponderously inefficient."

Akinesia or Bradykinesia.
This symptom is characterized by poverty of spontaneous movements and slowness in initiation of movements.

Rigidity or Increased Muscle Tone.
There occurs rigidity or resistance to passive movements.

Loss of Normal Postural Reflexes.
This is the disorder of postural fixation and equilibrium.

OPPOSING ACTIONS OF ACETYLCHOLINE AND DOPAMINE IN THE CORPUS STRIATUM.
Comprehension of the mechanism of actions of drugs used in parkinsonism depends on thorough understanding of the concept that acetylcholine and dopamine have opposing actions in the corpus striatum. The former serves as an excitatory neurotransmitter while the latter functions as an inhibitory one.

The Parkinson syndrome, regardless of its etiology (idiopathic, postencephalitic, arteriosclerotic, manganese- or drug-induced) is neurochemically considered a "striatal dopamine deficiency syndrome." The main extrapyramidal symptoms—tremor, akinesia, and rigidity—are positively correlated with the degree of the striatal dopamine deficiency. Although eight separate neurotransmitters interact in the nigrostriatonigral loop, the basic therapeutic problem in parkinsonism has been to find suitable compounds that (1) increase the concentration of dopamine, (2) stimulate the dopamine receptor sites directly, or (3) depress the activity at cholinergic receptor sites. These drugs are discussed under two main headings: Agents That Increase Dopaminergic Functions and Agents That Inhibit Cholinergic Hyperactivity.

AGENTS THAT INCREASE DOPAMINERGIC FUNCTIONS.
There are several mechanisms by which the activity at dopamine receptor sites may be enhanced in the striatum:

Increasing the synthesis of dopamine (levodopa)
Inhibiting the catabolism of dopamine (L-deprenyl)
Stimulating the release of dopamine (amphetamine)
Stimulating the dopamine receptor sites directly (bromocriptine, pergolide)
Blocking the uptake and enhancing the release of dopamine (amantadine)

Of these possibilities, discussed individually, the most effective means of treating parkinsonism has been to enhance the synthesis of dopamine [4, 9].

Drugs That Increase the Synthesis of Dopamine: Summary Pharmacology of Levodopa.
Two major precursors of dopamine, L-tyrosine and L-dopa, have been investigated. L-Tyrosine has proved ineffective for two reasons: (1) Tyrosine hydroxylase is the rate-limiting enzyme, and it must be bypassed in order to raise the concentration of dopamine. (2) There is some evidence that tyrosine hydroxylase may be defective in parkinsonism. Levodopa is an inert chemical, but its metabolite, dopamine, is active pharmacologically. The amount of levodopa to be used depends on the severity of the parkinsonism. At the present time, levodopa is combined with carbidopa, a peripheral dopa-decarboxylase inhibitor.

The first signs of improvement are usually a subjective feeling of well-being with increased vigor. The symptoms yield according to the following sequence: akinesia, rigidity, and tremor, which disappears slowly and incompletely. On stopping the drug, the symptoms reappear in reverse order: tremor, rigidity, and akinesia.

EMETIC ACTION OF LEVODOPA. Among the adverse reactions encountered in the first months of therapy is nausea, usually without vomiting. The emetic action of levodopa is often troublesome and seems to be aggravated by coffee. Eliminating coffee, or replacing it with decaffeinated coffee, usually overcomes this annoying reaction. The use of phenothiazine antiemetic (such as chlorpromazine, which blocks the dopamine receptor sites in the brain and therefore nullifies the beneficial effects of levodopa) is discouraged.

The development of involuntary movements may limit the usefulness of levodopa. This peak-dose dyskinesia is usually manifested in choreatic movements involving the hands, arm, legs, and face. Ten percent of the patients develop oromandibular dystonia. In addition, increased oral activity, with constant chewing, biting, opening and closing of the mouth, and intermittent protrusions of the tongue, is the most frequent side effect. The abnormal involuntary movements ordinarily occur during the time of maximum benefit from levodopa, which is usually 1 to 2 hours after each dose, and may last from several minutes up to 1 or 2 hours. To avoid these involuntary movements, it is generally necessary to increase the frequency of drug administration and at the same time decrease the dose of levodopa.

The beneficial and side effects of levodopa may be mediated via different receptor sites. For example, the beneficial effects may be brought about by dopamine receptor 1 or D_1 whereas the dyskinesia may be brought about by dopamine receptor 2 or D_2. Dopamine receptor$_2$ blocking agents such as oxyperomide and tiapride are able to reduce levodopa-induced dyskinesia without exacerbating parkinsonian symptomatology. The conventional phenothiazines (such as chlorpromazine) and butyrophenones (such as haloperidol) block both dopamine$_1$ and dopamine$_2$ receptors. Therefore, these drugs are not suitable for the management of levodopa-induced dyskinesia.

Levodopa should be used with caution in various cardiovascular disorders. Peripheral decarboxylation of levodopa markedly increases the concentration of dopamine in blood. Dopamine is a pharmacologically active catecholamine that influences alpha- and beta-adrenergic receptors.

Therapeutic doses of levodopa produce cardiac stimulation by activating the beta$_1$ receptor site in the heart. In some elderly patients, this may produce cardiac arrhythmias. The cardiac stimulation is blocked by propranolol, the beta-adrenergic blocking agent. Propranolol has also been shown to be effective in suppressing tremor. Conditions that warrant careful attention to the use of levodopa are angina pectoris and history of cardiac arrhythmias.

PHARMACOLOGY OF A PERIPHERAL DOPA DECARBOXYL-ASE INHIBITOR. The orally administered L-dopa becomes metabolized substantially in the gut and tissues; very little penetrates into the brain to become converted to dopamine. If one administers L-dopa along with a peripheral dopa decarboxylase inhibitor, the formation of dopamine in the periphery is decreased substantially and that in the brain increases. The pharmacology of a peripheral dopa decarboxylase inhibitor given along with levodopa (e.g., Sinemet 1 : 10) is summarized:

The peripheral dopa decarboxylase inhibitors do not pass across the blood-brain barrier; hence the formation of dopamine in the brain is not affected.

Since the metabolism of levodopa in the periphery is reduced, the doses of levodopa and hence its peripheral side effects (hypotension and tachycardia) are reduced.

Levodopa, once converted to dopamine, stimulates the chemoreceptor trigger zone for emesis located in area postrema and causes nausea and vomiting. This side effect is reduced when levodopa is given with carbidopa.

Peripheral dopa decarboxylase inhibitors dramatically reduce the levodopa-induced tachycardia.

In the presence of carbidopa, vitamin B_6 will not be contraindicated. Added vitamin B_6 may even enhance the formation of dopamine in the brain.

Peripheral dopa decarboxylase inhibitor reduces the onset of the "off-on" phenomenon.

THE LEVODOPA-INDUCED OFF-ON PHENOMENON. The two major limitations of chronic levodopa therapy for parkinsonian patients are involuntary movement and the off-on phenomenon. The off-on phenomenon is a sudden loss of effectiveness with abrupt onset of akinesia "off" effects that may last minutes or hours, followed by an equally sudden return of effectiveness, "on" effects, that may even be accompanied by hyperkinesia. The action is so sudden that is has been compared to a light switch action.

Combined levodopa and carbidopa produces a frequency of 10 to 20 percent off-on reaction whereas levodopa by itself produces 50 percent off-on reaction.

The mechanism of off-on effects of levodopa is not known. Probably it has to do with the unavailability of dopamine to its receptor sites. For example, it has been shown that the off-on phenomenon is greatly relieved in patients who are on low-protein diets. Dietary amino acids compete with levodopa for absorption from the gut and for transport across the blood-brain barrier. During the off period, the plasma level of L-dopa is low.

Dopamine receptor agonists are able to correct the symptoms, indicating that the receptor site is active.

The off-on effect should be differentiated from "wearing off" or "end-of-dose response." The wearing-off effect is clearly related to the dosage and blood level of levodopa. As the disease progresses and the number of nigrostriatal neurons decreases, less dopamine storage is available in the striatum. The resultant need for constant replenishment from the blood means that the bioavailability of plasma levodopa plays an important role.

The true off-on phenomenon, the sudden random oscillations that are rarely seen before the second year of treatment, are probably more closely related to the pharmacodynamic properties of the receptors themselves. The receptor mechanisms are turned "off" suddenly as they are also turned "on" suddenly [8].

L-Deprenyl, a Drug That Inhibits the Catabolism of Dopamine. Dopamine is metabolized according to the following reactions:

$$\text{Dopamine} \xrightarrow[\text{Inhibited by deprenyl}]{\text{Monoamine oxidase}} X \longrightarrow$$

$$\text{3,4-dihydroxy-phenylacetic acid} \xrightarrow{\text{Catechol-}O\text{-methyltransferase}} \text{homovanillic acid}$$

Monoamine oxidase inhibitors are classified into A and B types. Monoamine oxidase A preferentially uses serotonin and norepinephrine as substrates and is inhibited by clorgyline and harmaline. Monoamine oxidase B preferentially uses dopamine and is inhibited by deprenyl.

Clinical evidence, primarily from European neurologists, indicates that 10 mg of L-deprenyl in combination with levodopa and carbidopa is superior to levodopa with carbidopa [1].

Amphetamine, a Drug That Releases Dopamine. Amphetamine has been used adjunctively in some parkinsonian patients. It is thought that amphetamine, by releasing dopamine and norepinephrine from storage granules, makes the patient more "mobile" and "motivated." It is felt that a less rigid and more motivated patient becomes a more active patient. Amphetamine may be used in combination with levodopa or along with anticholinergic drugs. Although amphetamine reduces rigidity and hypokinesia, it aggravates parkinsonian tremors.

Bromocriptine, a Direct Dopamine Receptor Agonist. As parkinsonism progresses, the activity of dopa decarboxylase may become so low that it cannot adequately decarboxylate dopa to dopamine. In this case, one could stimulate the dopamine receptor sites located postsynaptically by compounds such as bromocriptine. This drug is an ergot alkaloid that inhibits the secretion of prolactin by interfering with hypophyseal dopaminergic neurons, and it has been used in endocrine disorders such as Chiari-Frommel syndrome and Forbes-Albright syndrome. Low-dose bromocriptine has been found to be effective in some but not all patients. Bromocriptine has a longer duration of action than levodopa and is particularly useful in patients with high incidence of off-on phenomenon.

Bromocriptine is effectively used with submaximal doses of levodopa. It should be considered "a refinement rather than a replacement" for levodopa. The possibility exists that more effective dopamine receptor agonists such as pergolide or lisuride will replace bromocriptine [2, 3, 5, 7].

Amantadine, a Drug That Blocks Uptake and Releases Dopamine. Amantadine (Symmetrel) is an effective prophylactic agent for the prevention of respiratory infection caused by A_2 influenza (Asian flu) virus strains. Amantadine inhibits the penetration of viruses into cells. While the actions of amantadine are still not fully understood, there is some evidence that the drug can inhibit the uptake of dopamine into the synaptosomes. In addition, amantadine has an indirect amphetaminelike effect in that it releases dopamine.

ADVANTAGES AS COMPARED TO LEVODOPA.
The onset of action of amantadine is rapid (1 day) whereas that of levodopa is slow (1–2 weeks).
Amantadine is effective in drug-induced parkinsonism; levodopa is not.
No contraindication has been reported with the use of amantadine whereas the use of levodopa is contraindicated in psychiatric syndrome, cardiac diseases, peptic ulcer, and glaucoma.

Side effects with chronic usage of amantadine are rare whereas levodopa produces involuntary movements and off-on phenomenon.
The chief areas of usefulness of amantadine are in mild parkinsonism, in hemiparkinsonism, and in drug-induced parkinsonism.
Levodopa is effective in moderate to severe parkinsonism and in postencephalitic parkinsonism.
A state refractory to amantadine develops in some parkinsonian patients that disappears when the drug is withheld. When amantadine is reinstituted, the initially favorable therapeutic response returns.

AGENTS THAT INHIBIT CHOLINERGIC HYPERACTIVITY. In parkinsonian patients, the deficiency of dopamine results in hyperactivity of cholinergic receptors. Therefore, anticholinergic drugs may be used to mitigate some of the symptoms. These are:

Trihexyphenidyl (Artane)
Cycrimine (Pagitane)
Procyclidine (Kemadrin)
Biperiden (Akineton)
Orphenadrine (Disipal)
Benztropine (Cogentin)

Contraindications to anticholinergic drugs used in parkinsonism are identical to those cited for atropine and are:

Glaucoma
Prostatic hypertrophy
Myasthenia gravis
Stenosing peptic ulcer
Duodenal or pyloric obstruction

Urinary retention and tachycardia should be heeded and regarded as signs of impending toxicity.

QUESTIONS ON DRUGS FOR PARKINSON'S DISEASE

Select one answer that best completes the statement or answers the question.
_____ 61. In the management of a parkinsonian patient with central anticholinergic drugs, which side effects should alert the physician to reduce dosage?
A. Urinary retention and tachycardia.
B. Hypothermia and mydriasis.
C. Bradycardia and blurred vision.
D. Polyuria and dry mouth.
_____ 62. The incidence of off-on phenomenon has been shown to be reduced with which of the following drug combinations?
A. Anticholinergic drugs with levodopa.
B. Amphetamine with levodopa.
C. L-Deprenyl, carbidopa, and levodopa.
D. Bromocriptine with levodopa.
_____ 63. Levodopa-induced emesis may be reduced by administration of:
A. Apomorphine.
B. L-Deprenyl.
C. Bromocriptine.
D. Carbidopa.

____ 64. The nullification of the beneficial CNS effects of levodopa by vitamin B$_6$ is due to:
  A. Unavailability of dopamine to the area postrema.
  B. Reduced absorption of levodopa from the gastrointestinal tract.
  C. Enhanced excretion of levodopa by the kidney.
  D. Enhanced decarboxylation of levodopa in the periphery.
____ 65. The akinesia (poverty of movement) in parkinsonian patients is thought to be due to:
  A. Dopamine-mediated "positive disturbance."
  B. Serotonin-mediated "negative and positive disturbances."
  C. Dopamine-mediated "negative disturbance."
  D. Acetylcholine-mediated "negative disturbance."
____ 66. Tolerance with chronic treatment usually develops to levodopa-induced tachycardia. This effect is due to:
  A. Disappearance of beta receptor sites in the heart.
  B. Augmentation of cholinergic receptor sites in the heart.
  C. Down regulation of beta receptor sites in the heart.
  D. Lack of conversion of levodopa to dopamine in the heart.
____ 67. During the maintenance phase of levodopa therapy, the chief dose-limiting side effect is the development of:
  A. Choreiform movements.
  B. Nausea.
  C. Orthostatic hypotension.
  D. Insomnia.
  E. Sinus tachycardia.

ANSWERS AND EXPLANATIONS ON DRUGS FOR PARKINSON'S DISEASE

61. A.
62. C.
63. D.
64. D.
65. C.
  Explanation: The motor disturbances that result from destructive lesions in the basal ganglia take the following two forms:
  (1) *Negative disturbances* involve a loss of function that is normally performed by the basal ganglia. An example is the so-called poverty of movement in Parkinson's disease.
  (2) *Positive disturbances* refer to abnormal involuntary movements and rigidity that appear with lesions of the basal ganglia. Such manifestations cannot arise from destroyed structures; rather they are due to mechanisms that have been released from control by destruction of the basal ganglia. These release phenomena have the following two forms:
    a. *Static manifestations*, which present themselves with some degree of constancy (e.g., the rigidity of Parkinson's disease).
    b. *Involuntary movements*, which are intermittent (e.g., tremor and dyskinesias).
66. C.
67. A.

REFERENCES

1. Birkmayer, W., Riederer, P., and Youdin, M. B. H. (−)Deprenyl in the treatment of Parkinson's disease. *Clin. Neuropharmacol.* 5:195, 1982.
2. Calne, D. B. Dopaminergic agonists in the treatment of parkinsonism. *Clin. Neuropharmacol.* 3:153, 1978.
3. Grimes, J. D., and Hassan, M. N. Bromocriptine in the long-term management of advanced Parkinson's disease. *Can. J. Neurol. Sci.* 10:86, 1983.
4. Klawans, H. L. (ed.) Management of Parkinson's Disease at Different Stages of the Illness. *Clinical Neuropharmacology*, Vol. 5, Suppl. 1. New York: Raven Press, 1982.
5. LeWitt, P. O., Ward, C. D., and Larsen, T. A. Comparison of pergolide and bromocriptine therapy in parkinsonism. *Neurology* (N.Y.) 33:1009, 1983.
6. Rinne, U. K. Recent advances in parkinsonism. *J. Neural Transm.* 51:1, 1981.
7. Schneider, E., Hubener, K., and Fischer, P. A. Treatment of Parkinson's disease with 8-alpha-amino-ergoline, CU 32-085. *Neurology* (N.Y.) 33:468, 1983.
8. Weiner, W. J., and Bergen, D. Prevention and management of the side effects of levodopa. *Clin. Neuropharmacol.* 2:1, 1977.
9. Yahr, M. D. Overview of present day treatment of Parkinson's disease. *J. Neural Transm.* 43:227, 1978.

6. Anticonvulsants

Dignity does not consist in possessing honors, but in deserving them.

Aristotle

The word *epilepsy*, meaning to be "seized by forces from without," has been defined by John Hughlings Jackson as "occasional, sudden, excessive, rapid, and local discharges of gray matter of the brain." Convulsive seizures may result from a number of causes including acute cerebral anoxemia, disturbances of calcium metabolism, hypoglycemia, excessive hydration, the ingestion of drugs with convulsive activity, and metabolic disturbances. The period during which the seizure occurs is referred to as the ictal period. The time immediately following a seizure is called the postictal period, and the interval between seizures is named the interictal period. The aura, the premonitory signs, the warning signal, may occur early and is the only portion of the seizure the patient may remember [1].

The etiology of this disorder is only partially and incompletely understood. The ideal therapy for convulsive seizures, which may have to be given for life, has not been discovered [3].

THERAPEUTIC OBJECTIVE. The therapeutic objective in pharmacologic management of epilepsy is complete suppression of all seizures without impairment of CNS function.

Part One: Drugs Effective in Tonic-Clonic Seizures (Grand Mal) and Complex Partial Seizures

HYDANTOIN DERIVATIVES. The hydantoin derivatives are phenytoin (diphenylhydantoin) and mephenytoin (Mesantoin).

Pharmacokinetics of Phenytoin. Phenytoin, having a pK_a of 8.3 to 9.2, is insoluble at the pH of gastric juice and therefore is not absorbed to a significant degree from the stomach. On passage into the small intestine, where the pH is basic (7.0–7.5), phenytoin will exist in nonionized form, which favors its absorption. The absorption is highest from the duodenum and decreases rapidly as one descends to lower parts of the small intestine. Because phenytoin is not absorbed well from the large intestine, the rectal administration of phenytoin is of little therapeutic value and should not be encouraged.

Phenytoin, when it is to be used chronically, is always given orally. In status epilepticus, it should be given intravenously. Since the injectable form of phenytoin has a pH of 12, it should not be injected intramuscularly.

After absorption, phenytoin becomes bound to plasma proteins to the extent of 92 to 93 percent, allowing only 7 to 8 percent of the drug to remain free. Circumstances or drugs that may alter the degree of protein binding will significantly affect the therapeutic usefulness and the toxicity of phenytoin. For example, in uremic patients, in whom the free phenytoin may be as high as 30 percent, the dosage of phenytoin should be reduced. Similarly, in hypoalbuminemia resulting from numerous disorders, the doses of phenytoin should be adjusted downward.

Phenytoin becomes metabolized in the liver to hydroxyphenytoin, an inactive metabolite. Hydroxyphenytoin itself becomes conjugated with glucuronic acid and excreted by the kidneys. Hydroxyphenytoin inhibits the metabolism of phenytoin, and the half-life of phenytoin may become altered with greater than therapeutic doses of phenytoin, as shown in the following example:

Oral Dose of Phenytoin (mg/kg)	Plasma Level of Phenytoin (μg/ml)	Half-Life (hours)
4	10–15	24
12	> 25	60

Clinical evidence indicates that epileptic patients are either slow or rapid metabolizers of phenytoin.

In the slow metabolizer, 4 mg per kilogram of phenytoin may produce toxicity, whereas in the rapid metabolizer, 4 mg per kilogram of phenytoin may be a subtherapeutic dose.

Pharmacodynamics of Phenytoin. The mode of action of phenytoin has been attributed to its "membrane-stabilizing effects," in that phenytoin (1) limits the development of maximal seizure activity and (2) reduces the spread of seizure process from an epileptic focus. The precise mechanisms as to how the neuronal membrane is stabilized are uncertain [4]. Several concepts have been advanced.

PHENYTOIN'S INTERFERENCE WITH CALCIUM ACTION. Phenytoin inhibits the development of and reverses posttetanic potentiation or posttetanic facilitation. It is thought that posttetanic potentiation is an important mechanism in the development of high-frequency trains of impulses in cerebral excitatory feedback circuits and in the spread of such activity to neighboring loops resulting in maximal seizure activity. Phenytoin reduces calcium transport at the outer nerve membrane by blocking its high-affinity binding sites. By competing with calcium, phenytoin prevents the release of norepinephrine, which is necessary for the generation of posttetanic potentiation. In the absence of this action, the spread of the impending seizure process is curtailed.

PHENYTOIN'S INTERFERENCE WITH SODIUM MOVEMENT. In a hyperexcitable state, the intracellular concentration of sodium is elevated. Phenytoin decreases the inward sodium current. Furthermore, in circumstances in which the intracellular concentration of sodium is elevated, phenytoin is thought to stimulate $Na^+K^+ATPase$ to reestablish the ionic gradient. The activity of $Na^+K^+ATPase$ is reduced in the brain in epileptic patients.

The membrane-stabilizing effect of phenytoin is not limited to neurons but is also seen in other excitable tissues such as skeletal muscle and heart. Furthermore, phenytoin is effective in treating myotonia and cardiac arrhythmias.

PHENYTOIN-MEDIATED GABAERGIC TRANSMISSION. Chloride ion enhances the binding of phenytoin to a specific but unknown receptor site in the brain. It has been postulated that this binding may enhance GABA-mediated chloride conductance in the postsynaptic membrane.

Side Effects and Toxicity of Phenytoin. Phenytoin may cause nystagmus, diplopia, staggering, and ataxia. These side effects are generally regarded as dose dependent and usually appear whenever the plasma concentration of phenytoin exceeds 20 μg per milliliter. Similarly, they are often deliberately caused by a physician in order to make certain that maximum tolerable doses have been given. These side effects are reversible with dose reduction.

Phenytoin causes gingival hyperplasia, which occurs with much greater frequency in children (60%) than adults (40%), shows no race or sex predilection, and may appear 2 to 3 months after the initiation of therapy. Gingival hyperplasia, which does not occur in edentulous portions of the gum, regresses gradually upon discontinuation of medication.

Phenytoin causes hypertrichosis in 5 percent of the patients. It occurs several months after initiation of therapy and is either slowly reversible or irreversible in nature, even after discontinuation of medication.

Phenytoin may cause hypersensitivity reaction, characterized by rashes, Stevens-Johnson syndrome, lymphoid hyperplasia, blood dyscrasias, and serum sickness. When any of these reactions occur, the medications must be discontinued.

Chronic phenytoin therapy may impair cognitive functions.

Chronic phenytoin therapy may cause bilateral peripheral neuropathy characterized by decreased reflexes and sensory deficits.

Chronic phenytoin may cause hypocalcemia and osteomalasia resulting in acceleration in the metabolism of vitamin D [1].

Indications for Phenytoin. Phenytoin has been approved for tonic-clonic seizures (grand mal) and complex partial seizures. Although parenteral phenytoin is effective in tonic-clonic status epilepticus, it is not the first drug of choice.

Pharmacology of Mephenytoin (Mesantoin). Mephenytoin is demethylated to 5-ethyl-5-phenylhydantoin (Nirvanol), an active anticonvulsant. Mephenytoin binds to plasma protein to the extent of 40 percent with an elimination half-life of 7 hours. Mephenytoin causes sedation whereas phenytoin does not. The incidence of dose- and time-dependent side effects of mephenytoin is lower than that of phenytoin. On the other hand, the incidence of severe and fatal hypersensitivity reactions is far higher than that reported for phenytoin. Therefore, mephenytoin is not the first drug of choice.

Indications for Mephenytoin. Mephenytoin is used for treatment of tonic-clonic, simple partial, and complex partial seizures in patients who have become refractory to phenytoin or other drugs.

BARBITURATE DERIVATIVES. The barbiturate derivatives are mephobarbital (Mebaral), phenobarbital (Luminal), metharbital (Gemonil), and primidone (Mysoline).

In the body, mephobarbital is demethylated to phenobarbital (Fig. 6-1). Therefore, the antiepileptic effects of mephobarbital may be due in part to phenobarbital.

Primidone is not a barbiturate derivative. A replacement of C at position 2 by a CH_2 group changes the ring from barbiturate to that of a pyrimidine. In the body, primidone is converted to phenobarbital and phenylethylmalonamide (PEMA), which are both active anticonvulsants.

Fig. 6-1. *Catabolism of mephobarbital and primidone to phenobarbital.*

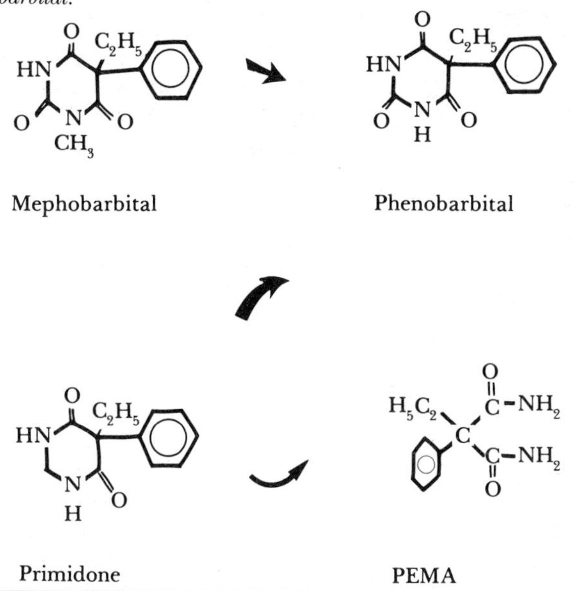

Mephobarbital   Phenobarbital

Primidone   PEMA

Pharmacokinetics of Phenobarbital. Phenobarbital is absorbed from the small intestine. Bound to albumin to the extent of 50 percent, phenobarbital is metabolized in the liver to hydroxyphenobarbital. Approximately 20 to 25 percent of phenobarbital is excreted in the urine unchanged. Phenobarbital has a very long elimination half-life of up to 140 hours. Therefore, it is administered orally in a dose of 2 to 3 mg per kilogram once a day. The renal excretion of phenobarbital is enhanced by alkalinization of urine, which favors ionization and excretion of phenobarbital. $NaHCO_3$ has been used in phenobarbital toxicity.

Phenobarbital induces hepatic microsomal drug-metabolizing enzymes. Its interaction with other drugs such as coumarin anticoagulants is discussed in Chapter 3 on drug-drug interactions. Since the sudden withdrawal of phenobarbital may cause withdrawal seizures, the doses should be tapered gradually whenever discontinuation of medication is contemplated.

Pharmacodynamics of Phenobarbital. The mode of action of phenobarbital is to inhibit posttetanic potentiation and especially to raise seizure threshold. The precise mechanism of action is not known. Two dissimilar mechanisms have been advanced.

PHENOBARBITAL AND ALDEHYDE REDUCTASE. By inhibiting aldehyde reductase, phenobarbital interferes with metabolism of aldehyde generated by biogenic amines such as dopamine, norepinephrine, and serotonin. The accumulation of these aldehydes in the CNS has depressing properties and reduces the neuronal sensitivity to excitation.

PHENOBARBITAL AND GABA. Phenobarbital is thought to enhance presynaptic release of GABA and at the same time reduce the postsynaptic uptake of GABA.

Side Effects and Toxicity of Phenobarbital. Compared to phenytoin, phenobarbital is a relatively safe compound. The occurrence of a morbilliform rash is rare. However, in some patients heavy sedation, reduction in activity, and impairment in cognition may be pronounced [1].

Indication for Phenobarbital. Phenobarbital has a broad spectrum of antiepileptic activity and efficacy. It is often used by itself or in combination with phenytoin.

Primidone (Mysoline). Primidone (Fig. 6-1) is a non-barbiturate compound that is structurally related to phenobarbital. Primidone is absorbed well and does not bind to plasma proteins extensively. It seems wise not to administer primidone to subjects with a history of adverse reaction to phenobarbital.

Side Effects and Toxicity of Primidone. The most frequent side effect of primidone is heavy sedation, which seems to be due to primidone itself and not its metabolite phenobarbital. Tolerance to sedation develops in a few days or weeks of continuous administration.

Indication for Primidone. Primidone is indicated in tonic-clonic and partial seizures. Since by administration of primidone essentially three anticonvulsants are present in the body, for some patients it may be superior to phenobarbital.

Mephobarbital (Mebaral). Mephobarbital, which is more lipid soluble than phenobarbital, becomes metabolized to phenobarbital (Fig. 6-1). Mephobarbital is similar to phenobarbital in pharmacology and is used as an alternative drug. It has been reported that mephobarbital causes fewer sedation and hypersensitivity reactions than phenobarbital.

IMINOSTILBENE DERIVATIVES—CARBAMAZEPINE (TEGRETOL). Carbamazepine is structurally related to phenytoin and to the tricyclic antidepressant imipramine.

Pharmacokinetics of Carbamazepine. The oral bioavailability of carbamazepine, which may depend on a particular pharmaceutic preparation, is 75 to 85 percent. After absorption, it is bound to plasma proteins to the extent of 60 to 70 percent. Carbamazepine is metabolized to 10,11-epoxide and 10,11-dihydroxide derivatives of carbamazepine, some of them excreted unchanged and others conjugated with glucuronic acid. The 10,11-epoxide derivatives are active anticonvulsants.

Pharmacodynamics of Carbamazepine. The mode and the mechanism of carbamazepine are similar but not identical to those of phenytoin. In high but therapeutic doses, carbamazepine decreases sodium and potassium conductances and depresses posttetanic potentiation. Furthermore, carbamazepine increases taurine, decreases glutamic acid, and enhances GABAergic transmission.

Side Effects and Toxicity of Carbamazepine. The most frequent side effects of carbamazepine are drowsiness (11%), diplopia (16%), ataxia (3%), and dizziness (3%). Blood dyscrasias occur on rare occasions.

Indications for Carbamazepine. Carbamazepine is used for trigeminal neuralgia and complex partial seizures with temporal lobe symptomatology. In addition to its antiepileptic effect, carbamazepine demonstrates sedative, anticholinergic, antidepressant, muscle relaxant, antiarrhythmic, antidiuretic, and neuromuscular transmission inhibitory actions. Therefore, it has been used in childhood episodic behavior disorder, multiple sclerosis, central diabetes insipidus, and dystonia. Additional clinical trials should clarify the usefulness of carbamazepine in these conditions [1].

Part Two: Drugs Effective in Absence (Petit Mal) Seizures

SUCCINIMIDE DERIVATIVES. The succinimide derivatives are ethosuximide (Zarontin), methsuximide (Celontin), and phensuximide (Milontin).

Since ethosuximide is a drug of first choice in the management of absence seizure, it will be discussed in more detail than trimethadione, an oxazolidine derivative, or valproic acid, a propyl pentanoic acid derivative. Drugs effective against pentylenetetrazol (Metrazol)-induced seizures have been shown to be effective against absence seizures. In this case, ethosuximide is more effective than either methsuximide or phensuximide.

Pharmacokinetics of Ethosuximide. Ethosuximide does not bind to plasma proteins. It appears in spinal fluid 30 to 60 minutes after its administration and crosses the placental barrier. Ethosuximide is metabolized primarily by hydroxylation, and the metabolite is not an active anticonvulsant. In addition to other minor metabolites, 20 percent of ethosuximide is excreted unchanged in the urine.

Pharmacodynamics of Ethosuximide. The precise mechanism of action of ethosuximide and other succinimide derivatives has not been established. However, it is thought that absence seizures may arise from paroxysmal activity of inhibitory cortical and subcortical pathways, and ethosuximide enhances these inhibitory processes by augmenting the functions of inhibitory transmitter such as dopamine and GABA [1].

Side Effects and Toxicity of Ethosuximide. The most common side effect of ethosuximide is gastrointestinal toxicity—anorexia, weight loss, or epigastric pain. Occasionally, CNS symptoms such as drowsiness, headache, fatigue, ataxia, irritability, and hiccups develop. The rare side effects of ethosuximide are blood dyscrasias such as leukopenia, eosinophilia, agranulocytosis, and pancytopenia.

Indication for Ethosuximide. The only indication for ethosuximide is the treatment of absence seizures.

OXAZOLIDINE DERIVATIVES. The oxazolidine derivatives are trimethadione (Tridione) and paramethadione (Paradione).

Trimethadione is rapidly absorbed orally. Its binding to plasma protein is negligible. Trimethadione is demethylated to dimethadione, which is an active anticonvulsant. The rate of conversion of trimethadione to dimethadione is rapid, but the rate of elimination of dimethadione is slow. As a result, the plasma ratio of dimethadione to trimethadione is 20:1. The toxicity of trimethadione consists in hematologic side effects (neutropenia, pancytopenia), hemeralopia (day blindness), photophobia, diplopia, dermatologic side effects (rash, erythema multiforme), CNS side effects (drowsiness, though tolerance develops to it), nephrotoxic syndrome (albuminuria), and teratogenic effect such as "fetal trimethadione syndrome." From this list of toxicities, it is apparent that trimethadione is indicated only for control of absence seizures that are not responsive or have become refractory to less toxic substances such as ethosuximide or valproic acid [1].

PROPYL PENTANOIC ACID DERIVATIVES— VALPROIC ACID (DEPAKENE). Valproic acid is absorbed rapidly and binds to plasma proteins to the extent of 85 to 90 percent. It is able to displace bound phenytoin or phenobarbital and is metabolized to metabolites that are not anticonvulsants. Valproic acid has a short half-life of 8 to 9 hours. The side effects of valproic acid are gastrointestinal in nature: transient and inconsequential nausea and vomiting. In addition, sedation occurs (50%), especially when the drug is taken in combination with phenobarbital. Furthermore, hepatic toxicity, pancreatitis, alopecia, and hematologic side effects have occurred on rare occasions [1, 2].

Indications for Valproic Acid. Valproic acid has a broad spectrum of anticonvulsant activity and is effective in absence seizures (with effectiveness equal to that of ethosuximide), myoclonic seizures, and tonic-clonic seizures, especially those occurring concomitantly with absence seizures.

Pharmacodynamics of Valproic Acid. The mechanism of action of valproic acid has been postulated to enhance GABAergic transmission.

Part Three: Drugs Effective in Status Epilepticus

BENZODIAZEPINE DERIVATIVES. The benzodiazepine derivatives are diazepam (Valium), clorazepate (Tranxene), and clonazepam (Clonopin).

Diazepam, when given intravenously, produces transient high serum and brain concentrations and is effective in persistent and uninterrupted tonic-clonic convulsions. Since the orally administered diazepam does not produce adequate plasma level, it is effective neither for status epilepticus nor for chronic management of epilepsies. The metabolites of diazepam, desmethyldiazepam, and oxazepam are active anticonvulsants.

Side Effects and Toxicity of Diazepam. Cardiorespiratory depression and hypotension occur especially in elderly patients or in individuals who have been pretreated with depressant drugs.

Clonazepam, a Broad-Spectrum Anticonvulsant. Clonazepam may be used by itself or in combination with other antiepileptic drugs for absence seizures (typical and atypical petit mal), infantile spasms (infantile myoclonic, massive spasms), myoclonic seizures, and atonic seizures (akinetic). It is also believed to be effective in tonic-clonic (grand mal) and complex partial (psychomotor–temporal lobe) seizures.

Side Effects and Toxicity of Clonazepam. Clonazepam causes drowsiness (increased by barbiturate) and a dose-dependent ataxia. In addition, behavioral abnormalities such as hyperactivity, irritability, and aggression may occur, mostly in children.

Diazepam and clonazepam interact with benzodiazepine receptor sites, which in turn enhance the postsynaptic GABAergic transmission.

QUESTIONS ON ANTICONVULSANTS

Select one answer that best completes the statement or answers the question.

_____ 68. At therapeutic doses, which one of the following anticonvulsants causes the least degree of sedation?
A. Phenytoin (Dilantin).
B. Primidone (Mysoline).
C. Phenobarbital (Luminal).
D. Clonazepam (Clonopin).

_____ 69. In an epileptic patient with both absence and tonic-clonic seizures, mephenytoin (Mesantoin) is _least likely_ to be used in combination with which one of the following drugs?
A. Ethosuximide (Zarontin).
B. Trimethadione (Tridione).
C. Valproic acid (Depakene).
D. Clonazepam (Clonopin).

_____ 70. All the following antiepileptic agents _except which one_ have one or more pharmacologically active metabolites?
A. Trimethadione (Tridione).
B. Phenytoin (Dilantin).

C. Carbamazepine (Tegretol).
D. Mephobarbital (Mebaral).

_____ 71. The use of clonazepam (Clonopin) as an antiepileptic drug is limited because:
A. It causes hemeralopia.
B. It causes hypertrichosis.
C. It produces heavy sedation, and tolerance develops to its antiepileptic effect.
D. It is not effective in status epilepticus.

_____ 72. When planning to use phenytoin (Dilantin) for a newly diagnosed patient with tonic-clonic seizures, a neurologist may use which one of the following side effects as a guiding factor for establishing doses?
A. Stevens-Johnson syndrome.
B. Ataxia.
C. Hypertrichosis.
D. Gingival hyperplasia.

_____ 73. Which of the following is an effective drug of choice by itself in complex partial seizures with temporal lobe symptomatology?
A. Valproic acid (Depakene).
B. Diazepam (Valium).
C. Paramethadione (Paradione).
D. Carbamazepine (Tegretol).

_____ 74. Phenytoin (Dilantin) is thought to exert its antiepileptic effect by:
A. Competing with the neuronal action of calcium.
B. Causing hypocalcemia.
C. Causing hypomagnesemia.
D. Causing both hypocalcemia and hypomagnesemia.

_____ 75. All of the following items characterize the pharmacokinetics of phenytoin _except_ which one?
A. It is bound to albumin to the extent of 93 percent.
B. It is hydroxylated in the liver.
C. It is absorbed entirely in the stomach.
D. Its doses should be reduced in uremia and hypoalbuminemia.

_____ 76. Phenytoin-induced gingival hyperplasia:
A. Occurs most often among elderly patients.
B. Occurs usually several months after initiation of therapy.
C. Occurs always in a toothless portion of the gum.
D. Is permanent in nature.

_____ 77. Alkalinization of urine by bicarbonate (causing pH > 10) will facilitate the excretion of which one of the following anticonvulsants?
A. Phenobarbital.
B. Phenytoin.
C. Ethosuximide.
D. Carbamazepine.

_____ 78. Which of the following two anticonvulsants become converted to phenobarbital?
A. Mephenytoin and carbamazepine.
B. Mephobarbital and primidone.
C. Ethosuximide and metharbital.
D. Mephobarbital and barbital.

_____ 79. One reason phenobarbital is administered only once a day may have to do with the fact that:
A. It is conjugated with glucuronic acid slowly.
B. It is excreted primarily by active tubular secretion.
C. It is converted to PEMA, which has anticonvulsant activity.
D. It is hydroxylated slowly.

_____ 80. In an epileptic patient, when the plasma concentration of phenytoin approaches 25 μg/ml, all of the following occur _except_ which one?
A. The half-life of phenytoin is lengthened.
B. The metabolism of phenytoin is inhibited.
C. The metabolism of phenytoin may switch to zero-order kinetics.
D. The therapeutic effectiveness of phenytoin is increased.

ANSWERS AND EXPLANATIONS ON ANTICONVULSANTS

68. A.
69. B.
     Explanation: Both trimethadione and mephenytoin cause blood dyscrasias and other hypersensitivity reactions.
70. B.
71. C.
72. B.
73. D.
74. A.
75. C.
76. B.
77. A.
78. B.
79. D.
80. D.
     Explanation: Hydroxyphenytoin inhibits the hydroxylation of phenytoin.

REFERENCES

1. Browne, T. R., and Feldman, R. B. _Epilepsy: Diagnosis and Management._ Boston: Little, Brown, 1983.
2. Chapman, A., et al. Mechanism of anticonvulsant action of Valproate. _Prog. Neurobiol._ 19:315, 1982.
3. Wilder, B. J., and Bruni, J. _Seizure Disorders. A Pharmacological Approach to Treatment._ New York: Raven Press, 1981.
4. Woodbury, D. M., Penry, J. K., and Pippenger, C. E. _Antiepileptic Drugs._ New York: Raven Press, 1982.

IV. Psychopharmacology

7. The Neuroleptics and Schizophrenia

It is the wounded oyster that mends its shell with pearl.
Ralph Waldo Emerson

Schizophrenia, "divided mind," has not been established as a single disease. Etiologic research has focused on genetic transmission, environmental influences, and biochemical abnormalities, especially in hyperactivity of mesolimbic dopaminergic neurons. The diagnosis of schizophrenia cannot be established by any single biochemical test and must be made on clinical criteria alone. The characteristic range of symptoms and behaviors are thinking or speech disturbances, catatonic motor behavior, paranoid ideation, auditory hallucinations, delusional thinking, blunted or inappropriate emotion, and disturbances of social behavior and interpersonal relations. The therapeutic approach to schizophrenia is based on empirical thinking and clinical diagnosis [11].

ANTIPSYCHOTIC DRUG THERAPY. In treating a patient with a neuroleptic, it is essential that diagnosis of schizophrenia be accurate. For example, in the manic phase of manic-depressive illness, patients often display acute or paranoid symptoms resembling schizophrenia. It should be understood that neuroleptics are not curative in nature, but they improve a patient's capacity for adjustive behavior. The patients should receive a single neuroleptic, and the maintenance dose should be a minimum amount. The predominant target symptoms that respond to drug treatment are overactivity, tension, hostility, combativeness, hallucination, negativism, and poor sleep. Symptoms such as lack of insight, poor judgment, impaired memory, and disorientation are less likely to improve [1, 9, 11].

THE NEUROLEPTICS. Neuroleptics (Fig. 7-1) are also referred to as neuroplegics, psychoplegics, psycholeptics, antipsychotics, and major tranquilizers. These are divided according to the following classification [4, 6]:

Phenothiazine derivatives (e.g., chlorpromazine)
Thioxanthene derivatives (e.g., thiothixene)
Butyrophenone derivatives (e.g., haloperidol)
Dihydroindolone derivatives (e.g., molindone)
Dibenzoxazepine derivatives (e.g., loxapine)
"Atypical" neuroleptics (e.g., sulpiride, pimozide, and clozapine)

PHENOTHIAZINE DERIVATIVES. The phenothiazine derivatives are classified according to their chemical structures:

Propylamino derivatives, which include chlorpromazine (Thorazine), promazine (Sparine), and triflupromazine (Vesprin)
Propylpiperazine derivatives, which include fluphenazine (Permitil, Prolixin), perphenazine (Trilafon), prochlorperazine (Compazine), trifluoperazine (Stelazine), and acetophenazine (Tindal)
Methylpiperidyl derivatives, which include thioridazine (Mellaril)

These agents differ in their potency but not their efficacy. Long-acting injectable drugs such as fluphenazine decanoate or fluphenazine enanthate, which need to be given only once every 2 or 3 weeks, are increasingly used in outpatients and in individuals who are uncooperative and noncompliant. Phenothiazine derivatives devoid of neuroleptic activity also exist. Promethazine (Phenergan) is an antihistaminic, and ethopropazine (Parsidol) has muscle-relaxant property and with its anticholinergic action may be used in parkinsonism. Methotrimeprazine (Levoprome) is claimed to be a nonaddictive analgesic that does not cause respiratory depression.

In discussing the pharmacology of neuroleptics,

Fig. 7-1. *Structures of neuroleptics.*

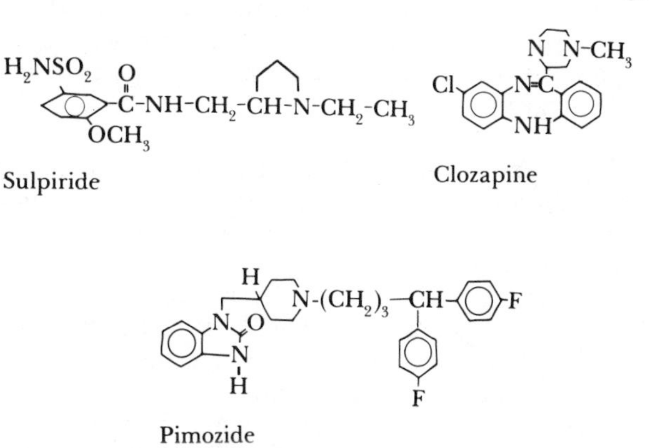

chlorpromazine will be regarded as a prototype drug, and all other drugs will be compared to it.

CNS Effects. Chlorpromazine produces a tranquility that is characterized by a "detached serenity without depression of mental faculties or clouding of consciousness." It depresses the CNS selectively by reducing input directed to the reticular formation through collaterals arriving from the sensory pathways. Chlorpromazine-induced sedation differs from sedation caused by barbiturates in that the patient can be easily aroused. In practice, often the more sedative drugs are prescribed for agitated, overactive patients, and the less sedative agents are used for apathetic, withdrawn patients. However, sedation is not necessary for antipsychotic action for two reasons: (1) Tolerance develops to the sedative effects, and (2) fluphenazine, prochlorperazine, and trifluoperazine are excellent neuroleptics lacking pronounced sedative effects. In general, chlorpromazine and other neuroleptics reduce spontaneous motor activity in proportion to their dosages. Chlorpromazine depresses conditioned avoidance behavior but not escape behavior. Barbiturates depress both avoidance and escape behaviors. Chlorpromazine inhibits defensive behavior defined as "automatization" or "utilization of formerly found solution" whereas amphetamine increases it. Chlorpromazine, given intravenously or intramuscularly, produces a dose-dependent electroencephalographic pattern associated with fatigue, drowsiness, or sleep. Phenothiazine derivatives reduce the seizure threshold [12].

Antiemetic Effects (Therapeutic Effects). Nausea and vomiting associated with circulating physical agents (radiation therapy, virus particles) or chemical agents (toxins, cancer chemotherapeutic agents) that stimulate the chemoreceptor trigger zone for emesis are treated with phenothiazine derivatives, such as chlorpromazine, perphenazine, prochlorperazine, promethazine, triethylperazine, and triflupromazine. With the exception of thioridazine (Mellaril), all have antiemetic effects. These agents depress the chemoreceptor trigger zone for emesis. Larger than therapeutic doses inhibit the vomiting center. Nausea and vomiting associated with emotion and anxiety, motion sickness, and pregnancy should be treated with sedatives and antihistaminics, and not with these potent agents. Nabilone, a synthetic cannabinoid, has been shown to be a more effective antiemetic agent than prochlorperazine in a random prospective double-blind study.

Hypothermic Effects. Phenothiazine derivatives are hypothermic in nature. The extent of hypothermia depends on the dosage and the environmental temperature [8].

Antiadrenergic and Hypotensive Effects. Phenothiazine derivatives cause postural or orthostatic hypotension. This effect may be more pronounced in patients with reduced vascular volume resulting from acute hemorrhage or from dehydration, and when the drugs are used with diuretic agents. Hypotension is more frequent with phenothiazine derivatives having on N_{10} an aliphatic substitution (e.g., chlorpromazine) or a piperidine substitution (e.g., mesoridazine or thioridazine). It occurs less often with compounds containing piperazine substitution (e.g., trifluoperazine). The hypotension is due to direct vasodilation and alpha-adrenergic receptor blocking effect. The pressor effects of epinephrine can be reduced, blocked, or reversed by appropriate doses of chlorpromazine. Surgical patients premedicated with chlorpromazine respond poorly to pressor drugs, requiring larger than anticipated doses. The inotropic (increase in the strength of muscular coordination) effect of epinephrine is reduced by chlorpromazine. The chronotropic (increase in the rate of contraction) effect of epinephrine is increased because chlorpromazine has anticholinergic properties. The local vasoconstrictor action of epinephrine (as used with a local anesthetic) is blocked by chlorpromazine whereas its hyperglycemic effect is not. The lethal effect of epinephrine or norepinephrine, when given in toxic doses, is blocked by chlorpromazine [8].

Anticholinergic Effects. Most phenothiazine neuroleptics have weak anticholinergic effects. However, the anticholinergic effects of thioridazine or ethopropazine are pronounced, and all cautionary items cited for atropine should be noted here. Indeed, fatal tachyarrhythmias and other electrocardiographic changes such as blunting and notching of T waves, prolongation of QT interval, increased convexity of the ST segment, and appearance of V wave have been caused by injudicious uses of thioridazine (1,500–3,600 mg/day), especially in elderly patients [8].

Gastrointestinal Effects. Nausea, which may be patient related, occurs frequently with psychotropic drugs. The incidence is also high in schizophrenic patients receiving placebos. Furthermore, the incidence of vomiting with thioridazine, which has no antiemetic effect, is high. Dry mouth, constipation, paralytic ileus, and decreased gastric secretion—all due to its anticholinergic effects—may occur [8].

Hepatotoxicity. Phenothiazine derivatives may cause jaundice in 5 percent of the patients. Jaundice is accompanied by intense pruritus, fever, chills, nausea, epigastric or right upper quadrant abdominal pain, and malaise. Jaundice is not dose-dependent and develops after a typical delay period of (usually) 2 to 3 weeks. Chlorpromazine-induced jaundice is a short and self-limited illness. With discontinuation of medication, the prognosis has been excellent [8].

Endocrine Effects. Phenothiazine derivatives (thioridazine, trifluoperazine, prochlorperazine, and fluphenazine) have caused reversible galactorrhea. This commonly occurs with large doses and long duration of treatment. Dopamine inhibits the release of prolactin, and neuroleptics, by blocking dopamine receptor sites, nullify this action. Thioridazine causes reversible ejaculation disorder. Patients have reported that erection and orgasms occur without ejaculation. Bromocriptine mesylate (Parlodel), a dopaminergic agonist (used in parkinsonism) has been shown to be effective in preventing postpartum lactation. Chlorpromazine, by preventing the release of insulin, may cause diabetes mellitus in a borderline individual or unstabilize a diabetic patient [8].

Hematologic Effects. Chlorpromazine and other phenothiazine derivatives (perphenazine, prochlorperazine, thioridazine, and triflupromazine) may cause agranulocytosis. The incidence is higher among female and elderly patients, whose bone marrows have lower proliferative potential. These agents inhibit DNA polymerase, thymidylate kinase, and incorporation of [^{3}H] thymidine into DNA. Since the phenothiazine-induced agranulocytosis is a toxic reaction, it may be prevented by careful monitoring of the status of peripheral blood [8].

Dermatologic Effects. The dermatologic reactions following use of phenothiazine derivatives may be divided into three categories:

1. Solar sensitivity, which occurs only in sun-exposed areas of the body, such as the hands and the face. This may be prevented by not exposing the patients to the sun.
2. Allergic dermatitis, which may be maculopapular, urticarial, or pruritic in character. This should be regarded as a hypersensitivity reaction and treated with discontinuation of the medication and initiation of other indicated supportive therapy.
3. Pigment retinopathy. This becomes manifest in deposition of dotlike particles in the anterior capsular and subcapsular portion of the lens, pupillary area, cornea, conjunctiva, and retina. It is thought that the highly reactive metabolites of phenothiazine in the presence of ultraviolet light form free radicals that undergo covalent linkage with melanin. It should be noted that the synthesis of melanocyte-stimulating hormone, like that of prolactin, is stimulated following treatment with phenothiazine derivatives. These side effects may be prevented by using the lowest maintenance doses of neuroleptics and by exercising "drug-free holidays" to reduce the endogenous concentrations of neuroleptics that have long and protracted half-life [8].

Extrapyramidal Side Effects. Phenothiazine derivatives cause the following extrapyramidal side effects:

Acute dystonic syndrome. This occurs particularly in children when they are treated with few doses of antiemetic agents such as prochlorperazine. This bizarre syndrome is best treated with substances having sedative and anticholinergic properties such as diphenhydramine (Benadryl).

Pseudoparkinsonism, which occurs weeks or months after treatment. This may be best treated by anticholinergic drugs such as trihexyphenidyl or benztropine.

Tardive dyskinesia, which involves often irreversible abnormal movements in virtually any part of the body. This is seen after several years of therapy with large doses of neuroleptics. The incidence and severity seem to be higher among patients who have received neuroleptics along with an anticholinergic medication intended as a prophylactic measure to avert parkinsonism. Unfortunately, no satisfactory treatment exists for this iatrogenic neurologic disease, which might have been prevented altogether. Furthermore, the concomitant usage of routine anticholinergics with neuroleptics should be avoided. Tardive dyskinesia is probably related to alteration in functional (denervation supersensitivity) and perhaps in structural integrity of the striatal dopaminergic neurons. Drugs that are partially effective in ameliorating the symptoms of tardive dyskinesia in some patients are [3, 5] reserpine (depletes dopamine), lithium (stimulates dopamine uptake and reduces dopamine receptor sensitivity), deanol or choline (raises acetylcholine), and diazepam (by enhancing GABAergic function, inhibits postsynaptic dopaminergic function).

Dopamine, Schizophrenia, and Neuroleptics. Dopamine receptors may play a role both in the etiology of schizophrenia and in the mechanism of action and side effects of neuroleptics. Dopaminergic hyperactivity in mesocortical and mesolimbic systems has been thought to contribute to schizophrenic symptomatology. Amphetamine (releasing dopamine) and levodopa (increasing dopamine) aggravate schizophrenia. Compounds blocking dopamine receptors in mesocortical and mesolimbic systems (chlorpromazine, haloperidol) are antipsychotic. The more potent a compound is in blocking dopamine receptor (haloperidol), the more potent it is as a neuroleptic. Compounds that do not block dopamine receptor sites (promethazine) are devoid of antipsychotic activity. Classic neuroleptics such as chlorpromazine block dopamine I and II (D_1 and D_2) receptor sites whereas atypical neuroleptics such as sulpiride block D_2 receptors only. Sulpiride causes negligible or no extrapyramidal side effects [2, 7].

Drug-Drug Interactions. Phenothiazine derivatives potentiate the CNS-depressing effects of alcohol and barbiturates and shorten the onset of action of anesthetics.

Pharmacokinetics. Chlorpromazine is well absorbed, mainly from the jejunum. It is extensively metabolized in the liver, producing several active metabolites. When given intramuscularly, the phenothiazine neuroleptics avoid metabolic degradation (first-pass metabolism) and therefore are more beneficial as long-acting depot antipsychotics.

ALTERNATIVE NEUROLEPTICS. Since the advent of psychotropic drugs in psychiatry 30 years ago, a number of innovative milestones have resulted in the more effective treatment of psychiatric patients and also in the production of fewer adverse reactions. Salient among these innovations has been the development of nonphenothiazine classes of neuroleptics: thioxanthenes (chlorprothixene and thiothixene), butyrophenones (haloperidol), diphenylbutylpiperidines (pimozide), dibenzoxazepines (loxapine), dihydroindole compound (molindone), and the benzamide compound (sulpiride). The development of

Table 7-1. *Comparative Pharmacology of Neuroleptics*

Pharmacologic Actions	Phenothiazine Derivative Chlorpromazine	Thioxanthene Derivative Thiothixene	Butyrophenone Derivative Haloperidol	Rauwolfia Alkaloid Reserpine*
Antipsychotic	Yes + +	Yes + +	Yes + + +	Yes +
Antiemetic	Yes + + +	Not tested	Yes + + +	No
Hypothermia	Yes +	Yes +	No	Yes + + + +
Hypotension	Yes + +	Yes + + +	+	Yes + + + +
Parkinsonism	Yes + +	Yes +	Yes + + +	Yes + +
Antiadrenergic	Yes + +	Yes + + +	+	No
Anticholinergic	Yes +	Yes +	Negligible	No
Antihistaminic	Yes +	Negligible	Negligible	No
Releases NE, DA	No	No	No	Yes + + + +
Blocks DA	Yes + +	Yes +	Yes + + +	No
Blocks NE	Yes + +	Yes + + +	Yes +	No
Central sympathetic suppressant	Yes + +	Yes +	Yes + +	Yes + +

Chlorpromazine, thiothixene, and haloperidol decrease the functional availability of dopamine (DA) and norepinephrine (NE) by blocking the dopamine receptor sites in the basal ganglia and norepinephrine receptor sites in thalamic and hypothalamic areas. Reserpine simply reduces the concentrations of norepinephrine and dopamine in these areas. Both of these actions result in suppression of central sympathetic activity.
+ → + + + + indicates from very weak to very strong effects.
*Reserpine, which is no longer used as a neuroleptic, is given for comparison.

Table 7-2. *Comparative Pharmacology of Newer Antipsychotics*

Drug	Sedation	Adrenergic Blockade	Extrapyramidal Reaction
Chlorpromazine	High	Moderate to high	Moderate
Chlorprothixene	High	High	Low to moderate
Haloperidol	Low	Low	High
Molindone	Moderate	Moderate	Moderate to high
Loxapine	High	Low to moderate	High

these compounds has resulted in drugs with greater specificity and lessened toxicity. The pharmacology of these agents is summarized in Tables 7-1 and 7-2.

COMPARATIVE PHARMACOLOGY OF ATYPICAL NEUROLEPTIC SULPIRIDE. Sulpiride is a benzamide derivative widely used in Europe as an antipsychotic, antidepressant, and antiemetic, and especially in the treatment of somatic complaints in neurotic patients. Sulpiride has several characteristics in common with typical neuroleptics but differs from the latter in many other respects.

Like the typical neuroleptics, sulpiride antagonizes certain effects of dopaminomimetic drugs, such as the emetic effect of apomorphine, the sedative effect of apomorphine and L-dopa, and the hypotensive response to apomorphine in humans. Moreover, like classic neuroleptics, sulpiride increases dopamine turnover in the nigrostriatal, mesolimbic, and mesocortical dopaminergic systems and displaces [^{3}H]dopamine and [^{3}H]haloperidol from caudate membranes.

Finally, like typical neuroleptics, sulpiride increases prolactin secretion in humans. However, sulpiride lacks other typical characteristics of neuroleptics in various animal models. In fact, sulpiride, except in toxic doses, does not produce catalepsy or major extrapyramidal deficits, does not antagonize apomorphine stereotypy, and does not reduce conditioned-avoidance responses.

An important difference between sulpiride and typical neuroleptics is that the former does not block dopamine-sensitive adenylate cyclase [10].

QUESTIONS ON NEUROLEPTICS AND SCHIZOPHRENIA

Select one answer that best completes the statement or answers the question.

___ 81. Which one of the following phenothiazine derivatives has neuroleptic properties?
A. Ethopropazine (Parsidol).
B. Thioridazine (Mellaril).
C. Promethazine (Phenergan).
D. Methotrimeprazine (Levoprome).

___ 82. All of the following statements are true about fluphenazine enanthate *except* which one?
A. It is given intramuscularly.
B. It is the antiemetic of first choice in viral diseases of children.
C. It has a duration of action of 2 weeks.

D. Its antipsychotic properties are identical to those of fluphenazine.

_____ 83. Which one of the following actions of chlorpromazine (Thorazine) contributes least to its antipsychotic properties?
  A. Blockade of dopamine receptors in the mesocortical system.
  B. Blockade of dopamine receptors in the mesolimbic system.
  C. Depression of the gamma motor efferent system.
  D. Depression of sensory input directed toward the reticular formation.

_____ 84. Prochlorperazine (Compazine)-induced acute dystonic syndrome is best treated with:
  A. Atropine sulfate.
  B. Imipramine HCl (Tofranil).
  C. Diphenhydramine (Benadryl).
  D. Tranylcypromine (Parnate).

_____ 85. Chlorpromazine-induced pseudoparkinsonism is best treated by:
  A. Dose reduction and the use of benztropine (Cogentin).
  B. Dose elevation and the use of physostigmine.
  C. Dose maintenance and the use of physostigmine.
  D. Dose reduction and the use of levodopa.

_____ 86. The incidence of neuroleptic-induced tardive dyskinesia may be reduced by:
  A. Simultaneous use of an anticholinergic drug with neuroleptics.
  B. Simultaneous use of physostigmine with neuroleptics.
  C. Simultaneous use of a neuroleptic with levodopa.
  D. Using neuroleptics at their lowest maintenance doses and giving "drug-free holidays."

_____ 87. Prochlorperazine (Compazine) should be used to combat nausea or vomiting associated with all of the following conditions *except* which one?
  A. Nausea and vomiting associated with cancer chemotherapy.
  B. Nausea and vomiting associated with radiation therapy.
  C. Nausea and vomiting associated with viral and bacterial infection.
  D. Nausea and vomiting associated with pregnancy.

_____ 88. Thioridazine (Mellaril) and chlorpromazine (Thorazine) have dissimilar pharmacologic actions (quantitatively and qualitatively) on all of the following systems or functions *except* which one?
  A. Chemoreceptor trigger zone for emesis.
  B. Aspermia and lack of ejaculation.
  C. Cholestatic hepatitis.
  D. Anticholinergic effect.

_____ 89. Chlorpromazine-induced allergic dermatitis is due to:
  A. Blockade of dopamine receptor sites in the hypothalamopituitary axis.
  B. Increased synthesis of melanin.
  C. A hypersensitivity reaction.
  D. Diminished synthesis of histamine.

_____ 90. In managing dopamine receptor–related extrapyramidal reactions, which disorder is *improperly* matched with the indicated medication?
  A. Acute dystonic syndrome—diphenhydramine (Benadryl).
  B. Pseudoparkinsonism—trihexyphenidyl (Artane).
  C. Tardive dyskinesia—trihexyphenidyl (Artane).
  D. Huntington's chorea—haloperidol (Haldol).

ANSWERS AND EXPLANATION ON NEUROLEPTICS AND SCHIZOPHRENIA

81. B.
82. B.
83. C.
84. C.
85. A.
86. D.
87. D.
88. C.
89. C.
90. C.
   Explanation: Anticholinergic drugs such as trihexyphenidyl not only are not helpful but also aggravate tardive dyskinesia.

REFERENCES

1. Bernstein, J. G. *Clinical Psychopharmacology.* Littleton, Mass.: PSG Publishing, 1978.
2. Cattabeni, F., et al. Long-term effects of neuroleptics. *Adv. Biochem. Psychopharmacol.* 24:275, 1980.
3. Deveaugh-Geiss, J. *Tardive Dyskinesia and Related Involuntary Movement Disorders. The Long-Term Effects of Antipsychotic Drugs.* London: John Wright, 1982.
4. Forrest, J. S., Carr, C. J., and Usdin, E. Phenothiazines and structurally related drugs. *Adv. Biochem. Psychopharmacol.* 9:1, 1974.
5. Klawans, H. L. Symposium on tardive dyskinesia. *Clin. Neuropharmacol.* 6:75, 1983.
6. Lipton, M. A., Dimascio, A., and Killam, K. F. *Psychopharmacology. A Generation of Progress.* New York: Raven, 1978.
7. Rodright, R. Schizophrenia: Some current neurochemical approaches. *J. Neurochem.* 41:12, 1983.
8. Shader, R. I., and Dimascio, A. *Psychotropic Drug Side Effects.* Baltimore: Williams & Wilkins, 1970. (Case histories)
9. Simpson, L. L. *Drug Treatment of Mental Disorders.* New York: Raven, 1976.
10. Spano, P. F., et al. *Sulpiride and Other Benzamides.* Italian Brain Research Foundation Monograph Series. New York: Raven, 1979.
11. Usdin, E., et al. *Clinical Pharmacology in Psychiatry.* New York: Elsevier North-Holland, 1981.
12. Valzelli, L. *Psychopharmacology.* New York: Spectrum Publications, 1972.

8. Anxiolytic Agents

The mind is its own place, and in itself can make a heaven of hell, a hell of heaven.

John Milton

Anxiety has been defined as "an unpleasurable state of tension which indicates the presence of some danger to the organism," or as "the apprehensive tension which stems from the anticipation of imminent danger, in which the source is largely unknown or unrecognized." The body's response to intense anxiety and to fear is identical. Persistent anxiety or fear may produce palpitation, tachycardia, sweating, pallor, urinary frequency, virtigo, headache, chest pain, anorexia, nausea, abdominal cramps, acid-pepsin disease, insomnia, muscular weakness, and inability to concentrate [2]. Benzodiazepine derivatives are the most widely used drugs in the treatment of anxiety and other psychiatric and neurologic disorders.

Numerous benzodiazepine derivatives have been synthesized (Fig. 8-1) and are used throughout the world [4]:

Fig. 8-1. *Structure of selected benzodiazepine derivatives. (Modified from B. Weidler and G. Hempelmann, Intravenous Use of Benzodiazepines. In E. Costa [ed.], The Benzodiazepines: From Molecular Biology to Clinical Practice. New York: Raven, 1983.)*

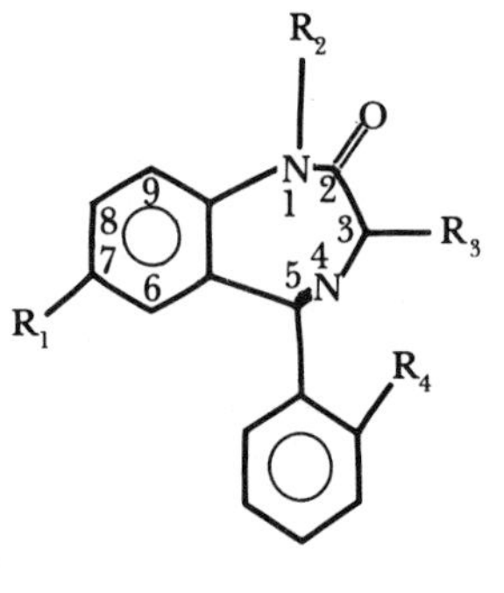

Active Compound	R_1	R_2	R_3	R_4
Chlordiazepoxide (Librium)	Cl	—	—	—
Diazepam (Valium)	Cl	CH_3	—	—
Oxazepam (Serax)	Cl	—	OH	—
Lorazepam (Tavor)	Cl	—	OH	Cl
Prazepam (Demetrin)	Cl	CH_2—◁—	—	—
Nitrazepam (Mogadon)	NO_2	—	—	—
Flunitrazepam (Dalmane)	NO_2	CH_3	—	F
Clonazepam (Clonopin)	NO_2	—	—	Cl
Clorazepate (Tranxene)	Cl	—	COOK	—

PHARMACOKINETIC PROPERTIES OF BENZODIAZEPINE DERIVATIVES. Chlordiazepoxide.
Chlordiazepoxide, a weakly basic substance, is unstable both in solution and when exposed to ultra-violet light. Thus, oral preparations are protected with opaque capsules, and solution for parenteral injection must be prepared freshly and used immediately. The absorption of chlordiazepoxide from an intramuscular site is erratic and unpredictable. Thus, the oral and the intravenous routes are used when reliable or rapid effects are expected. The peak plasma concentration of chlordiazepoxide is reached in 4 hours [7].

Diazepam. Diazepam is a lipid-soluble and water-insoluble substance. The solvent for parenteral diazepam consists of 40% propylene glycol, 10% ethyl alcohol, 5% sodium benzoate, and 1.5% benzyl alcohol. Injection site complications such as phlebitis may result from injudicious administration of these compounds. Like chlordiazepoxide, diazepam should be given either orally or intravenously. The peak plasma concentration of orally administered diazepam is reached in 2 hours. The short duration of action of diazepam when given intravenously is caused by its tissue redistribution and not metabolism. In this case, diazepam behaves identically to ultra-short-acting barbiturates such as thiopental. As a matter of fact, diazepam is metabolized slowly, its reported half-life varying from 25 to 50 hours. Since some of the metabolites are also active pharmacologically, steady-state concentrations develop slowly and usually 7 to 10 days after initiation of oral therapy.

Oxazepam. Oxazepam, which is available only in oral preparations, is metabolized rapidly and hence has a relatively shorter disposition half-life of 5 to 15 hours. Oxazepam's metabolite is inactive.

Lorazepam. Lorazepam resembles oxazepam in that it has a short disposition half-life of 10 to 20 hours. Lorazepam's metabolite is inactive. Oxazepam and lorazepam are considered safe drugs for the elderly or for patients with liver impairment.

Prazepam. Prazepam is dealkylated slowly to nordiazepam, which is also the metabolite of diazepam and clorazepate. Nordiazepam itself becomes converted to oxazepam, and oxazepam becomes metabolized to lorazepam. Therefore, it is apparent that prazepam has several active metabolites.

Nitrazepam, Clonazepam, and Flunitrazepam. Nitrazepam, clonazepam, and flunitrazepam undergo reduction of the nitro group in R_1 position of the A ring. The elimination half-life is approximately 20 to 30 hours. In addition to reduction of the nitro group, flunitrazepam is also demethylated in R_2 position.

Clorazepate. In the acidic environment of the stomach, clorazepate is rapidly hydrolyzed to nordiazepam, in which form it is rapidly absorbed orally. It should be recalled that diazepam is also slowly metabolized to nordiazepam.

PHARMACOLOGIC PROPERTIES OF BENZODIAZEPINE DERIVATIVES.

The pharmacology of benzodiazepine derivatives differs significantly from that of the neuroleptics in that the benzodiazepines have no psychoplegic (antipsychotic) activity, cause no extrapyramidal, autonomic, or endocrine side effects, and, unlike neuroleptics, which lower seizure threshold, are anticonvulsants. In addition, they are anxiolytics, muscle relaxants, and mild sedatives. Although the benzodiazepine derivatives do not produce pronounced autonomic or cardiovascular side effects, they are able to reduce or to block the emotionally induced changes in cardiovascular functions, probably through actions on the limbic systems [1, 3, 7, 8].

In considering the pharmacodynamic profiles of benzodiazepine derivatives, several points need reemphasis.

Compounds such as oxazepam and lorazepam, whose metabolites are inactive, are relatively short-acting drugs whereas compounds such as prazepam, with several active metabolites, have longer disposition half-lives. Consequently, it may be necessary to reduce the doses of benzodiazepines with active metabolites.

Benzodiazepines may display two- or three-compartment disposition kinetics. For example, a benzodiazepine derivative given in suitable dose at night may have dose-dependent effects. The concentration attained at night may be in the hypnotic range whereas the concentration of the drug or its active metabolite(s) may be sufficient to produce antianxiety effects during the following day [6].

It is generally accepted that the pharmacology of benzodiazepine derivatives is identical qualitatively but varies quantitatively. In other words, the sedative, hypnotic, anticonvulsant, muscle relaxant, and anxiolytic properties reside to various degrees in all of them. Nevertheless, pharmacologic specificity does occur and necessitates selection of a particular drug for a desired therapeutic effect.

PHARMACODYNAMICS OF BENZODIAZEPINE DERIVATIVES.

Benzodiazepine derivatives enhance GABAergic transmission [4, 5]. GABA and benzodiazepine sites are separate but coupled to chloride ionophore. In the presence of GABA, the permeability to chloride ion and chloride conductance increases. When both the benzodiazepine and GABA receptor sites are occupied, the transport of negatively charged ion is greatly facilitated, resulting in hyperpolarization and facilitation of GABA-mediated inhibition (see Fig. 1-3D).

Experimental evidence indicates that [³H]GABA binds to two populations of receptor sites, one of high affinity (20–30 nM) and one of low affinity (120–200 nM). The high-affinity population of binding sites is thought to down regulate by "GABA-modulin," an endogenous peptide, through an allosteric mechanism. Furthermore, GABA recognition sites have been classified into GABA A and GABA B. GABA A recognizes isoguvacine, muscimol, and bicuculline and requires no Ca^{2+} for binding. GABA B recognizes GABA and baclofen and requires 1 to 5 nM of Ca^{2+} for maximal binding. GABA B binding site is thought to represent the physiologic receptor site for GABA (see Fig. 1-3D).

GABA coexists with other putative neuromodulators such as motilin. A nerve expulse will release not only GABA but also other substances coexisting with it. The effects of GABA may be modified by these cotransmitters or comodulators. Furthermore, the nature and functions of these substances may vary in different regions of the brain [11, 12].

The released GABA may modulate by inhibiting the function(s) of other neurons such as noradrenergic, cholinergic, dopaminergic, and serotonergic neurons. Since benzodiazepine facilitates GABAergic functions, it is easily seen that the anticonvulsant, muscle relaxant, sedative, hypnotic, and antianxiety effects of benzodiazepine may be brought forth by GABAergic neurons and other neurons inhibited by GABA. Moreover, the nature of this inhibition may vary in different regions of the brain [10].

MODE OF ACTION OF BENZODIAZEPINE DERIVATIVES. Antianxiety Effects.

Benzodiazepines, by facilitation of GABAergic actions, are thought to exert their anxiety-reducing effects by selectively depressing the hyperactivity of neuronal circuits in limbic system. In addition to facilitation of GABAergic action, they may inhibit the hyperexcitability of hippocampal cholinergic and serotonergic neurons.

Muscle Relaxant Activity. Benzodiazepines enhance presynaptic inhibition in the spinal cord by releasing GABA from interneurons.

Sedative Effects. The sleep-promoting effects of benzodiazepines may relate to reduction of hyperarousability and emotional tension. The anterograde amnesia produced by high doses may be due to interference with hippocampal functions.

Anticonvulsant Activity. Benzodiazepine derivatives are thought to exert their anticonvulsant activity by facilitating GABAergic transmission. Substances that inhibit the synthesis of GABA (e.g., isoniazid) or block GABA recognition sites (e.g., bicuculline) cause convulsions.

THERAPEUTIC USES OF BENZODIAZEPINES. Treatment of Neurotic Anxiety State.

Benzodiazepines are of value in "anxious depressions," in "anxiety tension" associated with schizophrenia, and during psychotherapy. They should be used only when the symptoms are disabling. The use of these drugs to alleviate stress is not justified.

Treatment of Neuromuscular Disorders. Benzodiazepines are of value in cerebral palsy, in spasticity from degenerative disorders such as multiple sclerosis, in tetanus, in stiff-man syndrome, and in backache and muscle strain. The effective doses are generally large and may be increased as the disease progresses (e.g., multiple sclerosis) [13].

Intractable Seizures. In epileptic seizure, diazepam is a drug of choice, for intravenous administration. Clonazepam is also effective.

Alcohol Withdrawal. During acute withdrawal from alcohol, intravenous diazepam is indicated. This is usually followed by chlordiazepoxide given orally.

Sleep Disorders. Diazepam and flunitrazepam are often used as sedatives. These agents are also effective in somnambulism, enuresis, and night terrors.

Preanesthetic, Premedication, and Diagnostic Procedures. Intravenous diazepam may be used for induction prior to maintaining anesthesia with other agents, in endoscopic procedures, and in cardioversion. In general, these agents cause amnesia, relieve anxiety, and reduce or eliminate the use of narcotic analgesics. During labor and delivery, only a short-acting benzodiazepine such as oxazepam should be used [9].

UNWANTED SIDE EFFECTS AND HAZARDS.

The more troublesome side effects are drowsiness and postural hypotension, which may be especially pronounced in elderly patients. In children, benzodiazepines should be used only in convulsive disorders. Since benzodiazepines are metabolized extensively, they should be used with extreme caution in liver diseases. Other complications that may rarely occur are paradoxic excitement and self-destructive ideation, injection site complications (phlebitis), and congenital malformation (cleft lip or palate). Psychologic and physical dependence occurs if benzodiazepines are given in excess doses over a prolonged period of time.

In general, the dose should be adjusted to maximize symptomatic relief and minimize daytime over-sedation. The patients may be educated and encouraged to adjust the dosage to their subjective and perceived needs but to remain within prescribed upper allowable limits.

QUESTIONS ON ANXIOLYTIC AGENTS

Select one answer that best completes the statement or answers the question.

____ 91. Benzodiazepine may be useful during the "probing phase" of psychotherapy because this phase may be associated with:
   A. Paradoxic rage reaction.
   B. Augmented anxiety.
   C. Unmitigated amnesia.
   D. Unabashed hostility.

____ 92. The intravenous uses of diazepam (Valium) may be justified for the following conditions *except* which one?
   A. Alcohol-related delirium tremens.
   B. Somnambulism and enuresis.
   C. Status epilepticus.
   D. Cardioversion.

____ 93. Which one of the following drugs is an active metabolite of diazepam (Valium)?
   A. Oxazepam (Serax).
   B. Chlordiazepoxide (Librium).
   C. Clorazepate (Tranxene).
   D. Clonazepam (Clonopin).

____ 94. Which one of the following actions or reactions of diazepam (Valium) probably does *not* involve an interaction with GABAergic transmission?
   A. Anxiety reducing—limbic system.
   B. Muscle relaxation—presynaptic inhibition.
   C. Anticonvulsant action.
   D. Physical dependence—medulla oblongata.

____ 95. Diazepam (Valium) is a drug of choice in treating tetanus because diazepam produces muscle relaxation by:
   A. Enhancing presynaptic interneuronal inhibitory functions.
   B. Abolishing postsynaptic excitatory functions.
   C. Reducing presynaptic excitatory functions.
   D. Uncoupling the interactions of tetanus toxin with postsynaptic receptor sites.

____ 96. Which one of the following benzodiazepine derivatives is the shortest acting and does not accumulate in the body?
   A. Chlordiazepoxide (Librium).
   B. Oxazepam (Serax).
   C. Diazepam (Valium).
   D. Clorazepate (Tranxene).

____ 97. The antianxiety effects of chlordiazepoxide (Librium) are thought to result from inhibition of:
   A. Amygdalohippocampal transmission.
   B. Occipitotemporal transmission.
   C. Nigrostriatal transmission.
   D. Cerebelloreticular transmission.

____ 98. Valium and thiopental, when injected intravenously, have short duration of CNS action because they are:
   A. Metabolized rapidly.
   B. Excreted rapidly.
   C. Redistributed from brain to other tissues.
   D. Bound rapidly to protein and hence become inactive.

ANSWERS AND EXPLANATION ON ANXIOLYTIC AGENTS

91. B.
   Explanation: Antianxiety agents are useful in psychotherapy. They may be administered (1) initially to facilitate communication between patients and physicians, (2) during probing phase, where anxiety may increase from gaining insight into one's problem, and (3) during discharge, where once more anxiety may increase.
92. B.
93. A.
94. D.
95. A.
96. B.
97. A.
98. C.

REFERENCES

1. Bellantuono, C., et al. Benzodiazepines: Clinical pharmacology and therapeutic use. *Drugs* 19:195, 1980.
2. Branch, C. H. *Aspects of Anxiety*. Philadelphia: Lippincott, 1972.
3. Classen, H. G., and Schramm, V. New perspectives in benzodiazepine therapy. *Arzneimittelforsch.* 30:851, 1980.
4. Costa, E. *The Benzodiazepines: From Molecular Biology to Clinical Practice*. New York: Raven, 1983.
5. Costa, E., and Greengard, P. Mechanism of action of benzodiazepines. *Adv. Biochem. Psychopharmacol.* 14:131, 1975.
6. Dettli, L. Benzodiazepines in the Treatment of Insomnia: Pharmacokinetic Considerations. In E. Costa (ed.), *The Benzodiazepines: From Molecular Biology to Clinical Practice*. New York: Raven, 1983. Pp. 201–223.
7. Greenblatt, D. J., et al. Clinical pharmacokinetics of the newer benzodiazepines. *Clin. Pharmacokinet.* 8:233, 1983.
8. Greenblatt, D. J., and Shader, R. I. *Benzodiazepines in Clinical Practice*. New York: Raven, 1974.
9. Greenblatt, D. J., Shader, R. I., and Abernathy, D. R. Current status of benzodiazepines. *N. Engl. J. Med.* 309:354, 410, 1983.
10. Haefely, W., et al. Neuropharmacology of Benzodiazepines: Synaptic Mechanisms and Neural Basis of Action. In E. Costa (ed.), *The Benzodiazepines: From Molecular Biology to Clinical Practice*. New York: Raven, 1983. Pp. 21–66.
11. Lippa, A. S., Meyerson, L. R., and Beer, B. Molecular substrates of anxiety: Clues from the heterogeneity of benzodiazepine receptors. *Life Sci.* 31:1409, 1982.
12. Tallman, J. F., et al. Receptors for the age of anxiety. Pharmacology of the benzodiazepines. *Science* 207:274, 1980.
13. Young, R. R., and Del Waide, P. J. Drug therapy: Spasticity. *N. Engl. J. Med.* 304:28, 96, 1981.

9. The Pharmacology of Depression —the Thymoleptics

In every winter's heart there is a quivering spring, and behind the veil of each night there is a smiling dawn.

Kahlil Gibran

Depressive disorders are the most prevalent of psychiatric illnesses, occurring more often among women (16%) than men (8%). Depression, a recurrent but self-limiting disorder, is classified as exogenous or reactive depression and endogenous depression. Furthermore, depression is classified as unipolar and bipolar. Unipolar patients display one type of affective disorder, most commonly depression, whereas bipolar patients usually experience mania and depression. Depression is characterized by anxiety, agitation, motor retardation, psychologic retardation, delusions, depersonalization, physical complaints, sleep disturbances, sexual disturbances, and suicidal ideations, especially in poorly treated or untreated patients [4, 5].

CLASSES OF DRUGS USED IN DEPRESSION.

Drugs used in depression are referred to as thymoleptics, thymoanaleptics, psychoanaleptics, psychic energizers, and antidepressants.

Part One: Classification of Antidepressants

Antidepressants are divided into the following classes:

1. Dibenzazepine derivatives. The agents in this class, called tricyclic antidepressants, are imipramine (Tofranil), desipramine (Norpramin), amitriptyline (Elavil), nortriptyline (Aventyl), protriptyline (Vivactyl), and doxepin (Adapin).
2. Monoamine oxidase inhibitors. These agents are used occasionally. The hydrazine derivatives are isocarboxazid (Marplan) and phenelzine sulfate (Nardil). The nonhydrazine derivatives include tranylcypromine (Parnate).
3. Monoamine precursors. L-Tryptophan is the only monoamine precursor.
4. Newer, novel, or atypical antidepressants. These include bupropion (Wellbatrin), zimelidine and norzimelidine, sulpiride, trazodone, mianserin, nomifensine, and caroxazone.

Since the tricyclic antidepressants are the most often investigated and used drugs, they will be discussed in detail.

DIBENZAZEPINE DERIVATIVES. The three-ring nucleus characteristic of these drugs has given them the epithet *the tricyclics*. They resemble the phenothiazine derivatives both in structures and in functions (Fig. 9-1).

Imipramine is demethylated to desipramine, and amitriptyline is demethylated to nortriptyline. Both metabolites are active antidepressants. Tricyclic antidepressants bind to plasma proteins to the extent of 90 percent, and because of their extensive "first-pass metabolism" in the liver, they have very low and variable bioavailability. In circumstances in which the measurement of plasma concentrations of these drugs is desirable, the concentrations of their active metabolites should also be measured.

Pharmacologic Properties. Tricyclic antidepressants, like some phenothiazine derivatives, are sedative in nature. Those compounds containing a tertiary amine (imipramine, amitriptyline, and doxepin) are most sedative. Those compounds containing a secondary amine (nortriptyline and desipramine) are less sedative whereas protriptyline is devoid of any

Fig. 9-1. *Structures of tricyclic antidepressants.*

Chlorpromazine

Amitriptyline

Imipramine

Nortriptyline

Desipramine

Protriptyline

Doxepin

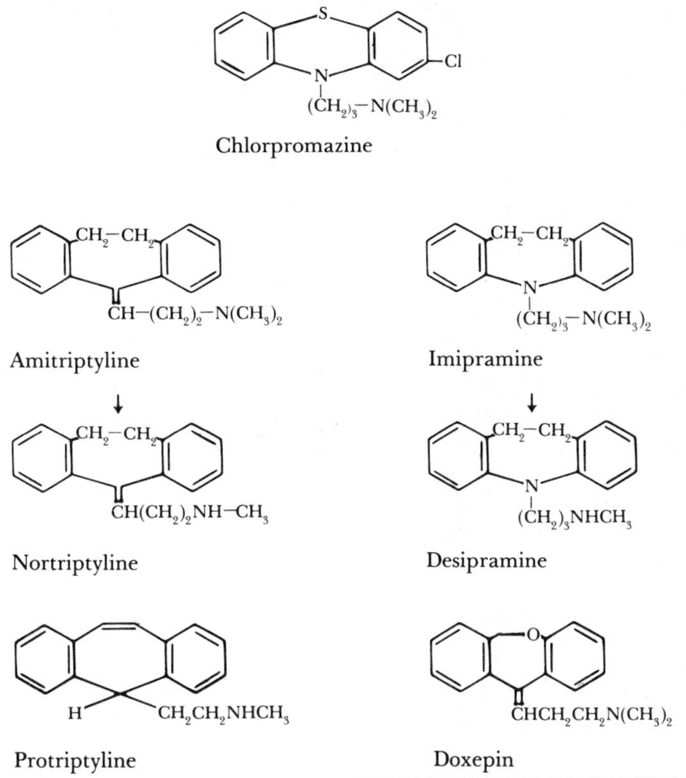

sedative property.

Tricyclic antidepressants, again like some phenothiazine derivatives (e.g., thioridazine) have anticholinergic property. Amitriptyline is the strongest, desipramine the weakest.

Like ouabain and cocaine, tricyclic antidepressants block the uptake of norepinephrine and serotonin. They tend to potentiate the effectiveness of sympathomimetic amines whereas the phenothiazine derivatives, by blocking the receptor sites, tend to attenuate these effects.

Tricyclic antidepressants cause orthostatic hypotension by obtunding the various reflex mechanisms involved in maintaining blood pressure. The following chart compares the effects of chlorpromazine with those of imipramine on various amine-mediated cardiovascular functions.

	Chlorpromazine	Imipramine
Cardiovascular effects of sympathomimetic amines	Reduced	Enhanced
Thyroxine-induced potentiation of actions of biogenic amines	Reduced	Enhanced
Cyclopropane-induced potentiation of amine-related cardiac effects	Reduced	Enhanced

Pharmacodynamics of Tricyclic Antidepressants.
The mechanisms of action of tricyclic antidepressants

have not been established. Furthermore, the possibility exists that different antidepressants exert their effects through dissimilar mechanisms. The following mechanisms of actions have been postulated [1, 2, 8, 9, 11, 12].

The tricyclic antidepressants block the uptake of serotonin and norepinephrine according to the following scale:

Drugs	Serotonin Uptake	Norepinephrine Uptake
Imipramine	Moderate	Moderate
Amitriptyline	High	Slight
Desipramine	None	High
Nortriptyline	Slight	Moderate

It should be noted that the blockade of uptake$_1$ sites takes place prior to appearance of antidepressant effects, which usually occur between 7 and 10 days after treatment.

Antidepressant such as mianserin enhances the release of norepinephrine from the presynaptic neurons by interacting with presynaptic alpha$_2$-adrenergic receptors.

Antidepressants such as amitriptyline increase serotonergic activity by enhancing postsynaptic sensitivity to this indoleamine.

Antidepressants such as norzimelidine are potent inhibitors of [^{3}H]imipramine binding, a receptor to which the endogenously existing antidepressants may bind.

Therapeutic Indications. ENDOGENOUS DEPRESSION. In treatment of an endogenous depression, it should first be differentiated from sadness. Disabling depression and its vegetative symptoms generally respond to tricyclic antidepressants. On the other hand, sadness does not respond to antidepressants but does respond to changes in environmental events. The effective dose of tricyclic antidepressants, which are equivalent drugs, is chosen empirically. Furthermore, the less sedative agents are chosen for apathetic and withdrawn patients. Moreover, since the margin of safety of these agents is very narrow, they should not be prescribed in large supply for a depressed patient, who may use them to commit suicide.

ENURESIS. The anticholinergic effect of imipramine has been used successfully in managing enuresis.

DISEASES PRODUCING PAIN. Pain associated with diabetic peripheral neuropathy, trigeminal neuralgia, or cancer may predispose the patient to depression. Tricyclic antidepressants have been shown to be effective adjuncts in these and other similar conditions.

PHOBIAS. Some episodic phobias are regarded as "masked" depression and respond to treatment with tricyclic antidepressants.

TOXICITY. The potent anticholinergic effects of tricyclic antidepressants produce pronounced sinus tachycardia, choreiform movements, hyperreflexia, and epileptiform seizures. These symptoms can be effectively managed by intravenous administration of physostigmine. The long duration of action of tricyclic antidepressants may necessitate the repeated administration of physostigmine, which has a short duration of action.

MONOAMINE OXIDASE INHIBITORS.

Monoamine oxidase can metabolize monoamines by oxidative deamination and convert them to inactive acidic derivatives. Monoamine oxidase inhibitors seem to compete with physiologically active monoamine for the active site of the enzyme (electrostatic interaction between the positively charged ammonium ion of the drug and the negatively charged group of the enzyme). In general, these agents inhibit not only oxidase that metabolizes amines but also oxidase that metabolizes drugs and essential nutrients. Hence, the incidence of drug-drug interaction and drug-food interaction is extremely high with these agents. Monoamine oxidase inhibitor may be local anesthetic (cocaine), antihistaminic (diphenylhydramine), or antidepressant (tranylcypromine). Monoamine oxidase inhibitors have been used in hypertension (direct blockade of sympathetic ganglion), angina pectoris (coronary dilatation), narcolepsy (stimulating reticular activating system), and depression (increasing norepinephrine pool of the brain). Needless to say, these agents should be used with extreme caution with sympathomimetic amines, ganglionic blocking agents, procaine, and anesthetic agents. They are contraindicated in hyperthyroidism and along with tricyclic antidepressants. In case of poisoning, adrenergic blocking agents such as phentolamine may be effective to combat the hypertensive crisis.

Indications for Monoamine Oxidase Inhibitors. The high incidence of drug-food and drug-drug in-

teractions does not make the monoamine oxidase inhibitors antidepressants of first choice. However, in some circumstances these agents may be used effectively and successfully:

When a patient has not responded to a tricyclic antidepressant for an adequate trial period and with an appropriate dosage

When a patient has developed allergic reactions to tricyclics

When a patient has had previous depressive episodes that responded well with monoamine oxidase inhibitors

MONOAMINE PRECURSORS. Tryptophan alone or tryptophan in combination with a monoamine oxidase inhibitor or with a tricyclic antidepressant has been shown to be effective in some depressed patients who are believed to be deficient in serotonin.

NEWER, NOVEL, OR ATYPICAL ANTIDEPRESSANTS.

These recently manufactured antidepressants, which may become available for clinical uses, are worthy of consideration [3].

Bupropion. Bupropion has minimal effects on blocking reuptake of norepinephrine or serotonin. Furthermore, it does not inhibit monoamine oxidase, has no anticholinergic effect, and is devoid of any cardiovascular action.

Zimelidine and Norzimelidine. Zimelidine and its metabolite norzimelidine strongly inhibit the reuptake of serotonin. The onset of action of zimelidine is faster than that of amitriptyline.

Sulpiride. Sulpiride is a dopamine receptor antagonist. It is an effective neuroleptic and thymoleptic. Sulpiride's disinhibitory effects in depression may be due to its presynaptic action on adrenergic neurons, and its antischizophrenic effects may be due to its postsynaptic action on dopaminergic neurons.

Trazodone. Trazodone inhibits serotonin uptake without modifying norepinephrine or dopamine uptake. It has no anticholinergic action nor does it cause cardiotoxicity.

Mianserin. Mianserin does not inhibit the uptake of dopamine, norepinephrine, or serotonin. It increases the turnover of norepinephrine and has no anticholinergic action.

Nomifensine. Nomifensine strongly inhibits the uptake of dopamine and norepinephrine. Furthermore, it releases dopamine.

Caroxazone. Caroxazone inhibits monoamine oxidase and increases the concentrations of dopamine, norepinephrine, and serotonin. It has no anticholinergic action.

Part Two: Control of Manic Episodes in Manic-Depressive Psychosis with Lithium

PHARMACOKINETICS OF LITHIUM. Absorption. Lithium is given orally as a salt, and the particular salt does not affect therapeutic action. Lithium's anionic partner—be it carbonate, chloride, acetate, citrate, or sulfate—serves only as an inert vehicle. The carbonate is by far the most widely used lithium salt. In addition, lithium carbonate contains more lithium, weight for weight, than the other lithium salts.

Distribution. Since lithium is not bound to any plasma or tissue proteins, it becomes distributed widely throughout the body.

Elimination. Lithium ions are eliminated mainly by the kidneys. There is a direct relationship between the amount of sodium chloride ingested and the fraction of filtered lithium resorbed. More lithium will be retained if sodium intake is low. The contraindications are significant cardiovascular or renal diseases, which would compromise its excretion.

SIDE EFFECTS. Lithium is unique among psychopharmacologic compounds in that it rarely produces any undesirable effects on emotional and intellectual functioning. A few unwanted effects are seen in the somatic sphere; they fall into three overlapping categories [6, 7, 10].

Initially, when the maintenance dose of lithium is being established, the patient may develop gastrointestinal discomfort such as nausea, vomiting, diarrhea, stomach pain, muscular weakness, thirstiness, frequent urination, and slight feeling of being dazed, tired, and sleepy. These early side effects disappear when the patient is stabilized on lithium.

From the beginning of treatment with lithium, the patient develops slight and barely noticeable hand tremors, which do not respond to antiparkinsonian agents.

After several months of continuous therapy with lithium, the patient may develop diabetes insipidus and goiter. The kidney tubules become insensitive to the action of antidiuretic hormone (ADH), and its administration is ineffective. Dose reduction or discontinuation of lithium corrects the side effect without leaving any residual pathology. In the presence of goiter, the patient remains euthyroid. It has been reported that administration of small amounts of thyroxine may also obviate this side effect.

PHARMACODYNAMICS OF LITHIUM. Lithium is thought to exert its effect by interfering with the Ca^{2+}-mediated release of norepinephrine, increasing the uptake of norepinephrine, and decreasing the sensitivity of postsynaptic receptor sites to norepinephrine.

THERAPEUTIC USES OF LITHIUM. The uses of lithium fall into two categories.

Established Uses. Lithium salts are used in acute mania and as a prophylactic measure to prevent the recurrence of bipolar manic-depressive illness [13].

Innovative Uses. Lithium salts have been used with certain success in the following illnesses or conditions:

In combination with tricyclic antidepressants, lithium is used in recurrent endogenous depression.
In combination with neuroleptics, lithium is used in schizoaffective disorders.
In combination with neuroleptics, lithium is used in schizophrenia.
Lithium is used in alcoholism associated with depression.
Lithium has been investigated to subdue aggressive behaviors in nonpsychotic but possibly "brain-damaged" patients.
Lithium has been investigated in the management of inappropriate secretion of antidiuretic hormone.
Lithium has been used to correct neutropenia seen in cancer chemotherapy.

QUESTIONS ON THYMOLEPTICS

Select one answer that completes the statement or answers the question.

_____ 99. Which one of the following drugs is a monoamine oxidase inhibitor?
    A. Zimelidine.
    B. Tranylcypromine.
    C. Nortriptyline.
    D. Doxepin.

_____ 100. Imipramine resembles chlorpromazine in all of the following aspects *except* which one? Both compounds:
    A. Interfere with the action of norepinephrine.
    B. Have the same therapeutic index.
    C. Have structural similarities.
    D. Have sedative properties.

_____ 101. Physostigmine may be used to overcome the toxicity of all of the following compounds *except* which one?
    A. Amitriptyline.
    B. Thioridazine.
    C. Ethopropazine.
    D. Edrophonium.

_____ 102. On theoretic grounds, which one of the following compounds may be used to antagonize the amine pump–related toxicity of desipramine?
    A. Reserpine.
    B. Amphetamine.
    C. Tranylcypromine.
    D. Tryptophan.

_____ 103. Which one of the following agents shows the least amount of binding to albumin?
    A. Digoxin.
    B. Lithium.
    C. Chlorpromazine.
    D. Protriptyline.

_____ 104. Which one of the following is not an indication for a tricyclic antidepressant?
    A. Enuresis in school children.

B. Phobia.
C. Trigeminal neuralgia.
D. Temporal lobe epilepsy.

_____ 105. Tricyclic antidepressants have been shown to cause interactions with all of the following drugs *except* which one?
A. Guanethidine.
B. Alcohol.
C. Thyroid preparations.
D. Lithium carbonate.

ANSWERS AND EXPLANATIONS ON THYMOLEPTICS

99. B.
100. B.
Explanation: Tricyclic antidepressants including imipramine have a very narrow margin of safety. The patients should not be oversupplied with tricyclics, since they have been used successfully to commit suicide.

101. D.
Explanation: Amitriptyline, thioridazine, and ethopropazine have anticholinergic properties. Both physostigmine and edrophonium are cholinesterase inhibitors.

102. A.
Explanation: Reserpine depletes the granule from serotonin and norepinephrine and catabolizes them presynaptically.

103. B.
104. D.
105. D.
Explanation: They nullify the antihypertensive effects of guanethidine. They cause paralytic ileus and CNS depression when given with alcohol. Their actions and especially cardiovascular effects are enhanced by thyroid drugs.

REFERENCES

1. Banki, C. M., and Arato, M. Amine metabolites and neuroendocrine responses related to depression and suicide. *J. Affective Disord.* 5:223, 1983.
2. Costa, E., et al. Molecular mechanisms in the action of imipramine. A mini-review. *Experientia* 39:855, 1983.
3. Costa, E., and Racagni, G. Typical and Atypical Antidepressants. *Advances in Biochemical Psychopharmacology*, Vol. 31. New York: Raven, 1982. P. 125.
4. Frangos, E., et al. Psychotic depressive disorder—a separate entity? *J. Affective Disord.* 5:259, 1983.
5. Freedman, A. M., Kaplan, H. I., and Sadock, B. J. *Comprehensive Textbook of Psychiatry* (2nd ed.). Baltimore: Williams & Wilkins, 1975. Pp. 1003–1054.
6. Gershon, S., and Shopsin, B. *Lithium. Its Role in Psychiatric Research and Treatment.* New York: Plenum, 1976.
7. Johnson, F. N. *Lithium Research and Therapy.* New York: Academic, 1975.
8. Kelwala, S., Jones, D., and Sitaram, N. Monoamine metabolites as predictors of antidepressant response—critique. *Prog. Neuropsychopharmacol. Biol. Psychiatry* 7:229, 1983.
9. Leonard, B. E. Current status of the biogenic amine theory of depression. *Neurochem. Int.* 4:339, 1983.
10. Mendels, J., and Secunda, K. *Lithium in Medicine.* London: Gordon & Breach, 1972.
11. Sugrue, M. F. Current concepts on the mechanisms of action of antidepressant drugs. *Pharmacol. Ther.* 13:219, 1981.
12. Sugrue, M. F. Do antidepressants possess a common mechanism of action? *Biochem. Pharmacol.* 32:1811, 1983.
13. Wood, K., and Coppen, A. Prophylactic lithium treatment of patients with affective disorders is associated with decreased platelet [^{3}H] dihydroergocryptine binding. *J. Affective Disord.* 5:253, 1983.

V. CNS Pharmacology

10. Narcotic Analgesics

All glory comes from daring to begin.

Eugene F. Ware

Analgesia means lack of pain, and analgesics are substances that obtund the perception of pain without the loss of consciousness. Analgesics should not be given until the cause of pain has been determined. If proper diagnosis has been made, the use of an analgesic may not become necessary. A few examples:

Stoker's cramp. Individuals who become dehydrated in hot weather, without fluid replenishment, develop painful muscular cramp. This condition may be prevented or corrected by administering sodium chloride and by replenishing the lost fluid.

Tetanus. The severe muscular spasm occurring in tetanus is managed by a muscle relaxant.

Acid-pepsin disease. The painful epigastric pain is managed by antacids and by other medications.

Gouty arthritis. The pain associated with gouty arthritis is managed by antiinflammatory drugs and by agents that reduce the synthesis and the pool of uric acid in the body.

Hypertension headache. The headache associated with malignant hypertension is managed by antihypertensive agents.

From these examples, it is clear that pain may be associated with an extensive number of pathologic conditions. Although analgesics may reduce the pain in all of the aforementioned conditions, they should not be used until the pathology has been discerned and appropriate rehabilitative measures have been instituted [3].

The opium alkaloids, which are obtained from *Papaver somniferum*, contain two groups of compounds:

Compounds with phenanthrene derivatives consisting of morphine (1–10%), codeine (0.7–2.5%), and thebaine (0.5–1.5%)

Compounds with isoquinoline derivatives consisting of papaverine (1%) and noscapine (5–10%)

Narcotic alkaloids are divided into naturally occurring, semisynthetic, and synthetic derivatives (Fig. 10-1).

Naturally occurring analgesics: morphine and codeine (methylmorphine)

Semisynthetic analgesics: hydromorphone (Dilaudid) and hydrocodone (Dicodid)

Synthetic analgesics: meperidine (Demerol), alphaprodine (Nisentil), methadone (Dolophine), propoxyphene (Darvon), and pentazocine (Talwin)

The narcotic antagonists are nalorphine (Nalline) and naloxone (Narcan).

Dextromethorphan (Romilar) is used as an antitussive preparation.

Apomorphine is used as an emetic agent.

Narcotic analgesics may have high potency (morphine, hydromorphone, oxymorphone, methadone, meperidine, fentanyl, and levorphanol), or low potency (codeine, oxycodone, hydrocodone, propoxyphene, and diphenoxylate). These agents may be pure agonist (morphine), pure antagonist (naloxone), or mixed agonist-antagonist (pentazocine).

In discussion of the pharmacology of narcotic analgesics, morphine will be considered in detail as a prototype drug, and all other compounds will be compared to it [6, 8].

MORPHINE. Effects on CNS. Morphine depresses the cerebral cortex, the hypothalamus, and the medullary centers. These effects are responsible for decrease in pain perception, induction of narcosis, depression of the cough center, depression of the vomiting center, and depression of respiration.

Stimulation of Some Parts of CNS. In horses, morphine stimulates the spinal cord predictably. This effect is short-lived in humans, and is seldom seen with therapeutic doses. Initially, morphine stimulates the vomiting center, and emesis occurs early in intoxication. Depression of the vomiting center then ensues late in intoxication. Morphine stimulates the vagus, causing bradycardia, and also the nucleus of the third cranial nerve (oculomotor), causing miosis.

Analgesic Effects. The relief of pain by morphine is selective, and other sensory modalities such as touch, vibration, vision, hearing, and the like are not obtunded. Morphine does not reduce the responsivity of nerve endings to noxious stimuli, nor does it impair the conduction of nerve impulses along the peripheral nerves, an impairment that is seen following the administration of local anesthetics [1].

Morphine exerts its analgesic effects by elevating the pain threshold and especially by altering the patient's reactions to pain. Patients often report that the sensation of pain is often present, but under the influence of morphine they feel more at ease and comfortable. This euphoric "sense of well-being, rapture, exaltation" is present in 90 to 95 percent of the patients. In the remaining 5 to 10 percent of patients, morphine may cause dysphoria [6, 8, 9].

Therapeutic Uses. In relatively small doses of 5 to 10 mg, morphine relieves the constant but dull pain originating from the viscera, such as that of coronary, pulmonary, or biliary origin. In somewhat larger doses (10–20 mg), morphine relieves sharp, lancinating, and intermittent pain resulting from fracture of bones and other physically injurious traumas. Inop-

Fig. 10-1. *Structures of narcotic analgesics and their antagonists.*

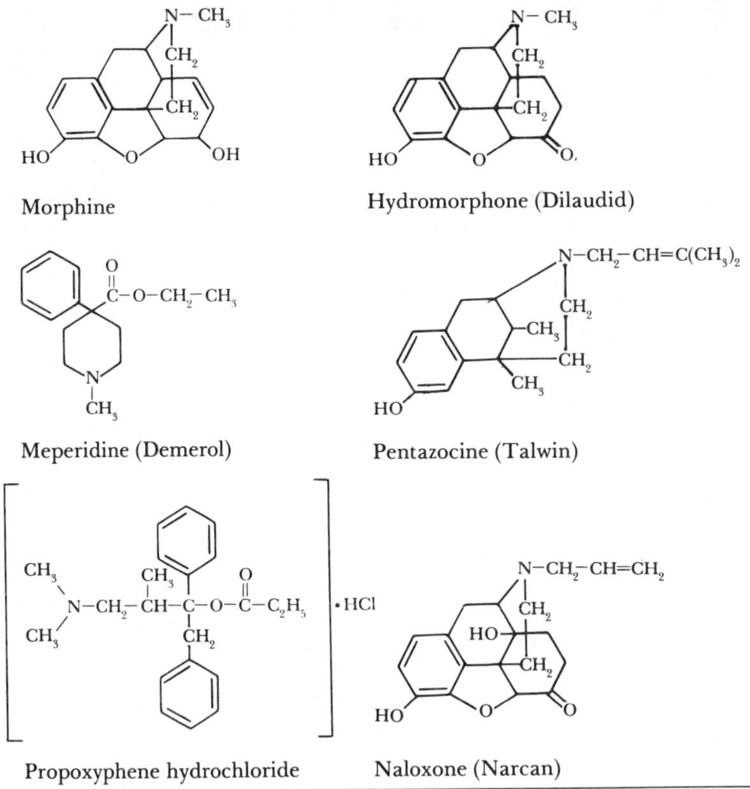

Morphine

Hydromorphone (Dilaudid)

Meperidine (Demerol)

Pentazocine (Talwin)

Propoxyphene hydrochloride

Naloxone (Narcan)

erable and terminal cases of neoplastic diseases usually require morphine or other narcotics in ever increasing doses, which will undoubtedly cause both tolerance and addiction [6].

Depression of Respiration. Morphine depresses all phases of respiration (respiratory rate, tidal volume, and minute volume) at subhypnotic and subanalgesic doses. In humans, overdosage of morphine causes respiratory arrest and death. Morphine and other narcotic analgesics should be used with extreme caution in asthma, emphysema, cor pulmonale, and where hypoxia may be present, as in chest wound, pneumothorax, or bulbar poliomyelitis [6, 8].

Effects on Cardiovascular System. Morphine releases histamine and may cause peripheral vasodilatation and orthostatic hypotension. The cutaneous blood vessels dilate around the "blush areas"—face, neck, and upper thorax. Morphine causes cerebral vasodilation (due to increased CO_2 retention secondary to respiratory depression), and hence it increases the spinal fluid pressure. Therefore, morphine should be used cautiously in meningitis and in recent head injury. When given subcutaneously, morphine will be absorbed poorly in either traumatic or hemorrhagic shock [6, 8].

Effects on Gastrointestinal System. Morphine reduces the activity of the entire gastrointestinal tract. It reduces the secretion of HCl, diminishes the motility of the stomach, and increases the tone of the up-

per part of the duodenum. These actions may delay the passage of the contents of the stomach into the duodenum. Both pancreatic and biliary secretions are also diminished. As a result, digestion may be hindered. In the large intestine, the propulsive peristaltic wave in the colon is reduced, the muscular tone, including that of the anal sphincter, is increased, and the activity of gastrocolic reflex (defecation reflex) is reduced. These actions, in combination, cause constipation, which seems to be a chronic problem among the addicts [6, 8].

Antidiarrheal Effects. Opiate preparations, usually given as paregoric, are effective and fast-acting antidiarrheal agents. They are also useful postoperatively to produce solid stool following ileostomy or colostomy. A meperidine derivative called diphenoxylate is usually dispensed with atropine and sold as Lomotil. Atropine is added to discourage the abuse of diphenoxylate by a narcotic addict who is tolerant to massive doses of narcotic but not to the CNS stimulant effects of atropine.

Oliguric Effect. Morphine causes oliguria resulting from (1) pronounced diaphoresis, (2) relative hypotension and decreased glomerular filtration rate, and (3) release of antidiuretic hormone from the neurohypophysis. In an elderly patient with prostatic hypertrophy, morphine may cause acute urinary retention. Morphine may reduce the effectiveness of a diuretic when both drugs are used in combination in congestive heart failure [6].

Morphine-Induced Tolerance. Tolerance is developed to the narcotic and analgesic actions of morphine so that increasingly larger doses are needed to render the patients pain free. Tolerance is acquired to many effects of morphine such as analgesia, euphoria, narcosis, respiratory depression, hypotension, and antidiuresis. Morphine-induced bradycardia is sometimes experienced. No tolerance develops to morphine-induced miosis or constipation. When the administration of morphine is discontinued, the tolerance is lost and the preaddiction analgesic doses of morphine will be once more effective [6].

Abstinence Syndrome. In subjects addicted to morphine, the initial symptoms of abstinence syndrome or withdrawal syndrome usually appear 6 to 12 hours after the last dose:

CNS irritability and feeling of fatigue
Autonomic hyperactivity such as tachycardia and hypertension
Gastrointestinal hyperactivity such as diarrhea
Autonomic supersensitivity such as insomnia and restlessness

CODEINE (ANALGESIC AND ANTITUSSIVE).
Codeine is methylmorphine and pharmacologically resembles morphine with the following exceptions:

The analgesic potency of codeine is approximately one-sixth that of morphine. Codeine raises the pain threshold without altering the patient's reaction to pain. Codeine produces very little euphoria. Therefore, 10 mg of morphine is far superior in alleviating pain to 60 mg of codeine.

Unlike morphine, codeine is effective orally. Side effects are exactly the same as described for morphine but are milder and far less frequent in incidence. Codeine produces miosis, respiratory depression, urinary retention, and constipation, but these are not of clinical and toxicologic significance.

Tolerance to codeine develops very slowly, and the addiction liability is far less than seen with morphine.

THE SEMISYNTHETIC ANALGESICS.
The semisynthetics are compared with morphine and codeine in Table 10-1.

THE SYNTHETIC ANALGESICS (TABLE 10-2).
Meperidine. The pharmacology of meperidine (Fig. 10-1) resembles that of morphine with the following exceptions: The antitussive and antidiarrheal effects of meperidine are minimum. Meperidine does not produce miosis and may even cause mydriasis. The duration of action of meperidine is extremely short; hence it is used as an analgesic during diagnostic procedures such as cystoscopy, gastroscopy, pneumoencephalography, and retrograde pyelography. It is also used as preanesthetic medication and as obstetric analgesic. Since meperidine has atropinelike action, toxic doses of meperidine produce a mixed picture

Table 10-1. *Comparative Pharmacologic Properties of Semisynthetic Derivatives of Opiates*

Agents	Properties
Dihydrocodeinone (Hycodan)	More potent than codeine
Dihydromorphinone (Dilaudid)	More potent than morphine
Methyldihydromorphinone (metopon)	Similar to morphine

Table 10-2. *Comparative Pharmacology of Synthetic Analgesics*

Agents	Properties
Alphaprodine (Nisentil)	More potent than meperidine
Anileridine (Leritine)	Resembles meperidine; shorter duration
Piminodine (Alvodine)	More potent than meperidine
Diphenoxylate (Lomotil)	Used in diarrhea
Fentanyl (Sublimaze)	Used in anesthesia; extremely potent; 500 times more potent than meperidine

of morphine and atropine poisoning. In a narcotic addict who has developed tolerance to depressant effects of morphine, meperidine poisoning resembles that of atropine, characterized by mydriasis, tachycardia, dry mouth, excitement, and convulsions. The atropinelike effects of meperidine are not reversed by naloxone, a narcotic antagonist [6, 8].

Methadone. Pharmacologically, methadone is very similar to morphine with the following exceptions: Methadone is effective orally. The onset of action and the duration of action of methadone are longer than those of morphine. Tolerance to methadone is acquired very slowly. On abrupt withdrawal of methadone, the abstinence syndrome develops more slowly, is less intense, and is more prolonged than the abstinence syndrome of morphine. The abuse potential of methadone is lower than is that of morphine [6, 8].

INDICATIONS FOR METHADONE. Like morphine, methadone is used in the management of pain. In addition, methadone is used in the detoxification from and treatment of narcotic addiction [7].

Dextropropoxyphene. Propoxyphene is structurally very similar to methadone. There are two stereoisomers of propoxyphene. Dextropropoxyphene is an analgesic with a potency two-thirds that of codeine. Levopropoxyphene is antitussive but lacks analgesic properties.

Adverse reactions include nausea, vomiting, sedation, dizziness, constipation, and skin rash with a frequency of incidence somewhat less than that of codeine. Although respiratory depression is a cardinal sign of acute dextropropoxyphene poisoning, the drug apparently does not affect respiration in the usual therapeutic doses of 32 to 65 mg.

Pentazocine (Talwin). The analgesia produced by pentazocine (30 mg), a mixed narcotic agonist and a weak antagonist, is comparable to that developed by morphine (10 mg). The onset and duration of action are shorter than morphine's. Pentazocine will antagonize some of the respiratory depression and analgesia of morphine and meperidine. However, the analgesic action and respiratory depression produced by pentazocine can be reversed by a narcotic antagonist. Pentazocine causes tolerance and addiction, but their emergence is very slow compared to that induced by morphine [6].

NARCOTIC ANTAGONISTS. Naloxone. Naloxone (Narcan) reverses the respiratory-depressant action of the narcotics related to morphine, meperidine, and methadone. It differs from the other narcotic antagonist in several respects. Naloxone does not cause respiratory depression, pupillary constriction, sedation, or analgesia. However, it antagonizes the actions of pentazocine. Naloxone neither antagonizes the respiratory-depressant effects of barbiturates and other hypnotics nor aggravates them. Like nalorphine, naloxone precipitates an abstinence syndrome when administered to patients addicted to opiatelike drugs [6].

ANTITUSSIVE PREPARATION. Dextromethorphan (Romilar). Dextromethorphan is the dextroisomer of the methyl ether of levorphanol. Unlike its levorotatory congener, it possesses no significant analgesic property, exhibits no depressant effects on respiration, and lacks addiction liability.

Dextromethorphan is an antitussive agent with a potency approximately one-half that of codeine.

Therapeutic doses of dextromethorphan (15–30 mg) produce little or no side effects whereas excessively high doses (300–1,500 mg) were reported to produce a state resembling intoxication accompanied by euphoria.

EMETIC AGENTS. Ipecac is a mixture of alcohol-soluble alkaloids and is obtained from the South American plant *Cephaëlis ipecacuanha*. It is solely used as syrup of ipecac. Apomorphine hydrochloride and copper sulfate are also emetics.

Syrup of ipecac and copper sulfate cause emesis by local irritation of the stomach whereas apomorphine stimulates the chemoreceptor trigger zone for emesis located in the caudal portion of the fourth ventricle (area postrema), which in turn stimulates the vomiting center in the lateral reticular formation of the medulla.

NEUROBIOLOGY OF ENDOGENOUS OPIATE PEPTIDES. For many years pharmacologists considered the possibility that opioids mimicked a naturally ongoing process. Investigations revealed opiatelike peptides from brain consisting of two similar pentapeptides with the following sequences:

Tyr-Gly-Gly-Phe-Met (met-enkephalin)
Tyr-Gly-Gly-Phe-Leu (leu-enkephalin)

Both met-enkephalin and leu-enkephalin behave as agonists and inhibit opiate receptor binding with affinities comparable to the affinity of morphine. The effects of met-enkephalin and leu-enkephalin are reversed by naloxone.

Met-enkephalin depresses all neurons depressed by morphine and many neurons excited by morphine. The mechanism of enkephalin-mediated inhibition may be indirect. It may block the release of excitatory neurotransmitters such as acetylcholine and glutamate.

THE EVIDENCE FOR MULTIPLE OPIATE RECEPTORS. The opiates produce a large variety of pharmacologic responses by interacting with multiple opiate receptors. The indirect evidence for the presence of these multiple receptors is as follows:

Nalorphine produces many of the pharmacologic effects of morphine, yet it blocks or reverses morphine's action.
Naloxone, which does not produce any of the pharmacologic effects of morphine, blocks or reverses morphine's action.
Subjects tolerant to psychomimetic effects of morphine are not cross tolerant to the psychomimetic effects of cyclazocine.
Abstinence syndrome caused by morphine is qualitatively different from abstinence syndrome caused by cyclazocine.
Agonist-antagonist nalorphine and cyclazocine can induce tolerance to their agonistic effects but not to their antagonistic effects.

CLASSIFICATION OF OPIATE RECEPTORS. Opiate receptor sites have been tentatively classified as

Morphinelike (mu receptor)
Enkephalinlike (delta receptor)
Nalorphinelike (kappa receptor)
N-Allylnormetazocinelike (sigma receptor)
Beta-endorphinlike (epsilon receptor)

The validity of occurrence of these opiate receptors needs to be confirmed, and their clinical significance and potential therapeutic usefulness needs to be established [2, 4, 5, 10].

QUESTIONS ON NARCOTIC ANALGESICS

Select one answer that best completes the statement or answers the question.

106. Naloxone has the following pharmacologic properties *except* which one?
   A. It antagonizes morphine-induced narcosis.
   B. It causes respiratory depression.
   C. It precipitates abstinence syndrome in a morphine-addicted person.
   D. It has short duration of action.

107. Which one of the following compounds is a pure narcotic antagonist?
   A. Nalorphine.
   B. Pentazocine.
   C. Naloxone.
   D. Phenazocine.

108. Which one of the following statements is not true about dextromethorphan?
   A. It is an antitussive agent.
   B. It has antitussive potency unequal to that of codeine.
   C. It is analgesic.
   D. It does not depress the respiration.

109. The pharmacology of pentazocine (Talwin) is characterized by the following *except* which one?
   A. It is structurally related to phenazocine.
   B. It is a mixed agonist-antagonist.
   C. It is effective when given orally.
   D. It should be administered with morphine for maximum effect.

110. Morphine can be used for the following therapeutic purposes *except* which one?
   A. To relieve pain of myocardial infarction.
   B. To provide sedation and analgesia as part of "balanced" anesthesia.
   C. To relieve postoperative pain of abdominal surgery.
   D. To relieve pain caused by a severe head injury.
   E. To relieve acute pulmonary edema caused by left side heart failure.

111. An abstinence syndrome may be relieved:
   A. By any narcotic analgesic.
   B. By any long-acting sedative.
   C. By any narcotic antagonist.
   D. With the drug to which the person is addicted.
   E. Only with methadone.

112. Morphine poisoning may be characterized by the following symptoms *except* which one?
   A. Dysphoria.
   B. Respiratory depression.
   C. Hypertension.
   D. Urinary retention.

ANSWERS AND EXPLANATIONS ON NARCOTIC ANALGESICS

106. B.
107. C.
108. C.
109. D.
   Explanation: Mixed narcotic agonist-antagonist such as pentazocine should not be administered with a pure agonist such as morphine since it may block the analgesic effects of morphine.
110.. D.
   Explanation: Morphine retains CO_2 and by causing vasodilation raises the cerebrospinal fluid pressure. Therefore, morphine should not be used in conditions such as meningitis or recent head injury where the cerebrospinal pressure may already be elevated.
111. A.
   Explanation: Narcotic analgesics show cross sensitivity. A morphine-addicted person may receive methadone.
112. C.

REFERENCES

1. Beers, R. F., and Bassett, E. G. *Mechanisms of Pain and Analgesic Compounds.* New York: Raven, 1979.
2. Bloom, F. E. The endorphins: A growing family of pharmacologically pertinent peptides. *Annu. Rev. Pharmacol. Toxicol.* 23:151, 1983.
3. Bonica, J. J., Lindblom, U., and Iggo, A. *Advances in Pain Research and Therapy*, Vol. 5. New York: Raven, 1983.
4. Cox, B. M. Endogenous opiate peptides. A guide to structures and terminology. *Life Sci.* 31:1645, 1982.
5. Frederickson, R. C. A., and Geary, L. E. Endogenous opioid peptides: Review of physiological, pharmacological and clinical aspects. *Prog. Neurobiol.* 19:19, 1982.
6. Jaffe, J. H., and Martin, W. R. Opioid Analgesics and Antagonists. In A. G. Gilman, L. S. Goodman, and A. Gilman (eds.), *The Pharmacological Basis of Therapeutics* (6th ed.). New York: Macmillan, 1980. Pp. 494–534.
7. Kissin, B., Lowenson, J. H., and Milman, R. B. Recent developments in chemotherapy of narcotic addiction. *Ann. N.Y. Acad. Sci.* 311:81, 1978.
8. Murphree, H. B. Narcotic Analgesics. In J. R. DiPalma (ed.), *Drill's Pharmacology in Medicine* (4th ed.). New York: McGraw-Hill, 1971. Pp. 324–349.
9. Sternbach, R. A. *The Psychology of Pain.* New York: Raven, 1978.
10. Udenfriend, S., and Kilpatrick, D. L. Biochemistry of the enkephalins and enkephalin-containing peptides. *Arch. Biochem. Biophys.* 221:309, 1983.

11. Nonnarcotic Analgesics and Therapeutics for Gout and Arthritis

Words of comfort, skillfully administered, are the oldest therapy known.

Louis Nizer

Salicylates and allied compounds have analgesic, antipyretic, uricosuric, and antiinflammatory properties. They are classified into the following categories:

Salicylate derivative
    Acetylsalicylic acid (aspirin)
Pyrazolone derivatives
    Phenylbutazone (Butazolidin)
    Oxyphenbutazone (Oxalid, Tandearil)
    Sulfinpyrazone (Anturane)
Para-aminophenol derivatives
    Acetaminophen (Tylenol, Datril)
    Phenacetin
Propionic acid derivatives
    Ibuprofen (Motrin)
    Naproxen (Naprosyn)
    Fenoprofen (Nalfon)
    Flurbiprofen (Ansaid)
Others
    Indomethacin (Indocin)
    Sulindac (Clinoril)
    Mefenamic acid (Ponstel)
    Tolmetin (Tolectin)

The pharmacology of acetylsalicylic acid (aspirin) will be discussed in detail as a prototype drug, and all other drugs will be compared to it [1, 3, 5].

SALICYLATE DERIVATIVES. Para-aminosalicylic acid has bacteriostatic activity against *Mycobacterium tuberculosis*. Methyl salicylate (oil of wintergreen) has been used in the past as a "counterirritant." Salicylic acid (20% solution) has keratolytic properties and is used to remove hornified epidermis (corn). Since salicylic acid itself is too toxic for systemic uses, the various salts of salicylate including acetylsalicylic acid (aspirin) are used.

Aspirin-Induced Analgesia. Unlike narcotic analgesics such as morphine, aspirin does not depress respiration, is a relatively nontoxic drug, and is without addiction liability. Aspirin is a weak or mild analgesic that is effective in short, intermittent types of pain as encountered in neuralgia, myalgia, toothache, and the like. It does not have the efficacy of morphine and fails to relieve the severe, prolonged, and lancinating pain associated with trauma such as burn or fractures. Like morphine, it produces analgesia by raising pain threshold in the thalamus, but unlike morphine, it does not alter the patient's reactions to pain. Since aspirin does not cause hypnosis or euphoria, its sites of action have been postulated to be subcortical [4]. In addition to raising pain threshold, the antiinflammatory effects of aspirin may contribute to its analgesic effects. However, no direct association between antiinflammatory and analgesic effects of aspirin compounds should be expected. For example, aspirin has both analgesic and antiinflammatory properties whereas acetaminophen is analgesic without having antiinflammatory capability. Furthermore, potent antiinflammatory agents such as phenylbutazone have only weak analgesic effects [3].

Aspirin-Induced Antipyresis. Aspirin does not alter normal body temperature, which is maintained by a balance between heat production and heat dissipation. In fever associated with an infection, increased oxidative processes enhance heat production. Aspirin causes cutaneous vasodilation, prompts perspiration, and enhances heat dissipation. This effect is mediated via hypothalamic nuclei since lesion in the preoptic area suppresses the mechanism through which aspirin exerts its antipyretic actions. The antipyretic effects of aspirin may be due to inhibition of the synthesis of hypothalamic prostaglandin. Although aspirin-induced diaphoresis contributes to antipyretic effects, it is not absolutely necessary because antipyresis takes place in the presence of atropine [6].

Uricosuric Effects of Aspirin. Small doses (600 mg) of aspirin cause hyperuricemia whereas large doses (> 5 gm) have uricosuric effect. Aspirin inhibits uric acid resorption by the tubules in the kidneys. Because of more effective uricosuric agents, aspirin is no longer used for this purpose.

Antiinflammatory Effects of Aspirin. Aspirin has antiinflammatory action, possesses antirheumatic and antiarthritic properties, and may be used in the treatment of rheumatic fever. The cardiac lesion and other visceral effects are not altered by aspirin. Aspirin is extremely effective in rheumatoid arthritis and allied diseases involving joints, such as ankylosing spondylitis and osteoarthritis. It is thought that aspirin and indomethacin exert their antiinflammatory effects by inhibiting prostaglandin synthesis, through inhibition of cyclooxygenase. The presynthesized prostaglandins are released in tissue injury, fostering inflammation and pain. Furthermore, aspirin reduces the formation of prostaglandin in the platelets and leukocytes, causing the reported hematologic effects associated with aspirin.

Effects of Salicylate on Respiration. Aspirin stimulates respiration directly and indirectly. In analgesic doses, aspirin increases oxygen (O_2) consumption and carbon dioxide (CO_2) production. However, since increased alveolar ventilation balances the higher CO_2 production, plasma PCO_2 does not change. In salicylate intoxication (e.g., 10–12 gm of aspirin given every 6–8 hours, and even smaller dosage in children, whose brains are far more sensitive to salicylate intoxication than are those of adults), salicylate stimulates the medullary centers directly, causing hyperventilation characterized by an increase in depth and rate of respiration. The PCO_2 level declines, causing hypocapnia, and the blood pH increases, causing respiratory alkalosis. The low PCO_2 decreases renal tubular resorption of bicarbonate and compensates for the alkalosis.

If the salicylate level continues to rise, the respiratory centers become depressed, the PCO_2 level becomes elevated, and the pH of blood becomes more acidic, causing respiratory acidosis. Dehydration, reduced bicarbonate, and the accumulation of salicylic acid, salicyluric acid (resulting from metabolism of aspirin), lactic acid, and pyruvic acid (resulting from derangement in carbohydrate metabolism) may cause metabolic acidosis.

Treatment of Poisoning. The supportive treatment may include gastric lavage (to prevent further absorption of salicylate), fluid replenishment (to combat dehydration and oliguria), alcohol-water sponge (to combat hyperthermia), vitamin K (to combat possible hemorrhage), sodium bicarbonate (to combat acidosis), and in extreme cases peritoneal dialysis and exchange transfusion.

Gastrointestinal Effect of Aspirin. Although innocuous in most subjects, therapeutic analgesic doses of aspirin may cause epigastric distress, nausea, vomiting, and bleeding. Aspirin will exacerbate the symptoms of peptic ulcer characterized by heartburn, dyspepsia, and erosive gastritis. An extensive number of salts have been synthesized from salicylate (e.g., calcium carbaspirin, choline salicylate, alloxiprin, and numerous buffered derivatives) with some degree of success in reducing the gastrointestinal toxicity of aspirin. However, other, unknown factors may contribute to this undesirable property of aspirin. In experimental animals, petechial hemorrhage of the gastric mucosa has been caused by intravenous administration of sodium salicylate or subcutaneous administration of methyl salicylate. Furthermore, it should be recalled that compounds possessing antiinflammatory properties (aspirin, phenylbutazone, oxyphen-butazone) cause higher incidence of gastrointestinal toxicity than compounds devoid of antiinflammatory properties (phenacetin and acetaminophen).

Hemopoietic Effect of Aspirin. Aspirin reduces the leukocytosis associated with acute rheumatic fever. Given on a chronic basis, it also reduces hemoglobin and hematocrit. Aspirin causes reversible hypoprothrombinemia by interfering with the function of vitamin K in prothrombin synthesis. Therefore, aspirin should be used with caution in vitamin K deficiency, in preexisting hypoprothrombinemia, in hepatic damage, in patients taking anticoagulants, and in patients scheduled for surgery. Aspirin causes hemolytic anemia in individuals with glucose 6-phosphate dehydrogenase deficiency. Aspirin tolerance test is used diagnostically in von Willebrand's disease (it further prolongs bleeding time). Aspirin prevents platelet aggregation and may be helpful in thromboembolic disease. In addition to aspirin, indomethacin, phenylbutazone, sulfinpyrazone, and dipyridamole prevent platelet aggregation whereas epinephrine, serotonin, and prostaglandins promote platelet aggregation and hence are procoagulants. The therapy with aspirin gives a false-negative for the erythrocyte sedimentation rate that is often elevated in infections and inflammations.

NONSALICYLATE ANALGESICS. The pharmacology of pyrazolone derivatives, para-aminophenol derivatives, propionic acid derivatives, and the remaining compounds is compared with that of aspirin in Table 11-1.

In addition to pharmacologic properties described for these drugs in Table 11-1, other items of interest about each drug will be cited.

Phenylbutazone. The antiinflammatory effect of phenylbutazone is greater than that of aspirin but less than that of steroidal antiinflammatory agents. Phenylbutazone causes sodium and chloride retention, and edema may result. In addition, fatal aplastic anemia and agranulocytosis have occurred following the use of phenylbutazone. Activation of and perforation of hemorrhagic ulcer takes place. Hypersensitivity reactions are common. Consequently, phenylbutazone should be used only in inflammatory conditions (rheumatoid arthritis, ankylosing spondylitis, or osteoarthritis) where the safer antiinflammatory agents are no longer effective.

Phenacetin. Phenacetin and its deethylated metabolite, acetaminophen, are superior to aspirin in that they do not cause hypoprothrombinemia, gastrointestinal irritation, or disturbances of acid-base balance. The serious, but rare, side effects of phenacetin are methemoglobinemia and hemolytic anemia. The serious, but rare, side effects of acetaminophen are fatal hepatic necrosis and hypoglycemic coma. Interstitial nephritis and renal papillary necrosis are caused by both phenacetin and acetaminophen. The less toxic acetaminophen should be used only in pa-

Table 11-1. *Pharmacologic Efficacy of Various Compounds Possessing Analgesic, Antipyretic, Uricosuric, and Antiinflammatory Actions*

Specific Group	Specific Drug	Analgesic	Antipyretic	Antiinflammatory	Uricosuric
Salicylate derivatives	Acetylsalicylic acid (aspirin)	*	*	*	*
Pyrazolone derivatives	Phenylbutazone	*	*	*	*
	Oxyphenbutazone	*	*	*	*
	Sulfinpyrazone	0	0	0	*
Para-aminophenol derivative	Acetaminophen	*	*	0	0
Propionic acid derivatives	Ibuprofen	*	*	*	0
	Naproxen	*	*	*	0
	Fenoprofen	*	*	*	0
	Flurbiprofen	*	*	*	0
	Ketoprofen	*	*	*	0
Others	Indomethacin	*	*	*	0
	Sulindac	*	0	*	0
	Mefenamic acid	*	0	*	0
	Tolmetin	*	*	*	0

*indicates that it possesses the property assigned.
0 indicates that it lacks the property assigned.

tients who cannot tolerate aspirin or in whom aspirin is contraindicated.

Propionic Acid Derivatives. Propionic acid derivatives (ibuprofen, naproxen, fenoprofen, flurbiprofen, and ketoprofen) are all aspirinlike compounds that are allegedly better tolerated by patients in whom aspirin has caused troublesome side effects. These agents, but especially flurbiprofen, are potent inhibitors of cyclooxygenase involved in the synthesis of prostaglandins. Naturally, all hematologic side effects reported for aspirin, including inhibition of platelet aggregation, may occur with these compounds. These agents are advocated for symptomatic treatment of rheumatoid arthritis, juvenile rheumatoid arthritis, osteoarthritis, and ankylosing spondylitis.

Indomethacin. Indomethacin may cause high incidence of gastrointestinal toxicity and hematopoietic reactions such as neutropenia or thrombocytopenia. Therefore, it should not be used routinely and chronically as an analgesic and an antipyretic substance. However, in some cases (e.g., Hodgkin's disease), when fever does not respond to aspirin or chemotherapy, indomethacin is very effective. In addition, indomethacin and phenylbutazone are equally efficacious in the treatment of ankylosing spondylitis and gouty arthritis.

Sulindac. Sulindac is used mainly for the treatment of rheumatoid arthritis, osteoarthritis, and ankylosing spondylitis.

Mefenamic Acid and Tolmetin. Mefenamic acid is used mainly in rheumatology. Tolmetin is used solely in the treatment of juvenile arthritis and rheumatoid arthritis.

In the management of arthritic conditions, drugs are chosen on an empiric basis, the least toxic substance usually being selected and tried first. The following schedule may be used in drug selection:

First choice—nonsteroidal antiinflammatory agents
  Aspirin
  Ibuprofen, tolmetin, naproxen, fenoprofen, or sulindac
  Indomethacin or phenylbutazone
Second choice—disease-modifying agents
  Gold salts
  D-Penicillamine
  Hydroxychloroquine
Third choice
  Steroids
  Immunosuppressive agents

PHARMACOLOGIC MANAGEMENT OF GOUT.
Gout is a hyperuricemic state (> 6 mg/100 ml) that is effectively diagnosed by detecting the presence of monosodium urate crystal in synovial fluid of the involved joint. Conditions causing hyperuricemia are as follows:

Excessive synthesis of uric acid
Excessive synthesis of purine—precursor to uric acid
High dietary intake of purine (shellfish, organ meat, anchovies, wild game)
Diminished renal excretion of uric acid
Tissue destruction following injury or therapeutic irradiation

In addition, numerous agents when used in therapeutic doses cause hyperuricemia. These include analgesic dose of aspirin, thiazide diuretics, nicotinic acid, alcohol consumed on a chronic basis, and antineoplastic agents.

The untreated hyperuricemic state may precipitate an acute attack of gout (first appearing in a painful metatarsal phalangeal joint) and produce tophaceous deposits in joints and soft tissue such as kidneys. The hyperuricemic state may be corrected by (1) inhibiting the synthesis of uric acid by allopurinol or (2) enhancing the elimination of uric acid by uricosuric agents.

Allopurinol (Zyloprim). Allopurinol reduces the synthesis of uric acid by inhibiting the activity of xanthine oxidase according to the following scheme:

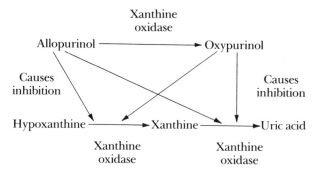

The reduction in uric acid pool occurs slowly. Since xanthine and hypoxanthine are more soluble than uric acid, they are easily excreted.

Allopurinol is used not only in hyperuricemia associated with gout but also in secondary hyperuricemia associated with the use of antineoplastic agents. It should be recalled that allopurinol may interfere with the metabolism of antineoplastic agents such as azathioprine and 6-mercaptopurine.

Uricosuric Agents. The most commonly used uricosuric agents are probenecid (Benemid) and sulfinpyrazone (Anturane). In low doses these agents block tubular secretion whereas at higher doses they also block the tubular resorption of uric acid. Since the solubility of uric acid is increased in alkaline urine, the administration of sodium bicarbonate may at times be advantageous. Furthermore, one should be cognizant of the fact that probenecid and sulfinpyrazone do also inhibit the excretion of agents such as aspirin, penicillin, ampicillin, and indomethacin. Although probenecid and sulfinpyrazone may be coadministered, neither compound should be given with aspirin, since their uricosuric effects will be nullified [2].

Treatment of Acute Attack of Gout. Colchicine (an alkaloid obtained from meadow saffron or autumn crocus) may be used both diagnostically to ascertain the presence of gout and prophylactically to prevent the further occurrence of gout. Usually, 0.5-mg oral doses of colchicine are given hourly until either the therapeutic effects are seen or the side effects develop. In addition to colchicine, phenylbutazone, indomethacin, ACTH, and steroidal antiinflammatory agents may be used to treat the acute attack of gout.

QUESTIONS ON NONNARCOTIC ANALGESICS AND THERAPEUTICS FOR GOUT AND ARTHRITIS

Select one answer that best completes the statement or answers the question.

___ 113. Which one of the following compounds causes hyperuricemia?
  A. Hydrochlorothiazide.
  B. Acetylsalicylic acid.
  C. Phenylbutazone.
  D. Oxyphenbutazone.

___ 114. Acetaminophen is characterized by which one of the following actions?
  A. It causes hypoprothrombinemia.
  B. It causes gastric irritation.
  C. It disturbs acid-base balance.
  D. It is devoid of uricosuric effect.

___ 115. The poisoning with aspirin includes the following symptoms *except* which one?
  A. Dehydration.
  B. Hypothermia.
  C. Oliguria.
  D. Metabolic acidosis.

___ 116. The hematologic effects or uses of aspirin include the following items *except* which one?
  A. It reduces leukocytosis in rheumatic fever.
  B. It reduces hemoglobin and hematocrit.
  C. It causes polycythemia vera in patients with glucose 6-phosphate deficiency.
  D. It is used diagnostically in von Willebrand's disease.

___ 117. All of the following agents prevent platelet aggregation *except* which one?
  A. Aspirin.
  B. Indomethacin.
  C. Dipyridamole.
  D. Epinephrine.

___ 118. Allopurinol inhibits the metabolism of which compound(s)?
  A. Azathioprine.
  B. 6-Mercaptopurine.
  C. Sulfinpyrazone.
  D. Both A and B.
  E. Both B and C.

___ 119. Agents inhibiting the synthesis of prostaglandin include:
  A. Aspirin.
  B. Indomethacin.
  C. Glucocorticoids.
  D. All of the above.
  E. A and B.

___ 120. Prostaglandins are involved in all the following actions of aspirin *except* which one?
  A. Patency of ductus arteriosus.
  B. Mediating inflammation.
  C. Homeostasis and thrombosis.
  D. Uricosuric effect.

ANSWERS AND EXPLANATIONS ON NONNARCOTIC ANALGESICS AND THERAPEUTICS FOR GOUT AND ARTHRITIS

113. A.
  Explanation: Thiazide diuretics cause hyperglycemia, hyperuricemia, and hypokalemia.
114. D.

115. B.
116. C.
117. D.
118. D.
119. E.
120. D.
Explanation: Prostaglandin (PGE_2) is responsible for keeping the ductus arteriosus patent in the newborn. Inhibitors of prostaglandin synthesis are used to close a persistent ductus in prematurely born infants.

REFERENCES

1. Barnett, H. J. M., Hirsch, J., and Mustard, J. F. *Acetylsalicylic Acid. New Uses for an Old Drug*. New York: Raven, 1982.

2. Flower, R. J., Moncada, S., and Vane, J. R. Analgesic-Antipyretics and Anti-Inflammatory Agents; Drugs Employed in the Treatment of Gout. In A. G. Gilman, L. S. Goodman, and A. Gilman (eds.), *The Pharmacological Basis of Therapeutics* (6th ed.). New York: Macmillan, 1980. Pp. 682–728.

3. Mandel, H. G., and Davison, C. Non-narcotic Analgesics and Antipyretics: Non Salicylates and Drugs Useful in Gout. In J. R. DiPalma (ed.), *Drill's Pharmacology in Medicine* (4th ed.). New York: McGraw-Hill, 1971. Pp. 404–426.

4. Sternbach, R. A. *The Psychology of Pain*. New York: Raven, 1978.

5. Tainter, M. L., and Ferris, A. J. *Aspirin in Modern Therapy*. New York: Sterling Drug, 1969.

6. Wolstenholme, G. E. W., and Birth, J. *Pyrogen and Fever*. London: Churchill Livingstone, 1971.

12. General, Spinal, and Local Anesthetics

> Arise, go forth and conquer.
> *Tennyson*

Part One: General Anesthetics

Anesthesia is a controllable and reversible depression of the central nervous system characterized by lack of perception of all sensations, analgesia, and amnesia. An ideal anesthetic is an inexpensive agent that has a fast rate of induction, has a rapid rate of emergence, is nonexplosive, is a good muscle relaxant, has analgesic properties, does not cause respiratory or myocardial depression, is nontoxic to liver and kidney, is inert metabolically, does not interact adversely with other pharmacologic agents used as preanesthetic and postanesthetic medications, and does not cause any postanesthetic complications. The search for this nonexistent ideal anesthetic agent continues.

PREANESTHETIC VISIT: ASSESSMENT OF PHYSICAL AND MENTAL STATUS OF THE PATIENT. A patient scheduled for surgery demonstrates discomfort and a high level of anxiety. The presurgery behavior may be characterized by thought of excessive and unrealistic danger of the anesthetics or the surgery and by repetitive and redundant inquiries about preanesthetic and postsurgical events. On the other hand, patients may show their anxiety by silence, avoidance of eye contact, lack of interest, or lack of communication. A visit by a caring physician or a nurse will be extremely useful and supportive. A reassured patient sleeps easier, requires less anesthetics, requires less analgesics, and shows less postanesthetic complications.

The choice of an anesthetic is always made by an anesthesiologist after consultation with the attending physician or the surgeon. It depends on many factors, including the patient's age, complicating and preexisting disease, the nature of the operation, the previous experience with anesthetics, and the nature of nonanesthetic medications to be taken by the patient.

Since general anesthetics do alter the cardiac and respiratory physiology, agents causing myocardial irritability, hypotension, circulatory depression, or tachyarrhythmias should be used with extreme caution. Furthermore, in preexisting cardiovascular problems, agents causing respiratory depression should be used with caution in bronchitis, in bronchospastic states, in emphysema, in patients with muscular dystrophy, and in myasthenia gravis. The use of skeletal muscle relaxants should be monitored in conditions of respiratory insufficiency such as ky-

phoscoliosis [7]. The opioids, which further depress respiration, should be employed with extreme care.

The preexisting endocrine disorders such as hypothyroidism, hyperthyroidism, or diabetes mellitus should dictate the choice of the general anesthetics. In hyperthyroidism, agents causing cardiac acceleration (atropine or sympathomimetic amines) should be used carefully.

Since the release of insulin is reduced by sympathomimetic amines and increased by their appropriate blockers, severe hyperglycemia or hypoglycemia may be caused in susceptible patients who have been given inappropriate anesthetics. Patients required to take medications on a chronic basis should be evaluated carefully, and the choice of anesthetics should be made judiciously.

Antihypertensive medications, diuretics causing hypokalemia that may predispose to cardiac irritability, and anticoagulants may have to be discontinued or have their regimens modified.

These cautionary notes, which might be extensively expanded on, should be taken into consideration in choosing an anesthetic for one's patient [1–4, 6].

PREANESTHETIC MEDICATIONS. The preanesthetic medications are given for the following reasons:

To sedate and reduce anxiety (secobarbital, diazepam)
To relieve pain, if present (opiates)
To reduce excess salivation (anticholinergics, such as atropine)
To prevent bradycardia during surgery (atropine)
To facilitate intubation (succinylcholine)

CLASSIFICATION OF GENERAL ANESTHETICS. Inhalation anesthetics are

Gases—nitrous oxide, cyclopropane (rarely used)
Volatile liquids—ether (rarely used), halothane, enflurane, isoflurane

The intravenous anesthetics are thiopental and ketamine.

Certain agents are used with or without general anesthetics in special circumstances:

Morphine in open heart surgery. Morphine in a dose of 0.5 to 3.0 mg per kilogram given intravenously over a 15- to 20-minute period produces unconsciousness. Morphine is supplemented with nitrous oxide and a muscle relaxant.

Dantrolene in malignant hyperthermia. In anesthetic-induced malignant hyperthermia, the offending anesthetics should be discontinued and dantrolene administered with an initial dose of 1 mg per kilogram [7].

Thiopental in carotid endarterectomy. In patients in whom carotid endarterectomy is contemplated, the maintenance of oxygen and nutrients to the brain during the temporary period of surgical occlusion of the common, internal, and external carotid arteries is essential. Thiopental, given as a bolus of 4 to 5 mg per kilogram or as an intravenous infusion of 10 mg per kilogram over a 20- to 30-minute period, protects the brain against ischemia. The general anesthetic may be 0.3 to 0.6 percent halothane in 50 to 60% nitrous oxide in oxygen.

MODE OF ACTION OF GENERAL ANESTHETICS.

The actions of general anesthetics do not depend on any specific structures, which vary vastly from compound to compound. Furthermore, no specific receptor site has been isolated for any of these drugs. In addition, although they alter the functions of various neurotransmitters, no specific transmitter is involved in the etiology of all anesthetic-induced depression of the CNS. Nevertheless, general anesthetics have the following common properties:

They decrease the activity of neurons by increasing their threshold to fire.
By interfering with sodium influx, they prevent the action potential from rising to a normal rate.

The various stages of anesthesia seem to be sponsored by a dose-dependent alteration of the physiology of different populations of neurons in the central nervous system. Furthermore, the various anesthetics do indeed show specificity in this respect.

Stage I (stage of analgesia) is due to a decrease in the activity of the dorsal horn of the spinal cord, interfering with the sensory transmission in the spinothalamic tract.

Stage II (stage of excitement or delirium) represents the anesthetic-mediated "disinhibition" and is due to blockade of inhibitory neurons (Golgi type II cells) and unleashing from control the actions of excitatory neurotransmitters.

Stage III (muscle relaxation and surgical stage) represents the attainment of a high concentration of anesthetic in the brain and depicts depression of the reticular activating system and suppression of spinal reflexes.

Stage IV (death) is due to depression of medullary neurons in the respiratory and vasomotor centers.

The general anesthetics depress the respiratory center only in higher than therapeutic doses whereas morphine depresses the respiratory center at a dose that does not cause narcosis.

MOLECULAR MECHANISM OF ANESTHESIA.

The mechanism of anesthesia is not known. The anesthetic-induced perturbation of membrane functions is so diversified that it militates against providing a unified mechanism encompassing all of the agents [5].

FACTORS AFFECTING THE DEPTH OF INHALATION ANESTHETICS.

The administration of anesthetics is arbitrarily divided into the following phases:

Induction—the time from the onset of administration of an anesthetic to a stage at which surgery becomes suitable
Maintenance—the duration of time a patient is kept in surgical anesthesia
Emergence—the time from discontinuation of an anesthetic agent until consciousness is regained by the patient

FACTORS INFLUENCING THE PHARMACOKINETICS OR PHARMACODYNAMICS OF ANESTHETICS. Concentration of Anesthetics.

The stage of anesthesia is directly related to and dependent on the concentration of an anesthetic in the brain; the higher the concentration, the deeper the stage of anesthesia. The stages, which are not always present with all anesthetics, are depicted in Table 12-1.

Stage I—analgesia
Stage II—excitement
Stage III—surgical stage, which is divided into four planes; plane 3 is the state of surgical anesthesia
Stage IV—respiratory paralysis

Premedication with opiate (causing miosis) or with anticholinergics (causing mydriasis) may make the pupillary signs unreliable. If both morphine and atropine have been administered, the miotic effect of morphine dominates. Reaction to light and pupillary signs are less reliable in patients aged 50 or over. The reaction to light is absent with halothane and enflu-

Table 12-1. *Stage of Anesthesia*

Stage	Pupil	Respiratory Rate	Pulse Rate	Blood Pressure
I. Induction	Constricted	Rapid	Irregular	Normal
II. Excitement	Constricted	Rapid	Irregular	High
III. Operative	Slightly dilated	Shallow and slow	Steady and shallow	Normal
IV. Danger	Extremely dilated	Very slow	Weak and thready	Very low

rane. The swallowing, retching, and vomiting reflexes decrease with the administration of anesthetics and return upon recovery.

FACTORS CONTROLLING THE CONCENTRATION OF ANESTHETICS. The concentration of anesthetic in the brain depends on the following:

Solubility of the anesthetic
Concentration of anesthetic in the inspired air
Rate of pulmonary ventilation
Rate of pulmonary blood flow
Concentration gradient of the anesthetic between arterial and mixed venous blood

The blood-gas partition coefficient is an index of the solubility of an anesthetic as depicted by the following examples:

Anesthetic Agents	Blood-Gas	Induction Time
Nitrous oxide	0.47	2–3 minutes
Isoflurane	1.4	5–10 minutes
Enflurane	1.9	5–10 minutes
Halothane	2.36	10 minutes

Similarly, the amount of an anesthetic needed to cause anesthesia is dependent on the relative lipid-solubility (oil-gas) of the compound as indicated by the following examples:

Anesthetic Agents	Oil-Gas	Minimal Anesthetic Concentration (vol %)
Nitrous oxide	1.4	101.00
Enflurane	98.0	1.68
Isoflurane	99.0	1.40
Halothane	224.0	0.76

Furthermore, the more lipid soluble an anesthetic, the lower the anesthetic tension needed to produce anesthesia. At equilibrium, the concentrations of an anesthetic in the brain and fat cells would be high and in the blood would be low. Finally, the potency of an anesthetic is inversely related to minimal anesthetic concentration (MAC), as exemplified in Table 12-2.

In addition to the physicochemical properties described, anesthetics have nonuniform actions on other physiologic parameters, summarized in Table 12-3.

Enflurane (Ethrane). The pharmacology of enflurane is similar to that of halothane. However, enflurane has a more rapid induction and emergence than halothane. It also possesses better analgesic and muscle relaxant properties. Enflurane causes less depression of cardiovascular and respiratory systems. In higher than anesthetic doses, it may cause CNS excitation.

Isoflurane (Forane). The physical properties of isoflurane are identical with those of enflurane. Although it causes greater respiratory depression than halothane, the functions of the cardiovascular system are maintained.

Ketamine (Ketalar, Ketaject). Ketamine, which is used for short procedures, produces analgesia and amnesia but is a poor muscle relaxant. As a substance causing a state of "dissociative anesthesia," it may produce psychic disturbances and hallucination during emergence. Ketamine does not depress the cardiovascular and the respiratory systems.

Droperidol and Fentanyl. Droperidol and fentanyl may be used alone or rarely in combination. Droperidol is a compound with neuroleptic property that produces tranquility, reduced motor activity, and indifference. Fentanyl is a potent meperidinelike analgesic, and when combined with droperidol, it induces a state called neuroleptic analgesia. These drugs may be used together with a muscle relaxant in short diagnostic procedures. Marked respiratory depression occurs.

Table 12-2. *Relationship Among Water-Solubility, Lipid-Solubility, Potency of Anesthetics, and Required Minimal Anesthetic Concentrations (MAC)*

	MAC	Potency	Oil-Gas		Blood-Gas
Methoxyflurane		Highest	Highest	Cyclopropane	
Halothane		↑	↑	Nitrous oxide	
Ether		↑	↑	Halothane	
Cyclopropane		↓		Ether	
Nitrous oxide	Highest			Methoxyflurane	Highest

Cyclopropane and N_2O have similar blood-gas partition coefficients. However, N_2O is not nearly as potent as cyclopropane. Therefore, in comparison to cyclopropane, a higher tension of N_2O must be administered to attain identical stage of anesthesia, but the time required for induction of anesthesia for the two anesthetics will be identical.

Table 12-3. *Summary Pharmacology of Nitrous Oxide, Cyclopropane, Halothane, and Ether*

Nature and Effect	N₂O	Cyclopropane	Halothane	Ether
Volatile anesthetic	No	No	Yes	Yes
Rate of induction	Fast (2–3 minutes)	Fast (1–2 minutes)	Slow (10 minutes)	Slow (10–20 minutes)
Potentially explosive anesthetic	No	Yes	No	Yes
Respiration	NC	Depressed	Depressed	Stimulates indirectly, depresses directly
Myocardial depression	NC	Yes	Yes	Yes
Myocardial depression compensated by increased sympathetic activity	—	Yes	No	Yes
Sensitizes heart to catecholamines	No	Yes	Yes	No
Produces excessive salivation and respiratory secretions	No	No	No	Yes
Potentiates neuromuscular blocking agents	No	Yes	Yes	Yes
Nausea and vomiting during emergence	Low	Frequent	Low	Frequent
Liver damage	No	No	Low?	No
Kidney damage	No	No	No	No
Heat regulatory center	NC	Depressed	Depressed	Depressed
Release of epinephrine from the adrenal gland	No	Increased	Decreased	Increased
Analgesia	Good	Good	Poor	Good
Muscle relaxation	NC	Adequate	Minimal	Good

NC = no change. Nitrous oxide (N₂O) is a nonexplosive and nonflammable gas.

Part Two: Spinal Anesthesia

Anesthesia of the lower extremities and abdomen may be induced by introduction of anesthetic drugs into the subarachnoid space. The drugs most often used are procaine and tetracaine.

Advantages of spinal anesthesia are ease of administration, rapid onset of anesthesia, good muscular relaxation, and the fact that the patient may remain awake.

Disadvantages of spinal anesthesia are hypotension (ephedrine and methoxamine may prevent this), nausea and vomiting (avoided by thiopental), respiratory depression (treated by artificial respiration), and postoperative headache (treated by increasing cerebrospinal pressure).

Part Three: Local Infiltration Anesthesia

GENERAL PHARMACOLOGY OF LOCAL ANESTHESIA. When a local anesthetic is injected near a nerve, it blocks the flow of electrons along the axons, it blocks pain without loss of consciousness, and the effects are reversible.

STRUCTURES OF LOCAL ANESTHETICS AND SENSITIVITY TO THEM. All local anesthetics contain a lipophilic group, an amino derivative, and an intermediate chain according to the following general structure:

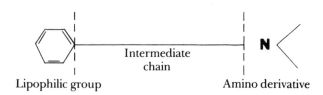

Lipophilic group   Intermediate chain   Amino derivative

The intermediate chain may be either an ester, as seen in compounds such as cocaine, procaine (Novocain), or tetracaine (Pontocaine); or an amide, as seen in compounds such as lidocaine (Xylocaine), mepivacaine (Carbocaine), bupivacaine (Marcaine), and dibucaine (Nupercaine). Cross sensitivity occurs among drugs in the same group (e.g., cocaine, procaine, and tetracaine) but not between compounds containing "ester" and "amide" linkages.

SUMMARY PHARMACOLOGY OF LOCAL ANESTHETICS.

Local anesthetics are unstable and insoluble in basic solution. If a local anesthetic lacks an amine, it will be insoluble in water and used only topically.

The larger the diameter of the nerve fiber, the more local anesthetic required to produce anesthesia.

Vascular Supply at Site of Injection. Epinephrine is used in combination with a local anesthetic to reduce its uptake, to prolong its duration of action, to produce a bloodless field of operation, and to protect against systemic effects. Local anesthetic solutions containing epinephrine should not be used in areas supplied by end arteries such as digits, ear, nose, and penis since ischemia and gangrene may occur. Furthermore, under no circumstance should anesthetic solutions containing epinephrine be used intravenously in patients with cardiac arrhythmias. In general, solutions designed for multiple doses should not be used for spinal or epidural anesthesia.

ADVERSE REACTIONS TO LOCAL ANESTHETICS. Allergic Reactions.

The ester-containing local anesthetics become metabolized to *p*-aminobenzoic acid derivatives with potential to cause hypersensitivity reactions. Allergic reactions to amide are extremely rare. In general, patients who have shown hypersensitivity reactions to ester compounds are treated with amide compounds. A patient who is sensitive to both ester and amide compounds is treated with certain antihistamines such as diphenhydramine, which also possesses local anesthetic properties.

Systemic Reactions. CARDIOVASCULAR EFFECTS. Local anesthetics block sodium channels, are cardiac depressants, and bring about ventricular conduction defect and block, which in toxic dosage may progress to cardiac and ventilatory arrest. In addition, they produce arteriolar dilatation. Circulatory failure may be treated with vasopressors such as ephedrine, metaraminol (Aramine), or mephentermine (Wyamine). Artificial respiration and cardiac massage may become necessary. Among local anesthetics, only cocaine blocks the uptake of norepinephrine, causes vasoconstriction, and may precipitate cardiac arrhythmias.

CNS EFFECTS. Overdosage of local anesthetics can produce dose-dependent CNS side effects such as insomnia, visual and auditory disturbances, nystagmus, shivering, tonic-clonic convulsions, and finally fatal CNS depression. The initial CNS excitation and convulsions may be treated by diazepam or thiopental.

QUESTIONS ON GENERAL, SPINAL, AND LOCAL ANESTHETICS

Select one answer that completes the statement or best answers the question.

_____ 121. In comparison to nitrous oxide, halothane (Fluothane):
   A. Exerts its anesthetic effects at lower concentration.
   B. Is less lipid soluble.
   C. Is less water soluble.
   D. Produces "dissociative anesthesia."

_____ 122. The rate of induction with halothane will be enhanced by:
   A. Giving it along with nitrous oxide.
   B. Decreasing the rate of respiration.
   C. Increasing the rate of blood flowing through the pulmonary artery.
   D. Decreasing the rate of blood flowing through the brain.

_____ 123. Local anesthetics:
   A. Block the release of neurotransmitter.
   B. Inhibit the efflux of Na from neurons.
   C. Block the influx of Na into the cell.
   D. Increase the release of inhibitory transmitter.

_____ 124. When a patient is allergic to tetracaine (Pontocaine), that patient will also be allergic to:
   A. Lidocaine (Xylocaine).
   B. Procaine (Novocain).
   C. Mepivacaine (Carbocaine).
   D. Bupivacaine (Marcaine).
   E. Dibucaine (Nupercaine).

_____ 125. In regard to the action of local anesthetic:
   A. Small nerve fibers are more susceptible than the large fibers.
   B. Myelinated fibers are more easily influenced than the nonmyelinated ones.
   C. Sensory but not motor fibers are blocked.
   D. All of the above.

_____ 126. Lidocaine:
   A. Is absorbed from gastrointestinal tract.
   B. Produces ventricular fibrillation in toxic doses.
   C. Causes sleepiness as a side effect.
   D. Is used intravenously as an antiarrhythmic agent.
   E. All of the above.

_____ 127. The mechanism of action of a general anesthetic probably includes which one of the following?
   A. It antagonizes specific neurotransmitter receptors in the brain.
   B. It blocks nerve transmission along the axon.
   C. It alters the fluidity of the nerve membrane.
   D. It stimulates Na^+K^+ ATPase.

_____ 128. All of the following statements are true about succinylcholine *except* which one?
   A. It is hydrolyzed by plasma cholinesterase.
   B. It is hydrolyzed to succinylmonocholine.
   C. It may be given intravenously.
   D. It has a long duration of action of 1 hour.

_____ 129. Which one of the following properties may be predicted about a very lipid-soluble anesthetic?
    A. It will be a potent anesthetic.
    B. It will not cause respiratory depression.
    C. It will have excellent analgesic activity.
    D. It will have excellent muscle relaxant property.

_____ 130. Halothane:
    A. Reduces arterial blood pressure.
    B. Reduces cardiac output.
    C. Alters the distribution of blood flow to various organs.
    D. All of the above.
    E. Only B and C.

ANSWERS AND EXPLANATION ON GENERAL, SPINAL, AND LOCAL ANESTHETICS

121. A.
122. A.
123. C.
124. B.
125. A.
    Explanation: The larger the diameter of the nerve fiber, the more local anesthetic is required. This is consistent with the order of nerve block: autonomic, pain, temperature, touch, and deep pressure. Recovery takes place in the reverse order, and autonomic neurons recover last.
126. E.
127. C.
128. D.
129. A.
130. D.

REFERENCES

1. Adriani, J. _The Chemistry and Physics of Anesthesia_ (2nd ed.). Springfield, Ill.: Thomas, 1970.
2. Benumof, J. L. _Clinical Frontiers in Anesthesiology._ New York: Grune & Stratton, 1983.
3. Brechner, V. L. _Pathological and Pharmacological Considerations in Anesthesiology._ Springfield, Ill.: Thomas, 1973.
4. Dripps, R. D., Eckenhoff, J. E., and Vandam, L. D. _Introduction to Anesthesia. The Principles of Safe Practice_ (5th ed.). Philadelphia: Saunders, 1977.
5. Fink, B. R. (ed.). _Molecular Mechanisms of Anesthesia._ Progress in Anesthesiology Vols. 1 and 2. New York: Raven, 1975, 1980.
6. Gray, T. C., and Nunn, J. F. (eds.). _General Anesthesia_, Vol. 1 (_Basic Sciences_) and Vol. 2 (_Clinical Practice_). New York: Appleton-Century-Crofts, 1971.
7. Hershey, S. G. _Refresher Courses in Anesthesiology,_ Vols. 4 and 6. Philadelphia: Lippincott, 1976, 1978.

13. The Skeletal Muscle Relaxants

One can never consent to creep when one feels an impulse to soar.

Helen Keller

Neuromuscular blocking agents may be used in the following ways:

To diagnose myasthenia gravis
To facilitate endotracheal intubation
To relieve laryngeal spasm
To provide relaxation during brief, diagnostic, or surgical procedures
To prevent bone fracture in electroconvulsive therapy
To produce apnea and controlled ventilation during thoracic surgery and neurosurgery
To reduce muscular spasticity in neurologic diseases (multiple sclerosis, cerebral palsy, or tetanus)
To reduce muscular spasm and pain resulting from sprains, arthritis, myositis, and fibrositis

CLASSIFICATION OF SKELETAL MUSCLE RELAXANTS.

1. Depolarizing agents
   a. Succinylcholine chloride (Anectine, Quelicin, Sux-Cert, Sucostrin)
2. Nondepolarizing or competitive blocking agents
   a. Tubocurarine chloride (Tubarine)
   b. Pancuronium (Pavulon)
3. Atypical competitive blocking agent
   a. Benzoquinonium (Mytolon chloride)
4. Direct-acting muscle relaxant
   a. Dantrolene sodium (Dantrium)
5. Centrally acting muscle relaxants
   a. Mephenesin carbamate (Tolseram)
   b. Chlorphenesin carbamate (Maolate)
   c. Carisoprodol (Soma)
   d. Metaxalone (Skelaxin)
   e. Cyclobenzaprine (Flexeril)
   f. Chlordiazepoxide (Librium)
   g. Diazepam (Valium)
   h. Baclofen (Lioresal)

MECHANISM OF ACTION OF MUSCLE RELAXANTS.
Succinylcholine has dual modes of action in that it depicts two phases of blocking action.

Phase I Block (Depolarization). Succinylcholine, like acetylcholine, interacts with the cholinergic receptors at the end-plate region of the muscle, resulting in depolarization of the chemically excitable membrane, creating local action potentials, spreading them to and depolarizing the adjacent excitable membranes, and finally culminating in a muscle contraction (fasciculation, an uncoordinated contraction of the muscle). However, unlike acetylcholine, succinylcholine is not metabolized by acetylcholinesterase and hence causes persistent depolarization of the end plate. The continuous presence of succinylcholine leads to inexcitability of the membrane adjacent to the end plate,

causing neuromuscular blockade, which is not reversed by the administration of cholinesterase inhibitors. As a matter of fact, agents such as neostigmine may even prolong neuromuscular blockade [2].

Phase II Block (Desensitization). In time and by repeated administration of succinylcholine, depolarization no longer contributes to neuromuscular blockade (desensitization), and neuromuscular blockade is changed in character. It is now antagonized by neostigmine, through an ill-defined mechanism very distinct from competitive blockade.

Agents such as tubocurarine or pancuronium compete with acetylcholine for the cholinergic receptors at the end plate. They combine with the receptors but do not activate them. Competitive or nondepolarizing agents are antagonized by neostigmine.

Benzoquinonium chloride (Mytolon), which is not used extensively, has a structure typical of neuromuscular blocking agents in that there are two quaternary ammonium centers joined by a bridge of two atoms. Although, like tubocurarine, it is a competitive neuromuscular blocking agent, its action and toxicity (respiratory paralyzing effect) is not blocked by neostigmine. The pharmacology of benzoquinonium chloride varies from that of *d*-tubocurarine; tubocurarine reduces blood pressure at curarizing doses whereas benzoquinonium may elevate the blood pressure slightly. Furthermore, unlike tubocurarine, benzoquinonium has a potent antiacetylcholinesterase effect.

Dantrolene, a hydantoin derivative, reduces the contraction of skeletal muscle directly on the muscle and not at the myoneural junction. It is thought to reduce the amount of calcium released and hence prevents excitation-contraction coupling. Its usefulness in the treatment of anesthetic-induced malignant hyperthermia may be due to its calcium-related uncoupling actions.

The centrally acting neuromuscular blocking agents such as mephenesin cause muscle relaxation by acting on internuncial spinal neurons to depress polysynaptic pathways. Chlordiazepoxide and diazepam enhance presynaptic inhibition by enhancing the release of GABA, an inhibitory transmitter. Baclofen interferes with the release of excitatory transmitter [2].

SEQUENCE AND ONSET OF NEUROMUSCULAR BLOCKADE.
The first muscles blocked are the rapidly contracting ones (eye, fingers, and toes), followed by the slowly contracting ones (diaphragm, limbs, and trunk). The onset and duration of action

of succinylcholine are 1 and 5 minutes respectively. The onset and duration of action of tubocurarine are 5 and 20 minutes respectively.

ADVERSE REACTIONS. Succinylcholine may cause tachycardia, cardiac arrhythmias, and hypertension (stimulation of sympathetic ganglia) or bradycardia (stimulation of muscarinic receptor sites in the sinus node of the heart). This effect is more pronounced when a second dose of succinylcholine is administered. The bradycardia may be blocked by thiopental, atropine, and ganglionic blocking agent.

Succinylcholine increases intraocular pressure transiently. It causes muscle pain, which may be due to fasciculation and uncoordinated muscle contraction. The prior administration of a competitive blocking agent may block both fasciculation and pain. Succinylcholine is metabolized according to the following scheme:

$$\text{Succinylcholine} \xrightarrow[\text{cholinesterase}]{\text{Plasma}} \text{succinylmonocholine}$$

$$\text{Succinylmonocholine} \xrightarrow[\text{Liver}]{} \text{succinate and choline}$$

Since cholinesterase is synthesized in the liver, the duration of action of succinylcholine is elevated in liver disease. Cholinesterase inhibitors dramatically increase the duration of action of succinylcholine. In patients with atypical cholinesterase, the intensity and duration of effects of succinylcholine are enhanced [3].

Patients with myotonia congenita and myotonia dystrophica respond differently to succinylcholine in that their muscles are contracted rather than relaxed. Succinylcholine increases serum concentration of potassium, and in susceptible patients such as those with renal failure, burns, infections, and closed head injury it may cause cardiac arrest. The potassium release may be blocked by prior administration of a competitive neuromuscular blocking agent.

TUBOCURARINE. Tubocurarine in large doses causes hypotension (ganglionic blockade and histamine release) and bronchospasm (histamine release). This effect is blocked by antihistaminic agent. Tubocurarine is inactive when given orally, is metabolized in the liver (35%), and is excreted by the kidney (65%) [1].

QUESTIONS ON THE SKELETAL MUSCLE RELAXANTS

Select one answer that best completes the statement or answers the question.

_____ 131. Pancuronium (Pavulon):
   A. Has a very short duration of action.

   B. Produces a phase II block if administered repetitively.
   C. Is antidoted by neostigmine.
   D. Produces hypertension.
   E. Produces fasciculations prior to the onset of muscle paralysis.

_____ 132. Dantrolene sodium (Dantrium) reduces muscular spasticity by:
   A. Decreasing the release of Ca^{2+} from the sarcoplasmic reticulum.
   B. Decreasing the release of GABA from internuncial neurons.
   C. Potentiating the action of GABA on the primary afferent nerve.
   D. Hyperpolarizing the nerve endings in the intrafusal muscle fiber.
   E. Abolishing the hippocampal after-discharges.

_____ 133. Baclofen (Lioresal) reduces muscular spasticity by:
   A. Interfering with the release of excitatory transmitters.
   B. Increasing the release of GABA from the internuncial neurons in the spinal cord.
   C. Decreasing the release of Ca^{2+} from the sarcoplasmic reticulum.
   D. Blocking the slow calcium channel.

_____ 134. The duration of action of succinylcholine depends on:
   A. Its metabolism by acetylcholinesterase.
   B. Its metabolism in the liver to succinate and choline.
   C. Its redistribution from synaptic clefts to mitochondria.
   D. Its excretion through the kidney.
   E. Its metabolism by plasma cholinesterase (pseudocholinesterase).

_____ 135. Tubocurarine has which main characteristic?
   A. Its effectiveness is dependent on the amount of acetylcholine in the synaptic cleft.
   B. Its actions are prolonged in patients with increased levels of plasma cholinesterase.
   C. Its effects are reversed by neostigmine.
   D. Its actions result in fasciculations prior to muscular paralysis.
   E. A and C.

ANSWERS ON THE SKELETAL MUSCLE RELAXANTS

131. C.
132. A.
133. A.
134. E.
135. E.

REFERENCES

1. Cheymol, J. *Neuromuscular Blocking and Stimulating Agents.* Vols. I and II. Oxford: Pergamon, 1972.
2. Miller, R. D. Skeletal Muscle Relaxants. In B. G. Katzung (ed.), *Basic and Clinical Pharmacology.* Los Altos, Calif.: Lange, 1982. Pp. 270–279.
3. Standaert, F. G. Interactions Among Neuromuscular Blocking Agents and Other Drugs. In S. G. Hershey (ed.), *Refresher Courses in Anesthesiology*, Philadelphia: Lippincott, Vol. 6. 1978. Pp. 111–125.

14. Sedatives and Hypnotics

The art of medicine consists of keeping the patient in a good mood while nature does the healing.

Voltaire

Sedatives and hypnotics depress the central nervous system. The degree of this reversible depression depends on the amount of drug ingested, causing effects according to the following scheme:

Sedation $\rightleftarrows$ hypnosis $\rightleftarrows$ anesthesia $\longrightarrow$ death

Sedation is the act of calming, reducing activity or excitement in an individual.

Hypnosis is a condition of artificially produced sleep or of a trance resembling sleep.

Anesthesia is loss of feeling or sensation.

Death is loss of life.

The degree of CNS depression including the loss of consciousness may be assessed according to the presence or absence of response to a painful stimuli, graded according to the following criteria:

Drowsy but responds to vocal command
Unconscious but responds to minimal stimuli
Unconscious and responds only to maximal painful stimuli
Unconscious and no response is evident

Contrary to general belief, the size and the activity of the pupils and the state of the limb reflexes are too variable to be useful indexes of degree of the CNS depression. However, absence of bowel sounds on auscultation of the abdomen is often associated with pronounced depression of the CNS.

Part One: The Pharmacology of Alcohol

LOCAL EFFECTS. Germicidal Effect. Application of alcohol to the unbroken skin has a disinfecting effect which is useful in presurgical scrubbing and as an antiseptic to prepare the injection site.

Astringent Effect. Alcohol is an astringent. These drugs are applied to the skin or mucous membranes for a local and limited protein denaturation in order to cause shrinkage of edematous tissues toward normal, to close off dilated blood vessels, and to form a protective coagulated protein preventing the excessive exudation.

Rubefacient Effect. Alcohol is used as a counterirritant in bed ridden patients to prevent bed sores, in that it cleanses and hardens the tissues.

SYSTEMIC EFFECTS. Central Nervous System. Alcohol is a central nervous system depressant obeying the law of "descending depression." It inhibits first the cerebral cortex, then cerebellum, the spinal cord, and lastly the medullary center.

ACUTE INTAKE OF ALCOHOL. In small quantities, "alcohol produces a feeling of well being and good fellowship. In large quantities, alcohol produces excitement characterized by laughter, loquacity, and gesticulation. Self control is lost and willpower is weakened. The sense of responsibility and the power of discrimination between the trivial and important are lost. The eyes become brighter and livelier, the speech may be brilliant but it often betrays the speaker. The movements are lively but they are often undignified" [2]. Alcohol depresses the inhibitory control mechanism and the reticular activating system. If a large amount of alcohol is consumed in a short period of time, unconsciousness and general anesthesia take place. Death will be due to respiratory and cardiac failure. Since numerous drugs in toxic doses produce ataxia and slurred speech (e.g., phenytoin), for medicolegal purposes the only acceptable means of proving intoxication is the determination of alcohol in any biologic fluid or in the expired air.

ALCOHOL AS AN APHRODISIAC. Alcohol is not an aphrodisiac, as is commonly believed. As Shakespeare said, it "provokes, and unprovokes; it provokes the desire, but it takes away the performance."

Cardiovascular Effects. Alcohol produces dilatation of the skin vessels, flushing, and a sensation of warmth. It also prevents the normal cutaneous vaso-constriction on exposure to cold. Heat is therefore lost very rapidly, and the internal temperature consequently falls. In toxic levels, the hypothalamic temperature-regulating mechanism becomes depressed, and the fall in the body temperature becomes pronounced. Consuming alcoholic beverages for the purpose of keeping warm in cold weather is irrational [2].

Gastrointestinal Tract. As a gastric secretagogue, alcohol stimulates the secretion of gastric juice, which is rich in acid and pepsin. Therefore, the consumption of alcohol is contraindicated in untreated acid-pepsin disease. In addition, alcohol releases histamine, which in turn releases gastric juice. This effect is not blocked by atropine.

In toxic doses (0.2%), gastric secretion is inhibited and peptic activity is depressed. It can easily be discerned that small amounts of alcohol stimulate appetite and aid digestion whereas large amounts may produce indigestion. Alcohol is a carminative and facilitates the expulsion of gas from the stomach.

Liver. Alcohol enhances the accumulation of fat in the liver. In alcoholism, fat accumulation continues, and cirrhosis of the liver may ensue. However, the two phenomena are not interrelated.

Endocrine Glands. Alcohol may release epinephrine, causing a transient hyperglycemia and hyperlipemia. Alcohol may be contraindicated in a diabetic. Alcohol causes diuresis by increasing fluid intake and by inhibiting the secretion of antidiuretic hormone elaborated by the posterior pituitary gland.

PHARMACOKINETICS OF ALCOHOL. Alcohol is absorbed from stomach and very rapidly from small intestine. Patients who have undergone gastrectomy may become intoxicated faster than others. Absorption from unbroken skin is negligible. As a water-soluble substance with a small molecular weight, alcohol is distributed uniformly throughout all tissues and all tissue fluids. It passes across the placental barrier, is found in spinal fluid, and accumulates in the brain. Consequently, any physiologic fluids (urine, blood, spinal fluid, milk, saliva) are suitable to determine the concentration of alcohol. Alcohol is metabolized primarily by alcohol dehydrogenase with zero-order kinetics according to the following reactions:

$$\text{Ethanol} \xrightarrow[\text{dehydrogenase}]{\text{Alcohol}} \text{acetaldehyde} \xrightarrow[\text{dehydrogenase}]{\text{Acetaldehyde}} \text{acetic acid}$$

$$\text{NAD} \rightarrow \text{NADH} \qquad \text{NAD} \rightarrow \text{NADH}$$

In addition, alcohol may be metabolized to a negligible extent by catalase according to the following reaction:

$$H_2O_2 + CH_3CH_2OH \xrightarrow{\text{Catalase}} 2H_2O + CH_3CHO$$

Although ethanol is not metabolized by the microsomal drug-metabolizing system, it inhibits it and increases the rate of its synthesis. This effect may create a significant alcohol-drug interaction in nonalcoholics and in alcoholic patients taking medications [6, 7].

Acute Poisoning. Poisoning may be characterized by inebriation, muscular incoordination, blurred vision, impaired reaction time, excitement due to loss of inhibition, impairment of consciousness, coma, tachycardia, and slow respiration. A blood alcohol of 80 mg per deciliter will produce recognizable features of drunkenness; a level above 300 mg per deciliter is dangerous to life. In children, severe hypoglycemia and convulsions may also occur.

Treatment of acute poisoning are gastric aspiration and lavage, and intensive supportive therapy, such as assessment of the patient and prevention of respiratory failure. In very severe poisoning, peritoneal dialysis or hemodialysis may become necessary.

Chronic Toxicity. Chronic alcoholism produces pathologic changes: chronic gastritis, cirrhosis of the liver, alcoholic cardiomyopathy, Korsakoff's syndrome, bloated look, flabby muscles, fine tremors, impaired physical capacity and stamina, diminished willpower, and impairment of memory [4].

Delirium Tremens. Delirium tremens usually occurs in a chronic alcoholic. The clinical features may include hallucinations, intense fear, sleeplessness, restlessness, agitation, delirium, and sometimes grand mal convulsions. Tachycardia, hypotension, and clover-shaped ST changes in the electrocardiogram are also evident.

Treatment of patient during delirium tremens includes the intravenous administration of another CNS depressant (usually diazepam) during the acute phase, followed by oral administration of chlordiazepoxide or oxazepam. In addition, other medications or dietary management, or both, may become essential.

TOXICOLOGY OF METHYL ALCOHOL. Methyl alcohol is used as an industrial solvent and as an adulterant added to ethyl alcohol to prevent its consumption. Methyl alcohol is metabolized to formaldehyde and formic acid according to the following reactions:

$$\text{Methanol} \xrightarrow[\text{dehydrogenase}]{\text{Alcohol}} \text{formaldehyde} \xrightarrow[\text{dehydrogenase}]{\text{Aldehyde}} \text{formic acid}$$

Besides producing all the CNS effects discussed, methyl alcohol causes acidosis and blindness. Treatment of methyl alcohol poisoning may include water and electrolyte replacement, sodium bicarbonate to combat acidosis, and intravenous administration of ethyl alcohol, which is a preferred substrate of liver alcohol dehydrogenase, allowing methyl alcohol to be excreted unmetabolized in the urine.

Part Two: Sedatives and Hypnotics

General uses of drugs in this category are to treat convulsions, to produce sedation, to produce hypnosis, and to produce anesthesia.

CLASSIFICATION. Sedatives and hypnotics may be divided into barbiturates and nonbarbiturates. The most commonly used barbiturates are:

Thiopental (Pentothal)
Methohexital (Brevital)
Secobarbital (Seconal)
Pentobarbital (Nembutal)
Amobarbital (Amytal)
Phenobarbital (Luminal)

Barbiturates are classified according to their duration of action:

Ultrashort-acting—thiopental, methohexital
Short- to intermediate-acting—pentobarbital, secobarbital, amobarbital
Long-acting—phenobarbital

In general, the more lipid soluble a barbiturate derivative is, the greater its plasma and tissue binding, the extent of its metabolism, and its storage in adipose tissues. In addition, very lipid-soluble substances have faster onset of action and shorter duration of action.

Barbiturates do not raise the pain threshold and have no analgesic property. They depress all areas of the CNS including the hypothalamic thermoregulatory system, respiratory center, and vasomotor centers at anesthetic doses. They depress the polysynaptic pathways in the spinal column at anesthetic doses. Some (e.g., phenobarbital) but not all are anticonvulsants. In toxic doses, barbiturates cause oliguria.

PHARMACOKINETICS OF BARBITURATES. Barbiturates are absorbed orally and distributed widely throughout the body. They are metabolized in the liver by aliphatic oxygenation, aromatic oxygenation, and N-dealkylation.

The inactive metabolites are excreted in the urine. The administration of bicarbonate enhances the urinary excretion of barbiturates whose pK_a is 7.4 (phenobarbital and thiopental). This generalization is not true with other barbiturates. The chronic administration of barbiturates induces the cytochrome P450 drug-metabolizing system.

ACUTE TOXICITY FROM BARBITURATES. Acute toxicity is characterized by automatism, a state of drug-induced confusion in which a patient forgets having taken the medication and ingests more. Death results from respiratory failure. The treatment of poisoning includes supporting respiration, preventing hypotension, forcing diuresis, doing hemodialysis, and giving sodium bicarbonate for phenobarbital poisoning. Tolerance does not develop to the lethal dose of barbiturates [5].

ADDICTION TO BARBITURATES. The abrupt withdrawal from barbiturates may cause tremors, restlessness, anxiety, weakness, nausea and vomiting, seizures, delirium, and cardiac arrest.

SELECTION OF DRUGS. Selection of a barbiturate is determined in part by the duration of action of the drug and the clinical problem at hand. When one is inducing anesthesia, an ultrashort-acting drug is used. In epilepsy, a long-acting barbiturate is chosen whereas in sleep disorders a short-acting or an intermediate-like drug is used depending on whether the patients have difficulty falling asleep or they fall asleep but have difficulty staying asleep [1, 3].

NONBARBITURATE SEDATIVES AND HYPNOTICS.

1. Chloral hydrate (Noctec, Somnos). This agent is a general hypnotic and sedative, used in the treatment of delirium tremens and of withdrawal from other drugs.
2. Paraldehyde (Paral). Therapeutic uses of paraldehyde resemble those of chloral hydrate.
3. Glutethimide (Doriden). Glutethimide is used to cause daytime or preoperative sedation, or in simple insomnia. It is useful too in patients who cannot tolerate barbiturates.
4. Flurazepam (Dalmane.) Flurazepam is used in simple insomnia.
5. Methaqualone (Quaalude, Sopor). Methaqualone is used in daytime sedation and simple insomnia. Furthermore, it is useful in patients who cannot tolerate barbiturates.
6. Methyprylon (Noludar). Methyprylon is used in simple insomnia. It is also useful in patients who cannot tolerate barbiturates.

QUESTIONS ON SEDATIVES AND HYPNOTICS

Select one answer that best completes the statement or answers the question.

____ 136. Both barbiturates and alcohol are able to:
  A. Raise the pain threshold.
  B. Depress the thermoregulatory center.
  C. Increase the secretion of the antidiuretic hormone.
  D. Depress the vasomotor center.
  E. Do both B and D.

____ 137. The catabolism or action of ethyl alcohol is:
  A. Inhibited by disulfiram (Antabuse).
  B. Potentiated by diazepam.
  C. Nullified by phenobarbital.

  D. Exemplified by both A and B.
  E. Exemplified by both B and C.

____ 138. Which of the following statement(s) is true about alcoholics?
  A. They metabolize phenobarbital at a slower rate when the plasma concentration of alcohol is high.
  B. They metabolize phenobarbital at a faster rate when sober.
  C. They use a larger dose of barbiturates to obtain sedation.
  D. All of the above.

____ 139. Which of the following statements is not true?
  A. Secobarbital is completely metabolized in the body.
  B. Alcohol is mostly metabolized in the body.
  C. Phenobarbital is completely metabolized in the body.
  D. Ethyl alcohol may inhibit the metabolism of methyl alcohol.

____ 140. Withdrawal syndrome occurs following addiction from:
  A. Morphine.
  B. Secobarbital.
  C. Meperidine.
  D. Ethyl alcohol.
  E. All of the above.

____ 141. Thiopental varies from phenobarbital in what respect(s)? Thiopental:
  A. Crosses the blood-brain barrier more rapidly.
  B. Exhibits a higher degree of protein binding.
  C. Is metabolized more completely.
  D. All of the above.

____ 142. In comparing the pharmacology of phenobarbital and morphine, which statement is not true?
  A. Both are addictive.
  B. Both cause grand mal seizures during their abstinence syndromes.
  C. Both depress respiration.
  D. They are catabolized in the liver by different enzymatic reactions.

ANSWERS ON SEDATIVES AND HYPNOTICS

136. E.
137. D.
138. D.
139. C.
140. E.
141. D.
142. B.

REFERENCES

1. Ganten, D., and Pfaff, D. *Sleep. Clinical and Experimental Aspects.* Berlin: Springer-Verlag, 1982.
2. Grollman, A. *Pharmacology and Therapeutics.* Philadelphia: Lea & Febiger, 1962.
3. Karmanova, I. G. *Evolution of Sleep. Stages of the Formation of the "Wakefulness-Sleep" Cycle in Vertebrates.* Basel: Karger, 1982.
4. Kissin, B., and Begleiter, H. (eds.). *Biology of Alcoholism:*

Physiology and Behavior. Vol. 2. New York: Plenum, 1972.

5. Matthew, H. *Acute Barbiturate Poisoning.* Amsterdam: Excerpta Medica, 1971.

6. Roach, M. K., McIsaac, W. M., and Creaven, P. J. *Biological Aspects of Alcohol.* Austin: University of Texas, 1971.

7. Wallgren, H., and Barry, H., III. *Actions of Alcohol.* Vols. I and II. Amsterdam: Elsevier-North-Holland, 1970.

VI. Diuretics and Cardiovascular Pharmacology

15. Cardiac Glycosides

We see, then, how far the monuments of wit and learning are more durable than the monuments of power or of the hands. For have not the verses of Homer continued twenty-five hundred years or more, without the loss of a syllable or letter; during which time infinite palaces, temples, castles, cities, have been decayed and demolished?

Francis Bacon

When the heart is no longer able to pump an adequate supply of blood to meet the metabolic needs of the tissues or in relation to venous return, cardiac failure may ensue. The causes of cardiac failure are complex but include (1) mechanical abnormalities (e.g., pericardial tamponade), (2) myocardial failure (e.g., cardiomyopathy, inflammatory), and (3) arrhythmias. In high-output failure, the cardiac output, which may be normal or even higher than normal, is not sufficient to meet the metabolic requirement of the body. Cardiac failure may predispose to congestive heart failure, which is a state of circulatory congestion.

Failure of only one ventricle is not common. In a hypothetic event, should it occur, the circulatory congestion resulting from failure of the left and right ventricles may be sequentially outlined [4].

Failure of the Left Ventricle

Backward Effects	Forward Effects
Decreased emptying of the left ventricle	Decreased cardiac output
Increased volume and pressure in left ventricle (end-diastolic pressure rises)	Decreased perfusion of tissues of body
Increased volume (pressure) in left atrium	Increased resorption of sodium- and water-retaining hormones
Increased volume in pulmonary veins	Increased extracellular fluid volume
Increased volume in pulmonary capillary bed (PCB)	Increased total blood volume
Transudation of fluid from capillaries to alveoli	
Rapid filling of alveoli spaces	
Pulmonary edema	

Therefore, it is apparent that in congestive heart failure the patient's cardiac compensatory mechanisms will be fully activated:

Cardiac dilatation and hypertrophy (taking advantage of the Frank-Starling relationship to utilize more contractile elements)
Sympathetic stimulation (increasing heart rate to maintain contractility and cardiac output)
Increasing oxygen consumption through arterial venous oxygen difference (increasing extraction of oxygen from limited blood flow)
Production of aldosterone (increasing Na+ and fluid retention), which may not be advantageous to the organism

Failure of the Right Ventricle

Backward Effects	Forward Effects
Decreased emptying of right ventricle	Decreased volume from right ventricle to lungs
Increased volume and increased end-diastolic pressure in right ventricle	Decreased return to left atrium and subsequent decreased cardiac output
Increased volume and pressure in right atrium	All the forward effects of left heart failure
Increased volume and pressure in the great veins	Expansion of blood volume
Increased volume in the systemic venous circulation	
Increased volume in distensible organs (liver, spleen)	
Increased pressure at capillary line	
Hepatomegaly, splenomegaly	
Dependent edema and serous effusion	

CARDIAC GLYCOSIDES. The most important and often used drugs in the treatment of congestive heart failure are the cardiac glycosides. Unfortunately, the margin of safety of these drugs is very narrow (therapeutic index = 3). Toxicity will develop readily, and careful attention to pharmacokinetic principles is absolutely crucial. In addition to cardiac glycosides, agents such as catecholamines, glucagon, angiotensin, atropine, and amrinone are able to stimulate the heart, but their usefulness is limited.

In chronic congestive heart failure, vasodilators may be effective. Some drugs and their uses are cited here [3]:

Drugs	Uses
Vasodilators—nitrates	In pulmonary congestion
Arteriodilators—hydralazine	In fatigue secondary to low left ventricular output
Arteriodilators and venodilators—prazosin	In pulmonary congestion and reduced cardiac output

Cardiac glycosides are obtained from numerous sources in nature including *Digitalis lanata* and *Digitalis purpurea* (white and purple foxglove), squill

Fig. 15-1. *The structure of digoxin.*

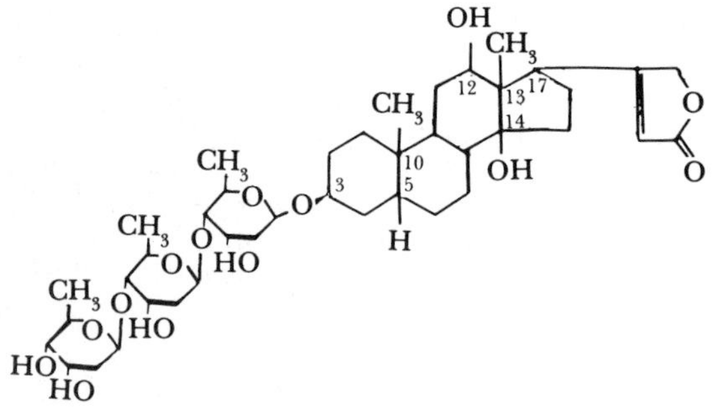

Table 15-1. *Comparison of the Pharmacokinetic Profiles of Digoxin and Digitoxin*

Property	Digoxin	Digitoxin
Lipid-solubility	Low	High
Gastrointestinal absorption	Good	Excellent
Protein binding	Low (25%)	High (90%)
$T_{1/2}$	Short (1–2 days)	Long (6–9 days)
Enterohepatic recycling	Minimal	High
Liver metabolism	Low	High
Excretion	Active drug	Inactive metabolites
Onset of action (intravenous)	Fast (5–30 minutes)	Slow (4–8 hours)

(Mediterranean sea onion), oleander, lily of the valley, and other plants. Among the useful available cardiac glycosides are the following [2]:

Digitalis purpurea	*Digitalis lanata*	*Strophanthus gratus*
Digitoxin	Digoxin	Ouabain
Digoxin	Lanatoside C	
Digitalis leaf	Deslanoside	

Among these, only digoxin (Fig. 15-1) and digitoxin and, to a certain extent, ouabain are used extensively.

Examination of the structures of cardiac glycosides, including digoxin, reveals three structural components:

A steroid nucleus (aglycones or genins)
A series of sugar residues in the C_3 position
A five- or six-membered lactone ring in the C_{17} position

The sugar residue in digoxin and digitoxin is -O-digitoxose-digitoxose-digitoxose. Digoxin varies from digitoxin by having a hydroxy group at C_{12}. It should be recalled that glycosides possess both lipophilic residues (steroid nucleus) and hydrophilic residues (lactone ring and OH group). These residues and other factors strongly influence the pharmacokinetic profiles of these cardiac glycosides. Digitoxin is more lipid soluble than digoxin and, compared to it, is absorbed better when given orally, has a longer half-life, depicts a higher protein binding, and is more extensively metabolized by the liver. Digoxin is excreted extensively unchanged by the kidney. Renal insufficiency alters its half-life and safety. An elevation of blood urea nitrogen (BUN) should signal diminished capacity to eliminate digoxin. A direct relationship exists between the clearance of digoxin and that of creatine, which, in addition to BUN, may be used in assessing the patient's ability to excrete digoxin. Table 15-1 compares the pharmacokinetic profiles of digoxin and digitoxin [3].

Since a drug may require four to five half-lives to attain a steady-state (maintenance) level, it is logical to assume that approximately 1 week will be required for digoxin and 4 weeks for digitoxin to reach their maintenance levels.

MODES OF ACTION OF CARDIAC GLYCOSIDES. Cardiac glycosides increase cardiac output by having a positive inotropic effect. They slow heart rate by relieving the sympathetic tone and having vagotonic effects. They reduce the heart size by relief of the Frank-Starling relationship (Fig. 15-2). They increase cardiac efficiency by increasing cardiac output and decreasing oxygen consumption (decreased heart size and rate).

The blood pressure remains unchanged following administration of cardiac glycosides. In congestive heart failure, the cardiac output is reduced, but the total peripheral resistance is increased. These effects are reversed by cardiac glycosides. Increasing cardiac output diminishes the total peripheral resistance.

Cardiac glycosides cause diuresis by increasing cardiac output and by increasing renal blood flow, which in turn reverses the renal compensatory mechanism activated in congestive heart failure. Consequently, the production of aldosterone is reduced, the retention of Na^+ is reversed, and the excretion of edematous fluid is enhanced.

MECHANISM OF POSITIVE INOTROPIC ACTION OF CARDIAC GLYCOSIDES (DIGITALIS). Cardiac glycosides potentiate the process of coupling of electrical excitation with mechanical contraction, and, by augmenting the myoplasmic concentration of calcium, they cause a more forceful contraction.

ELECTROPHYSIOLOGIC EFFECTS OF CARDIAC GLYCOSIDES (DIGITALIS). Cardiac glycosides have a vagotonic effect and may decrease impulse formation in the SA node. Although automaticity is not directly influenced by digitalis, conduction velocity is decreased. This effect of digitalis on the AV node is more prominent in congestive heart failure, where the vagal tone is low and adrenergic tone is high. Digitalis shortens the refractory period. This reduction is in part due to enhanced in-

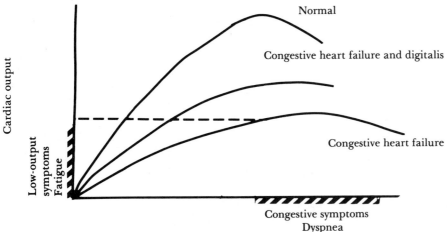

Fig. 15-2. *Use of the Frank-Starling mechanism to compensate for congestive heart failure. (Adapted from* Am. J. Cardiol. *32:437, 1973.)*

tracellular calcium, decreasing membrane resistance, and increasing membrane potassium conductance, leading to shortening of action potential and contributing to shortening of atrial and ventricular refractoriness. The electrophysiologic properties of digitalis make it a useful compound in atrial arrhythmias (vagotonic effect), in atrial flutter (depressant effect on atrioventricular conduction), and in atrial fibrillation (vagotonic effect).

DIGITALIS TOXICITY. Toxic effects of digitalis are frequent and may be fatal. It may result from (1) overdosage, (2) decreased metabolism and excretion, and (3) hypokalemia caused by thiazide diuretics, diarrhea, and vomiting. Digitalis toxicity has several manifestations [1].

Cardiac Effects. The most commonly reported cardiac signs of toxicity are dysrhythmias such as ventricular ectopic depolarization, second- and third-degree heart block, junctional tachycardia, atrial tachycardia with block, ventricular tachycardia, sinoatrial block, and sinus arrest.

Gastrointestinal Effects. Anorexia is seen, followed by nausea and vomiting.

Visual Effects. The most common visual side effects are blurring, dimness, flickering or flashing lights, color vision (yellow, green, red, and white), cycloplegia, and diplopia.

NEUROPSYCHIATRIC SYMPTOMS. A few of the neuropsychiatric symptoms reported are agitation, apathy, aphasia, ataxia, belligerence, changes in affect or personality, combativeness, confusion, delirium, delusions, depression, disorientation, dizziness, drowsiness, euphoria, excitement, fatigue, giddiness, hallucinations, headache, insomnia, irritability, lassitude, mania, muscle pain, nervousness, neuralgias, nightmares, paresthesias, restlessness, somnolence, vertigo, violence, and weakness.

TREATMENT OF DIGITALIS TOXICITY. General Treatment. The administration of digitalis and diuretics should be stopped. Furthermore, the patient should be monitored closely for any alteration in pharmacokinetic profile of the cardiac glycoside administered.

Specific Treatment. Potassium and magnesium may be indicated. Potassium is recommended for patients with digitalis-induced ectopic beat or tachycardia provided the patient is neither hyperkalemic, uremic, nor oliguric. It is the drug of choice if the patient is hypokalemic.

In the treatment of digitalis-induced arrhythmia, lidocaine with its fast onset of action and short duration of action is the first drug of choice. Since lidocaine is metabolized, it should be used carefully in liver diseases. Phenytoin may be used if potassium or lidocaine is ineffective. Propranolol is effective in ventricular tachycardia. Atropine is effective if digitalis-induced conduction delay is at the AV node and is mediated via the vagus. Calcium channel blocking agents such as verapamil are effective if arrhythmia is due to reentry or to increased diastolic depolarization in the Purkinje fibers or in oscillatory afterpotential. In addition to these drugs, a temporary pacemaker may be indicated. The following interventions are contraindicated. Quinidine should not be used since it displaces digoxin from binding sites. Bretylium should not be used since it releases norepinephrine. Carotid sinus stimulation should be discouraged since ventricular fibrillation may ensue [1].

QUESTIONS ON CARDIAC GLYCOSIDES

Select one answer that best completes the statement or answers the question.

_____ 143. In congestive heart failure, one of the patient's compensatory mechanisms is:
   A. Enhanced sympathetic stimulation.
   B. Enhanced parasympathetic stimulation.
   C. Decreased aldosterone secretion.
   D. Pronounced bradycardia.

_____ 144. The pharmacokinetics and pharmacodynamics of digoxin and digitoxin differ in all aspects *except* which one?
   A. Extent of renal excretion in unchanged forms.
   B. Extent of hepatic metabolism.
   C. Half-lives.
   D. Therapeutic index and margin of safety.

_____ 145. The pharmacology of digoxin in congestive heart failure is associated with all of the following *except* which one?
   A. Vagotonic effect.
   B. Relief of Frank-Starling relationship.
   C. Reduction of aldosterone-driven Na^+ retention.
   D. Marked hypotension.

_____ 146. Which one of the following actions or situations does *not* involve an alteration in the pharmacodynamic manifestation of Ca^{2+} ion?
   A. Digitalis-induced AV block in a normal heart.
   B. Supraventricular tachycardia resulting from a physiologic or an anatomic block in a cardiac conduction system.
   C. Enhanced oscillatory afterpotential in digitalis toxicity.
   D. Digitalis-induced positive inotropic effect in congestive heart failure.

_____ 147. In digoxin-induced toxicity characterized by ventricular ectopic depolarization, a physician should do which one of the following?
   A. Discontinue digoxin and switch the patient to digitoxin.
   B. Discontinue digoxin altogether and provide appropriate supportive treatment as indicated.
   C. Discontinue digoxin and use a sympathomimetic drug possessing positive inotropic effect.
   D. Continue with digoxin but take immediate action to reduce extracellular K^+ level.

_____ 148. A patient with pheochromocytoma developed congestive heart failure and was treated with 2 mg of digoxin/day. Three weeks later the patient manifested dramatic ventricular tachycardia presumably predisposed by pheochromocytoma but aggravated by digitalis. At this time, the treatment of choice would be:
   A. Discontinue digoxin and give propranolol (Inderal).
   B. Continue with digoxin but add reserpine (Serpasil).
   C. Discontinue digoxin but add reserpine (Serpasil).
   D. Discontinue digoxin but add isoproterenol (Isuprel).

_____ 149. In digitalis-induced AV block one may treat the patient with:
   A. Atropine.
   B. Quinidine (Quinora).
   C. Propranolol (Inderal).
   D. Verapamil (Isoptin).

_____ 150. Quinidine (Quinora) is contraindicated in digoxin-induced arrhythmias because:
   A. It decreases the excretion of digoxin.
   B. It displaces digoxin from the binding site.
   C. It decreases the metabolism of digoxin.
   D. It possesses positive inotropic effects that will aggravate the arrhythmias further.

ANSWERS AND EXPLANATIONS ON CARDIAC GLYCOSIDES

143. A.
144. D.
145. D.
146. A.
   Explanation: The glycoside-induced ventricular dysrhythmias may be due to transient oscillations in diastolic membrane potential (oscillatory afterpotentials), which are produced by the slow influx of calcium and are blocked by verapamil, a calcium channel blocking agent.
147. B.
148. A.
   Explanation: Propranolol, a beta-adrenergic blocking agent, is effective in digitalis-induced tachydysrhythmias such as ventricular tachycardia. Similarly, it is known that propranolol is effective in catecholamine-driven arrhythmias.
149. A.
   Explanation: Some of the digitalis-induced conduction delay at the AV node is mediated via the vagus. Therefore, patients with digitalis-induced heart block often respond to intravenous administration of atropine sulfate (0.5–2.0 mg).
150. B.

REFERENCES

1. Ewy, G. A. Digitalis Intoxication: Diagnosis and Therapy. In G. A. Ewy and R. Bressler (eds.), *Cardiovascular Drugs and the Management of Heart Disease*. New York: Raven, 1982. Pp. 657–674.
2. Hoffman, B. F., and Bigger, J. T., Jr. Digitalis and Allied Cardiac Glycosides. In A. G. Gilman, L. S. Goodman, and A. Gilman (eds.), *The Pharmacological Basis of Therapeutics* (6th ed.). New York: Macmillan, 1980. Pp. 729–760.
3. MacLeod, S. M., and Piafsky, K. M. Cardiac Glycosides. In P. Seeman, E. M. Sellers, and W. H. E. Roschlau, *Principles of Medical Pharmacology*. Toronto: University of Toronto, 1980. Pp. 303–310.
4. Schlant, R. C. Altered Physiology of the Cardiovascular System in Heart Failure. In J. W. Hurst, et al. (eds.), *The Heart* (3rd ed.). New York: McGraw-Hill, 1974. Pp. 416–433.

16. Antidysrhythmic Drugs

Colors fade, temples crumble, empires fall, but wise words endure.

Edward Thorndike

Cardiac dysrhythmias may be caused by a damaged heart (e.g., myocardial infarction) resulting from an abnormality in blood supply to pacemaker cells or conducting tissues, or both. In addition, fatal dysrhythmias may be caused by injudicious use of numerous drugs including digitalis, anesthetics, antidepressants with anticholinergic effects (e.g., amitriptyline), and neuroleptics with anticholinergic effects (e.g., thioridazine). Fortunately, antidysrhythmic agents, electrical defibrillators, and pacers are able to reverse cardiac dysrhythmias effectively.

THE NATURE OF DYSRHYTHMIAS. At the sinoatrial (SA) node, electrical impulses generate a cardiac contraction at regular intervals and with a frequency of one beat per second. The impulse spreads rapidly through the atria and enters the atrioventricular (AV) node. The conduction through the AV node takes 0.2 second, which is relatively slow. The impulse then propagates over the His-Purkinje system and contracts the entire ventricular muscle in 0.1 second in an anatomically synchronous and a hemodynamically effective fashion. Dysrhythmias deviate from the above and result from abnormalities either in (1) impulse generation or in (2) impulse conduction, whereby the normal impulse conduction rate is slowed somewhere in the specialized conducting system of the heart. This disturbance is frequently, but not always, found in the AV node or in the bundles of His (heart block), or both.

The major electrophysiologic manifestations of these two causes of cardiac dysrhythmias are found in the properties of automaticity (slope of phase 4 or diastolic depolarization) and conduction velocity, respectively. Drugs that alter pacemaker automaticity will have a direct effect on the heart rate (Fig. 16-1). Rapid diastolic depolarization (dashed line) leads to rapid rate of firing whereas lowered slope of phase 4 diastolic depolarization (solid line) leads to fewer action potentials in the same time interval. Similarly, drugs that increase conduction velocity in the heart can help to alleviate heart block, while those that decrease conduction velocity may slow a rapid heart rate [1, 7].

MECHANISM OF TACHYARRHYTHMIAS. Tachyarrhythmias are generated by two mechanisms: increased automaticity and reentry due to unidirectional block in a conducting system. Reentrant arrhythmias are abolished by

Increasing conduction velocity in abnormal tissue, thus removing unidirectional block. Phenytoin and lidocaine accomplish this.

Decreasing conduction velocity, so as to obtain bidirectional block. Quinidine, procainamide, and propranolol accomplish this goal.

Increasing refractory period relative to action potential duration, so that the reentrant current becomes extinct in the refractory tissue. Most antiarrhythmic agents are able to do this [7].

REENTRANT SUPRAVENTRICULAR TACHYCARDIA. Paroxysmal supraventricular tachycardia with AV intranodal reentry has been attributed to the presence of dual conducting pathways within the AV node according to a scheme shown in Figure 16-2 [4].

The longitudinal dissociation of the AV node is ascribed to two pathways, designated as beta and alpha. Beta, a sodium-dependent system, depicts a fast conduction but a longer refractoriness. Alpha, a calcium-dependent pathway, depicts a slower conduction and a shorter refractory period. Abnormal impulses generated by SA nodes travel the beta pathway and depolarize the His-Purkinje system and the ventricle impulses. The impulse traveling down the slower alpha pathway is blocked.

A premature atrial depolarization may be blocked in the beta pathway, but creating an opportunity for the α pathway to conduct the impulse at a slower rate. The previously refractory beta pathway has time to recover and the impulse not only depolarizes the ventricles but will also travel back up to beta pathway producing an atrial echo beat (an inverted P wave and a prolonged PR interval). Because of tachycardia, the P wave is either fused or buried with the previous QRS complex. A single atrial echo beat results when the alpha pathway has not fully recovered. An earlier premature atrial depolarization will conduct even more slowly down the alpha pathway and will not only conduct back up the beta pathway, but will reenter the top of the alpha pathway that now had time to recover. The result may be a sustained reentrant AV nodal supraventricular tachycardia [4].

PAROXYSMAL SUPRAVENTRICULAR TACHYCARDIA WITH A CONCEALED ACCESSORY. "A characteristic of a concealed pathway is that it does not conduct from the atrium to the ventricle, but conducts from the ventricle to the atrium [according to the scheme depicted in Figure 16-3]. Since the majority of these concealed pathways are located in the left AV groove, the conduction is from the left ventricle to the left atrium (P wave is negative in lead)" [4].

Fig. 16-1. *A hypothetical action potential depicting steep (--) and shallow (—) slope of phase 4 diastolic depolarization. The spontaneous discharge rate of the "autonomic cells" may be altered by changing either (a) the slope of phase 4 spontaneous depolarization, (b) the resting membrane potential, or (c) the threshold potential.*

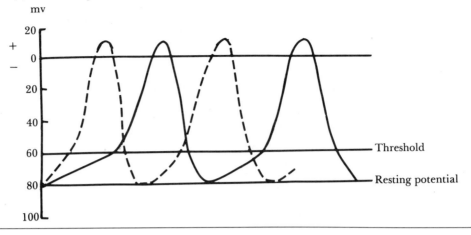

Fig. 16-2. *A proposed model depicting the mechanism of AV nodal reentry. The beta pathway is fast and sodium dependent whereas the alpha pathway is slow and calcium dependent. (From G. A. Ewy, Supraventricular Tachycardias: Diagnosis and Management. In G. A. Ewy and R. Bressler [eds.],* Cardiovascular Drugs and the Management of Heart Disease. *New York: Raven, 1982.)*

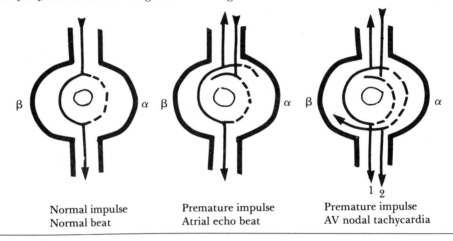

Normal impulse
Normal beat

Premature impulse
Atrial echo beat

Premature impulse
AV nodal tachycardia

Fig. 16-3. *Reentrant paroxysmal supraventricular tachycardia. (From G. A. Ewy, Supraventricular Tachycardias: Diagnosis and Management. In G. A. Ewy and R. Bressler [eds.],* Cardiovascular Drugs and the Management of Heart Disease. *New York: Raven, 1982.)*

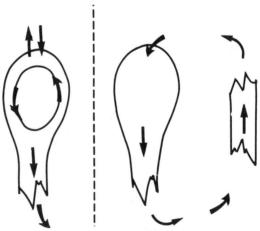

Atrioventricular nodal reentry   Reentry via concealed bypass tract

Cardiac dysrhythmias may be arbitrarily classified either by rate or by location. Some general guidelines for classification by rate are as follows:

Classification of Dysrhythmias by Rate (Beats/Minute)

	Atrial	Ventricular
Bradycardia	< 60	< 60
Normal	60–100	60–100
Tachycardia	140–200	130–175
Flutter	200–350	175–200
Fibrillation	>350	

Some of the more common dysrhythmias, identified by location, are classified as follows:

Classification of Common Dysrhythmias by Location

SA node
  Sinus bradycardia
  Sinus tachycardia
Atrial
  Atrial premature beats
  Paroxysmal atrial tachycardia (PAT)
  Atrial flutter
  Atrial fibrillation
AV node
  AV block (first, second, and third degree)
Ventricular
  Ventricular premature beats (VPB, PVC)
  Ventricular tachycardia
  Ventricular flutter
  Ventricular fibrillation

CLASSIFICATION OF ANTIDYSRHYTHMIC DRUGS.

Most of the major antiarrhythmic drugs are used to treat abnormally fast heart rates (tachyarrhythmias). Since several of these drugs have very similar electrophysiologic properties, they will be discussed together as a group and according to the following classification [2, 4–6, 8]:

Group I	Disopyramide
	Propranolol
	Procainamide
	Quinidine
Group II	Lidocaine
	Phenytoin

I and II are grouped together on the basis of some shared electrophysiologic features.

Group III	Bretylium
Group IV	Slow-channel calcium blocking agents
	Verapamil (Isoptin)
	Nifedipine (Procardia)
	Diltiazem (Cardizem)
Group V	Newer antidysrhythmic drugs
	Mexiletine
	Tocainide
	Encainide
Group VI	Others, e.g.:
	Atropine
	Catecholamines
	Digitalis
	Potassium

QUINIDINE AND PROCAINAMIDE. Quinidine and procainamide decrease automaticity by reducing the rate of phase 4 diastolic depolarization, probably mediated by a diminished membrane permeability to sodium, and decrease conduction velocity throughout the conducting system. They produce an indirect (vagolytic) effect that sometimes counteracts the direct effect at the AV node, causing a "paradoxic tachycardia" in some cases of atrial flutter or fibrillation. These agents terminate reentry arrhythmias by producing a bidirectional block in infarcted conducting tissues. They directly depress contractility, leading to a fall in cardiac output.

These agents are potent vasodilators, especially when given by the intravenous route. This effect is so great that quinidine is rarely given parenterally, and great care must be used when procainamide is used by this route. They depress blood pressure by their dual effects on cardiac output and peripheral resistance.

These agents produce widening of the QRS complex (by depressing ventricular conduction) and lengthening of the PR interval (by slowing AV conduction). A 25 to 30 percent widening of the QRS complex may be taken as the therapeutic limit when administering the drugs. They are excreted up to 50 percent unmetabolized in the urine. They commonly cause gastrointestinal disturbances as their major side effect. Emboli may be liberated from the atria during conversion of atrial flutter or fibrillation. Their toxicity involves a profound fall in blood pressure, resulting in a shocklike state accompanied by a variety of arrhythmias.

Quinidine and procainamide may also result in some unique but uncommon side effects. Quinidine may produce cinchonism (ringing in the ears, dizziness, visual disturbances, vertigo) and cutaneous hypersensitivity reactions. Procainamide may cause agranulocytosis during chronic therapy and a dose-dependent (> 2 gm/day) lupus erythematosus–like syndrome. These agents are mainly used in atrial (supraventricular) arrhythmias, although procainamide is also of value in PVCs and ventricular tachycardia. If either drug is used to convert atrial flutter or fibrillation, digitalis must be given first to protect against paradoxic tachycardia [3].

DISOPYRAMIDE. Disopyramide depresses automaticity primarily in the ventricular conducting system. It depresses conduction velocity throughout the heart but has less effect at the AV node than does either quinidine or procainamide. It does not have a vagolytic effect in the heart. Disopyramide terminates reentry by producing bidirectional block. It does not greatly depress blood pressure. Contractility and cardiac output are mildly depressed, but because the compound is not a vasodilator, a reflex increase in peripheral resistance tends to offset the fall in cardiac output. Like quinidine and procainamide, it is excreted 50 percent unmetabolized in the urine.

Disopyramide's side effects are primarily gastrointestinal in nature because of its peripheral anticholin-

Table 16-1. *Properties of Selected Antidysrhythmic Agents*

	Quinidine Procainamide (Pronestyl)	Disopyramide (Norpace)	Propranolol (Inderal)	Lidocaine (Xylocaine) Phenytoin (Dilantin)
Effects				
Automaticity	↓	↓	↓	↓
Conduction velocity	↓	↓	↓	0 or ↑
Inotropism	(−)	(−)	(−)	
Cardiac output	↓	↓	↓	0 or ↓
Blood pressure	↓	0 or ↓	↓	0 or ↓
Autonomic	Anticholinergic— heart	Anticholinergic	β-block	
Transference				
Route	Q—oral (IM) PA—oral, parenteral	Oral	Oral, IV	L—IV only PTY—oral, IV
Metabolism	~ 50% in liver	~ 50% in liver	Extensively in liver	90–100% in liver
Excretion	Kidney—50% unchanged	Kidney—40–60% unchanged	Kidney—inactive metabolites	Kidney—< 10% unchanged
Side effects	Hypotension N and V Emboli—atrial fibrillation	N and V Dry mouth, constipation, urinary hesitancy	Hypotension, bradycardia Bronchospasms (asthma)	L—sedation PTY—sedation, vertigo, nausea
Toxicity	Q—cinchonism PA—lupus syndrome, agranulocytosis (chronic R$_x$)	May → CHF	Cardiac depression → CHF	L—hearing dysfunction, convulsions PTY—ataxia
Contraindications	2° or 3° block Cardiac failure Renal dysfunction	2° or 3° block Cardiac failure Glaucoma Urinary retention Renal dysfunction	2° or 3° block Asthma Sinus bradycardia CHF Certain anesthetics	3° block, liver dysfunction Atrial flutter or fibrillation

From F. Dalske, *Review of Concepts in Cardiovascular Pharmacology*. Omaha: University of Nebraska, 1979.

ergic action causing dry mouth and urinary hesitancy. Disopyramide finds its major therapeutic use in treating PVCs and ventricular tachycardia. It does not appear particularly useful in atrial arrhythmias [3, 5].

PROPRANOLOL. Propranolol's antiarrhythmic effects are solely due to beta-adrenergic receptor site blocking action. A "quinidine-like action" does not occur at doses used in humans. This agent is a potent cardiac depressant, directly affecting contractility, cardiac output, and heart rate. It is extensively metabolized by the liver. Propranolol is generally a second-choice antiarrhythmic drug unless the arrhythmia is catecholamine mediated. It is best in atrial arrhythmias, as an addition to digitalis in the conversion of atrial flutter or fibrillation, or to treat digitalis-induced arrhythmias [3].

LIDOCAINE AND PHENYTOIN. Lidocaine and phenytoin depress automaticity almost exclusively in the Purkinje system. They do not depress conduction velocity and may actually increase AV conduction. These agents terminate reentry by producing bidirectional conduction through infarcted conducting tissue.

Lidocaine and phenytoin have little or no effect on contractility, cardiac output, or blood pressure at therapeutic doses. However, large doses or rapid intravenous administration will depress these parameters.

These agents do not produce significant ECG changes at therapeutic doses. They are extensively metabolized in the liver. Their side effects and toxicity are referable to the CNS: drowsiness, hearing dysfunction, convulsions (lidocaine), nystagmus and vertigo (phenytoin). They are both effective in treating any arrhythmia (including supraventricular) due to digitalis toxicity. Lidocaine, but not usually phenytoin, is routinely used in several ventricular arrhythmias, especially in MI patients. Both drugs may be given intravenously, but only phenytoin can be given orally.

The properties of agents in groups I and II—disopyramide, propranolol, lidocaine, and phenytoin—are summarized in Table 16-1 [3].

BRETYLIUM (BRETYLOL). Bretylium is not an antiarrhythmic of first choice. It is used intramuscularly or intravenously to treat ventricular tachycardia and ventricular fibrillation. It is excreted unmetabolized in the urine. The major side effect of bretylium is postural hypotension. Since it releases norepineph-

Table 16-2. *Treatment of Common Dysrhythmias*

Arrhythmia	Treatment of Choice	Alternative	Remarks
Atrial arrhythmias			
Atrial fibrillation	Cardioversion	Digitalis to control ventricular rate, verapamil	Propranolol may help slow ventricular rate; quinidine, disopyramide, or procainamide may be used for long-term suppression
Atrial flutter	Cardioversion	Digitalis, verapamil	Same as atrial fibrillation
Supraventricular tachycardia, paroxysmal atrial tachycardia (PAT)	Vagotonic	Digitalis, propranolol, edrophonium, verapamil	Choice of therapy depends on cardiac status during the arrhythmia; cardioversion is effective when necessary
Ventricular arrhythmias			
Ventricular premature contractions (VPB, VPC)	Lidocaine	Procainamide, others	Reduce lidocaine dosage in heart failure; quinidine, procainamide, disopyramide, propranolol, or phenytoin for prolonged suppression
Ventricular tachycardia	Cardioversion	Lidocaine, procainamide, bretylium	Same as VPC
Ventricular fibrillation	Cardioversion	Never drugs	Cardiopulmonary resuscitation essential
Digitalis-induced tachyarrhythmias	Phenytoin or lidocaine, KCl, verapamil	Procainamide, propranolol	Self-limited if short-acting digitalis stopped; avoid cardioversion; propranolol and procainamide can make heart block worse

Modified from *Medical Letter* 25:630, 1983.

rine, it should not be used in digitalis-induced arrhythmias.

CALCIUM CHANNEL BLOCKING AGENTS (VERAPAMIL).
Verapamil blocks activated and inactivated calcium channels, has marked effects on SA and AV nodes, and decreases oscillatory afterpotential resulting from digitalis toxicity. Its negative inotropic effects may lead to complete AV block (treatable with atropine, beta-adrenergic stimulants, or Ca^{2+}). It causes peripheral vasodilatation (beneficial in hypertension). Verapamil is extensively metabolized and should be used with caution in hepatic dysfunction.

Verapamil is indicated in reentrant supraventricular tachycardia (the drug is fast replacing propranolol, digoxin, edrophonium, and cardioversion) and in atrial fibrillation and flutter [2].

NEWER ANTIDYSRHYTHMIC DRUGS.
Mexiletine is comparable to procainamide and has efficacy against ventricular dysrhythmias of diverse etiology, especially myocardial infarction.

Tocainide, an analogue of lidocaine, is effective in suppressing chronic ventricular ectopy.

Encainide slows conduction in the His-Purkinje fibers selectively and is effective against ventricular ectopy [6].

MANAGEMENT OF BRADYDYSRHYTHMIAS AND CONDUCTION DISTURBANCES.
Epinephrine and isoproterenol (beta-adrenergic stimulants) may be used in severe bradycardia, heart block, and cardiac arrest. In addition, atropine (a cholinergic blocking agent) is used in sinus bradycardia and heart block. The treatment of common dysrhythmias is summarized in Table 16-2.

QUESTIONS ON ANTIDYSRHYTHMIC DRUGS

Select one answer that best completes the statement or answers the question.

____ 151. Quinidine (Quinora) is contraindicated in digoxin-induced arrhythmias because:
  A. It decreases the excretion of digoxin.
  B. It displaces digoxin from the binding site.
  C. It decreases the metabolism of digoxin.

D. It possesses positive inotropic effects that will aggravate the arrhythmias.

_____ 152. Bretylium (Bretylol) is contraindicated in digitalis-induced arrhythmias because:
A. It releases norepinephrine, complicating the management.
B. It aggravates the digitalis-induced hypokalemia state.
C. It increases oscillatory afterpotential.
D. It shortens the $t_{1/2}$ of digitalis.

_____ 153. Which one of the following pairs of drugs has been known to cause lupus syndrome?
A. Procainamide (Pronestyl) and hydralazine (Apresoline).
B. Lidocaine (Xylocaine) and phenytoin (Dilantin).
C. Propranolol (Inderal) and disopyramide (Norpace).
D. Guanethidine (Ismelin) and reserpine (Serpasil).

_____ 154. Which of the following antiarrhythmic drugs does *not* reduce automaticity?
A. Quinidine (Quinora).
B. Lidocaine (Xylocaine).
C. Propranolol (Inderal).
D. Digoxin.

_____ 155. Which one of the following antiarrhythmic agents does *not* alter the function of the autonomic nervous system?
A. Quinidine (Quinora).
B. Phenytoin (Dilantin).
C. Propranolol (Inderal).
D. Procainamide (Pronestyl).

_____ 156. Which one of the following antiarrhythmic drugs would *not* be contraindicated in glaucoma, theoretically or therapeutically?
A. Procainamide (Pronestyl).
B. Quinidine (Quinora).
C. Propranolol (Inderal).
D. Disopyramide (Norpace).

_____ 157. Prior to converting established atrial tachycardia to sinus rhythm with quinidine (Quinora), the patient should be treated with anticoagulants:
A. To prevent pulmonary embolism.
B. To protect against enhanced cardiac output causing hemostatic problems.
C. To prevent aggravation of renal dysfunction and hematuria.
D. To safeguard against pronounced hypotensive effect.

_____ 158. Antiarrhythmic drugs should be used very *cautiously, gingerly,* and *prudently* in third-degree heart block, because these agents:
A. Decrease automaticity in ectopic pacemakers.
B. Reduce conduction velocity.
C. Have negative inotropic effect.
D. Are cardiac depressants.

_____ 159. Which one of the following combinations relating to drug and disease is a mismatch?
A. Bretylium (Bretylol)—refractory arrhythmia.
B. Verapamil (Isoptin)—reentrant supraventricular tachycardia.
C. Atropine—bradyarrhythmias.
D. Pindolol—ventricular fibrillation.

_____ 160. In management of arrhythmia associated with myocardial infarction, the first antiarrhythmic of choice is:
A. Lidocaine, double intravenous bolus followed by continuous infusion.
B. Bretylium orally.
C. Quinidine intravenously.
D. Propranolol orally.

ANSWERS ON ANTIDYSRHYTHMIC DRUGS

151. B.
152. A.
153. A.
154. D.
155. B.
156. C.
157. A.
158. A.
159. D.
160. A.

REFERENCES

1. Bigger, J. T., Jr., and Hoffman, B. F. Antiarrhythmic Drugs. In A. G. Gilman, L. S. Goodman, and A. Gilman (eds.), *The Pharmacological Basis of Therapeutics* (6th ed.). New York: Macmillan, 1980. Pp. 761–792.
2. Comess, K. A., and Fenster, P. E. Calcium Channel Blocking Agents. In G. A. Ewy and R. Bressler (eds.), *Cardiovascular Drugs and the Management of Heart Disease.* New York: Raven, 1982. Pp. 179–190.
3. Dalske, F. *Review of Concepts in Cardiovascular Pharmacology.* Omaha: University of Nebraska, 1979.
4. Ewy, G. A. Supraventricular Tachycardias: Diagnosis and Management. In G. A. Ewy and R. Bressler (eds.), *Cardiovascular Drugs and the Management of Heart Disease.* New York: Raven, 1982. Pp. 395–413.
5. Fenster, P. E. Clinical Use of Antidysrhythmic Agents: Procainamide, Quinidine, Disopyramide. In G. A. Ewy and R. Bressler (eds.), *Cardiovascular Drugs and the Management of Heart Disease.* New York: Raven, 1982. Pp. 115–130.
6. Fenster, P. E., Comess, K. A., and Hanson, C. D. Newer Antidysrhythmic Drugs: Mexiletine, Tocainide and Encainide. In G. A. Ewy and R. Bressler (eds.), *Cardiovascular Drugs and the Management of Heart Disease.* New York: Raven, 1982. Pp. 131–146.
7. Sellers, E. M., Sunahara, F. A., and Piafsky, K. M. Antiarrhythmic Drugs. In P. Seeman, E. M. Sellers, and W. H. E. Roschlau (eds.), *Principles of Medical Pharmacology* (3rd ed.). Toronto: University of Toronto, 1980. Pp. 311–320.
8. Temkin, L. P. Lidocaine. In G. A. Ewy and R. Bressler (eds.), *Cardiovascular Drugs and the Management of Heart Disease.* New York: Raven, 1982. Pp. 103–114.

17. Diuretics

No wind favors him who has no destined port.

Michel de Montaigne

The volume and composition of urine are controlled by the kidneys. The governing factors include the following [4]:

Glomerular filtration, which is influenced by hydrostatic pressure applied and by the size of soluble molecules filtered. The glomerular filtration rate (GFR) may be influenced by blood pressure and renal blood flow. Filtration will cease when the mean blood pressure falls below 40 mm Hg. Furthermore, nephrotoxic substances such as aminoglycoside antibiotics (kanamycin or gentamicin) may reduce glomerular filtration rate.
Renal tubular resorption. Agents such as glucose and sodium are actively transported whereas lipid-soluble materials undergo simple passive diffusion.
Renal tubular secretion. Organic acids and bases and some drugs are eliminated by active processes of tubular secretion.

The major portions of sodium and water in the glomerular filtrate are resorbed in the nephron tubules. The filtered load of sodium is the product of its concentration in the filtrate times the glomerular filtration rate. Thus,

Filtered load = plasma concentration × GFR

The amount of sodium excreted in the urine is equal to the filtered load minus the amount resorbed in the tubules. The fractions of various substances filtered and resorbed in 24 hours are as follows:

Substances Undergoing Glomerular Filtration	Percent Resorbed
Sodium ion	99.4
Chloride ion	99.2
Bicarbonate ion	100.0
Urea	53.0
Glucose	100.0
Hydrogen ion	99.4
Potassium ion	100.0
H_2O	99.4

It is apparent that from approximately 180 liters of fluid undergoing glomerular filtration only 1 liter is not resorbed. The resorption of water from the tubule follows passively the resorption of sodium in the proximal tubule. Therefore, the tubular fluid is still isotonic with blood as it enters the loop of Henle. Within the medulla, however, a countercurrent exchange takes place so that the osmolarity of the tubular fluid changes. In the descending limb, the filtrate becomes more hypertonic, trying to establish equilibrium with the surrounding hypertonic interstitial fluid. The interstitial fluid becomes hypertonic because chloride and sodium are actively transported out of the thick ascending limb of the loop of Henle

to the surrounding tissue, while water is unable to follow because the entire ascending limb is impermeable to water. This property of the ascending limb of the loop of Henle (allowing the removal of Na^+ and Cl^- from the tubular filtrate, but not water) is an essential part of the renal mechanism for producing either a dilute or a concentrated urine.

The distal tubule and collecting duct are permeable to water only in the presence of antidiuretic hormone (ADH) (vasopressin). Consequently, when ADH is in abundance, water is resorbed from the collecting duct as it passes through the hyperosmolar interstitium of the medulla, and a low-volume, concentrated urine is formed. Without ADH, on the other hand, water cannot get through the walls of the collecting ducts and hence a large volume of dilute urine is produced, since the intratubular fluid became hyposmolar in the ascending limb of the loop of Henle.

The following data show the effect of vasopressin (ADH) on urine composition, assuming an osmotic load of 700 mOsm per day and a GFR of 125 ml per minute [2]:

	Maximal ADH Present	Urine Isotonic to Plasma	Patients with Diabetes Insipidus
Percentage of filtered water that is resorbed	99.7	98.7	88.0
Daily volume (liters) of urine produced	0.5	2.4	23.3
Concentration of solutes in urine (mOsm/liter)	1,400	290	30
Free water produced (liters/day)	−1.9	0	20.9

Major groups of diuretics and their sites of action are summarized in Table 17-1.

THIAZIDE DIURETICS. These agents are also called sulfonamide or benzothiadiazide diuretics (Fig. 17-1). The potency of hydrochlorothiazide (Hydrodiuril, Esidrix) is 10 times greater than that of chlorothiazide (Diuril), but the two drugs have equal efficacy. The duration of action of hydrochlorothiazide is equal to that of chlorothiazide—6 to 12 hours. On the other hand, chlorthalidone (Regroton) has a duration of action of 48 hours. Some thiazide derivatives inhibit carbonic anhydrase, which is unrelated to their diuretic activity. They cause moderate loss of sodium (5–10% of filtered load), chloride, and water.

Table 17-1. *Sites of Action of Diuretics*

Drug	Site of Action
Sulfonamide diuretics Hydrochlorothiazide Chlorthalidone	Thick ascending limb (cortical) of loop of Henle or distal tubule
Loop diuretics Furosemide Ethacrynic acid	Thick ascending limb (medullary) of loop of Henle
Potassium-sparing diuretics Spironolactone (Aldactone) Triamterene Amiloride	Distal tubules
Uricosuric diuretics Tienilic acid	Thick ascending limb (cortical) of loop of Henle
Osmotic diuretics Urea Mannitol	Proximal tubules, descending limb of loop of Henle, and collecting tubule
Carbonic anhydrase inhibitors Acetazolamide Ethoxzolamide Dichlorphenamide	Proximal tubules

From K. A. Conrad, Diuretics. In G. A. Ewy and R. Bressler (eds.), *Cardiovascular Drugs and the Management of Heart Disease.* New York: Raven, 1982.

The clearance of free water is impaired. They may cause metabolic alkalosis (resorption of bicarbonate and loss of hydrogen ions), hyperuricemia (enhanced resorption), and hyperglycemia (inhibit insulin release directly and because of hypokalemia).

Uses. EDEMA. Thiazide diuretics are used in edema of cardiac and gastrointestinal origin, causing a state of intravascular volume depletion. This depleted intravascular volume will be replenished from the interstitial (edematous) sites. Therefore, the thiazide diuretics should not be administered too frequently. For example, hydrochlorothiazide is given every other day, whereas chlorthalidone is given once every 2 to 3 days [3].

ESSENTIAL HYPERTENSION. Thiazide diuretics are extremely effective in small doses in essential hypertension. They exert their effects initially by volume depletion and then by reduction of peripheral resistance and sensitivity of vascular receptor sites to catecholamine. In addition, thiazide diuretics are used in conjunction with antihypertensive medications.

IDIOPATHIC HYPERCALCIURIA. Thiazides decrease urinary calcium (diminished glomerular filtration) and enhance urinary magnesium.

NEPHROGENIC DIABETES INSIPIDUS. In patients with diabetes insipidus, large amounts of free water are eliminated. Thiazide diuretics reduce free water formation [4].

Adverse Effects and Precautions. The loss of potassium can produce hypokalemia, which is particularly dangerous to patients receiving digitalis since it increases the risk of arrhythmias. Hypokalemia can be countered either by giving a K^+ supplement (KCl) or by concurrent use of a potassium-sparing diuretic, but not both measures because hyperkalemia would result. Hyperglycemia is a potential hazard for patients with diabetes mellitus. Hyperuricemia can produce an acute attack of gout, usually only in patients who already have gout or a propensity toward it. Since thiazides can cause a decrease in GFR, they should not be used in patients whose renal function is less than one-third of normal. The thiazide-induced hypercalcemia should be kept in mind in conditions such as malignancies or hyperparathyroidism in which hypercalcemia may exist [3].

LOOP DIURETICS. The major loop diuretics are furosemide (Lasix) and ethacrynic acid (Edecrin).

Furosemide is chemically related to the thiazide diuretics, but ethacrynic acid is not. These agents inhibit the active resorption of chloride (and sodium) in the thick, ascending, medullary portion of the loop of Henle and also in the cortical portion of the loop or the distal tubule. The diuresis, similar to that seen with the thiazides, causes predominantly a loss of Cl^-, Na^+, and K^+, but HCO_3 excretion is not increased. Although large volumes of fluid can be excreted, the ability of the kidney to produce either a dilute or a concentrated urine is greatly diminished. These agents are the most efficacious of diuretics now in use, usually causing loss of about 20 percent of filtered load of Na^+ (furosemide: 15–30%; ethacrynic acid: 17–23%).

Loop diuretics are ordinarily used orally but can be given intravenously for a very rapid onset of action, as in combinations of antihypertensive medications used in hypertensive crisis. Furosemide and ethacrynic acid undergo some active renal tubular secretion, as well as glomerular filtration. A minor portion is excreted by the liver.

Fig. 17-1. *The structures of selected diuretics.*

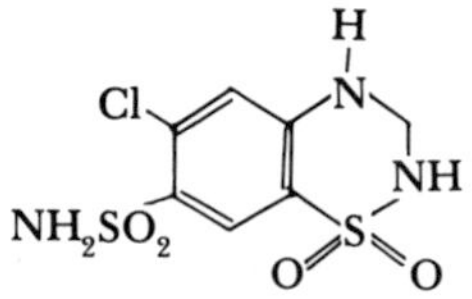

Hydrochlorothiazide

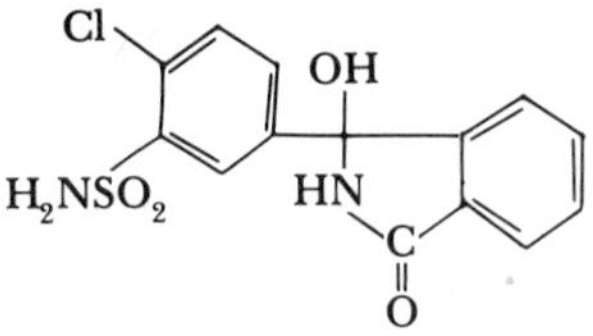

Chlorthalidone

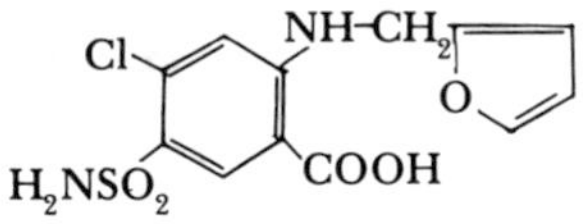

Furosemide

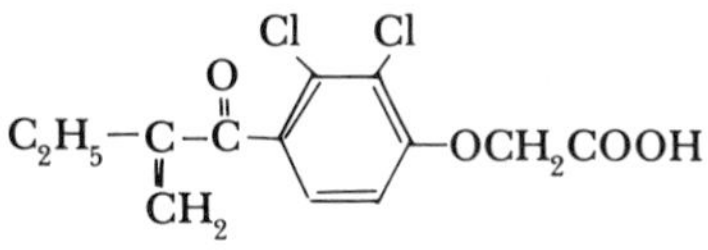

Ethacrynic acid

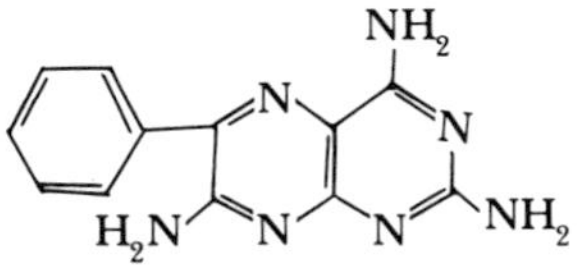

Triamterene

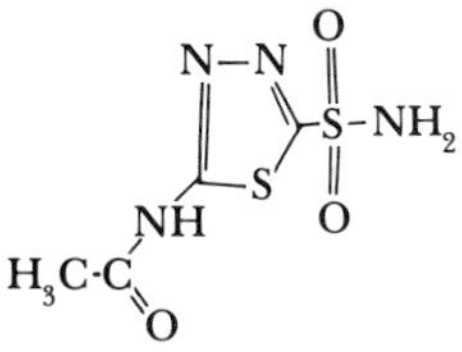

Acetazolamide

Uses. Loop diuretics are used in the following circumstances:

In edema of cardiac, hepatic, or renal origin, including acute pulmonary edema and hypertensive crisis.
In acute renal failure, to maintain urine flow. However, excessive loss of extracellular fluid volume can cause a decrease in GFR.
In treatment of hypercalcemia.

Adverse Effects and Precautions. In using loop diuretics, excessive volume depletion, hyponatremia, and hypotension are major risks. The side effects of hypokalemia, hyperuricemia, and hyperglycemia are ever present. Loop diuretics should not be used concurrently with ototoxic aminoglycoside antibiotics (e.g., streptomycin, gentamicin, kanamycin, tobramycin).

POTASSIUM-SPARING DIURETICS. Spironolactone (Aldactone) is an aldosterone antagonist.

Triamterene (Dyrenium) and amiloride (Midamor) exert their effects by a mechanism other than mineralocorticoid action.

All act in the distal tubule where resorption of Na^+ is accompanied by transfer of K^+ into the lumen contents. When resorption of Na^+ is hindered, excretion of K^+ is correspondingly reduced—i.e., more potassium is retained. The potassium-sparing diuretics are not very efficacious since they affect only 1 to 2 percent of filtered load of Na^+. All are given orally and eliminated in the urine, mostly by glomerular filtra-

tion, though some active tubular secretion may also occur.

Uses. A potassium-sparing diuretic may be concurrently given with a thiazide or a loop diuretic to prevent hypokalemia. Furthermore, spironolactone can be helpful in some patients with severe congestive heart failure or cirrhosis associated with ascites.

Adverse Reactions and Cautions. These agents should not be used concurrently with potassium supplements because the combination is likely to produce hyperkalemia. Poor renal function increases the risk of hyperkalemia. Gastrointestinal disturbances, rash, drowsiness, or dizziness can occur. Spironolactone can cause an elevation of blood urea nitrogen and menstrual irregularities.

URICOSURIC DIURETICS. Tienilic acid (Ticrynafen) is chemically related to ethacrynic acid, but pharmacologically it resembles the thiazide diuretics. Tienilic acid is as efficacious as hydrochlorothiazide but is superior in enhancing uric acid excretion, which is a problem with most effective diuretics [3]. The usefulness of this agent in medicine awaits confirmation.

OSMOTIC DIURETICS AND RELATED AGENTS. These drugs are mannitol (Osmitrol), urea (Urevert), glycerin (Glyrol, Osmoglyn), and isosorbide (Hydronol).

Mannitol and urea are nonelectrolytes that are freely filtrable and undergo very little or no metabolism or renal tubular resorption. Given in sufficient quantity, these drugs increase the osmolarity of plasma, the glomerular filtrate, and renal tubular fluid. The presence of such a drug in the lumen prevents the resorption of much of the water; hence urine volume is increased. Active resorption of sodium from the tubular fluid is not prevented, but some additional sodium is excreted as a normal constituent of the increased volume of urine. Osmotic diuretics are not effective in removing edematous fluid caused by sodium retention but are capable of maintaining the flow of urine even when the glomerular filtration rate is decreased. Osmotic diuretics are given by intravenous infusion (in a hypertonic solution), and they are excreted by glomerular filtration.

Uses. These agents may be used in any of the following conditions:

Congestive glaucoma, to reduce intraocular pressure
Neurosurgery, to reduce the pressure and volume of cerebral spinal fluid and hence decrease intracranial pressure
Acute renal failure, to maintain urine flow
Drug poisoning, to prevent nephrotoxicity

They should not be used in edematous states associated with diminished cardiac reserve, since any increase in extracellular fluid volume constitutes a hazard.

CARBONIC ANHYDRASE (CA) INHIBITORS.
These agents are acetazolamide (Diamox), ethoxzolamide (Cardrase), and dichlorphenamide (Daranide).

Acetazolamide is an old agent whereas ethoxzolamide and dichlorphenamide are newer preparations. Dichlorphenamide is the most potent carbonic anhydrase inhibitor in use today. The presence of the SO_2NH_2 (sulfonamide) causes such compounds to inhibit the enzyme carbonic anhydrase that catalyzes the hydration of carbon dioxide:

$$CO_2 + H_2O \xrightarrow{\text{CA}} H_2CO_3 \rightleftharpoons H^+ + HCO_3^-$$

These agents inhibit carbonic anhydrase in renal tubular cells in both proximal and distal tubules. When the rate of H^+ generation is reduced, HCO_3^- is lost in urine, and the patient tends to become acidotic. However, the plasma concentration of HCO_3^- is lowered, less is filtered, and the diuresis therefore becomes less effective. In addition, the sodium output is increased because its resorption in exchange for H^+ is limited by the decreased availability of H^+. With less H^+ available, the exchange of Na^+ for K^+ predominates, so the loss of K^+ is fostered. Chloride excretion is not altered significantly. Since aqueous humor has a high concentration of bicarbonate, carbonic anhydrase inhibitors are primarily used in

glaucoma. They are no longer used as diuretics or as antiepileptic agents [3, 4].

QUESTIONS ON DIURETICS

Select one answer that best completes the statement or answers the question.

____ 161. Thiazide diuretics may be used to treat all of the following conditions *except* which one?
  A. Hyperglycemia.
  B. Hypercalciuria.
  C. Hypertension.
  D. Nephrogenic diabetes insipidus.

____ 162. Which one of the following statements is *not* true about osmotic diuretics?
  A. They are used in glaucoma.
  B. They are used in neurosurgery.
  C. They are used in drug poisoning.
  D. They are resorbed extensively in the tubules.

____ 163. Which one of the following statements is *not* correct about triamterene?
  A. It is a potassium-sparing diuretic.
  B. It is used along with thiazide diuretics.
  C. Its effects are similar to those of amiloride.
  D. Its saluretic effect is greater than that of thiazides.

____ 164. Which one of the following statements is *not* correct about furosemide and ethacrynic acid?
  A. They are chemically related.
  B. They are the most efficacious diuretics in use today.
  C. They are active both orally and intravenously.
  D. They are able to decrease free water formation.

____ 165. Which one of the following statements is *false* about furosemide?
  A. It increases the excretion of sodium, chloride, and water.
  B. It increases the excretion of potassium.
  C. It increases the excretion of uric acid.
  D. It may have to be used in conjunction with diazoxide in hypertensive crisis.

____ 166. Which one of the following statements is *not* correct about chlorothiazide?
  A. It decreases free water formation.
  B. It is used in diabetes insipidus.
  C. It causes hypokalemia, hypercalcemia, and hyperuricemia.
  D. It causes severe hypoglycemia, since it is structurally related to sulfonylurea, an oral antidiabetic agent.

ANSWERS AND EXPLANATION ON DIURETICS

161. A.
162. D.
163. D.
164. A.
165. C.
  Explanation: Diazoxide may cause retention of water and salt. Occasionally, diazoxide may have to be combined with a diuretic such as furosemide in the management of hypertensive crisis.
166. D.

REFERENCES

1. Conrad, K. A. Diuretics. In G. A. Ewy and R. Bressler (eds.), *Cardiovascular Drugs and the Management of Heart Disease.* New York: Raven, 1982. Pp. 77–85.
2. Ganong, W. F. *Review of Medical Physiology* (7th ed.). Los Altos, Calif.: Lange, 1975.
3. Marquez-Julio, A. Diuretics. In P. Seeman, E. M. Sellers, and W. H. E. Roschlau (eds.), *Principles of Medical Pharmacology* (3rd ed.). Toronto: University of Toronto, 1980. Pp. 373–381.
4. Mudge, G. H. Drugs Affecting Renal Function and Electrolyte Metabolism. In A. G. Gilman, L. S. Goodman, and A. Gilman (eds.), *The Pharmacological Basis of Therapeutics.* New York: Macmillan, 1980. Pp. 885–915.

18. Antihypertensive Medications

The way to gain a good reputation is to endeavor to be what you desire to appear.

Socrates

Hypertension is defined as a condition of sustained elevated blood pressure. Hypertensive disease is a most serious affliction, producing premature sickness, disability, and death in the adult population. Furthermore, the hypertension-related morbidity and mortality are directly related to the level of blood pressure [10].

Since the blood pressure increases with age, the younger the patient is at the onset of hypertension, the shorter the life expectancy. In general, male patients show greater risk than female patients, and the incidence of hypertension in blacks is higher than in white populations [6].

Sustained elevated blood pressure may damage any organ, but especially the blood vessels of the heart, brain, eye, and kidney. In general, a direct relationship seems to exist between the extent of damage to these target organs and the cardiovascular mortality. Even minimally detectable damage increases risk threefold. Cigarette smoking, obesity, certain metabolic abnormalities (hyperlipidemia, diabetes), and life stresses also increase the risk of clinical disease. A history of relatively early death from a hypertensive complication (stroke, renal failure, or congestive heart failure) in a parent or sibling makes it more likely that a patient's own hypertension will progress to a more severe stage.

Hypertension may be caused by known factors such as Cushing's syndrome, pheochromocytoma, primary aldosteronism, trauma, tumor, aortic coarctation, and toxemia of pregnancy, to name only a few conditions. These conditions, most of which may be treated surgically, account for only 10 percent of all hypertensive patients. The other 90 percent fall into the category of essential or primary hypertension [11].

Primary arterial (essential) hypertension remains a vascular disorder of complex etiology. Available evidence indicates that neurogenic, endocrine, renal, vascular, hormonal, and probably other mechanisms, not yet identified, contribute to it. Since the precise etiology of primary arterial hypertension is unknown, current therapy is both empiric and nonspecific. Specific and curative therapy will become available only when its cause is discovered or the importance of each contributing factor is defined [11].

Although not entirely satisfactorily, in general, the severity of hypertension as a disease is judged by the degree of blood pressure according to the following classification:

Hypertension	BP (mm Hg)
Labile, borderline	140/90
Mild	140/90–160/100
Moderate	160/100–200/120
Severe	> 200/120
Malignant	Diastolic > 130
Crisis	*Rapid* rise to malignant levels

It would appear prudent to monitor carefully patients whose resting recumbent blood pressures repeatedly exceed 140/90 mm Hg, and to begin treatment when the resting diastolic pressure rises consistently to 95 mm Hg. Furthermore, it should be stated that the treatment of a young patient for life for a symptomless but ravaging disease requires understanding and compliance from the patient and caring and education from the physician. The full comprehension of a refined therapeutic regimen and judicious use of antihypertensive medications can enhance the quality and extent of life in a hypertensive patient.

STEPPED-CARE PROGRAM. In clinical practice, the treatment of hypertension involves a stepped-care program [13], which may consist in using several drugs sequentially in a predetermined regimen to be modified on a regular basis as clinical judgment dictates (Table 18-1).

The antihypertensive agents (Fig. 18-1) are classified according to their nature or site of action [2].

1. Diuretics
   Thiazide (like) diuretics
   Potassium-sparing diuretics
   Loop diuretics
2. Vasodilators
   Arteriolar
      Hydralazine
      Diazoxide
      Minoxidil
   Arteriolar and venular
      Nitroprusside
      Prazosin
3. Alpha-adrenergic blocking agent
   Phenoxybenzamine
4. Beta-adrenergic blocking agents
   Propranolol
   Nadolol
   Metoprolol

Table 18-1. *Management of Essential Hypertension by Antihypertensive Medications in a Sequential Care Program*

Stage one	Diuretics may be initiated in older patients whereas younger patients may receive beta-adrenergic blocking agents. The diuretic to be tried is thiazide or chlorthalidone. In renal insufficiency or diabetes mellitus, furosemide is appropriate.
Stage two	When a diuretic or a beta blocker given individually is ineffective, they should be used in combination.
Stage three	In addition to a diuretic and a beta blocker, a vasodilator (hydralazine) is used. If hydralazine is ineffective, minoxidil may be tried.
Stage four	Guanethidine may be added to the regimen discussed in stage three.

Modified from M. A. Weber and J. I. M. Drayer. Considerations in the Pharmacological Treatment of Hypertension. In G. A. Ewy and R. Bressler (eds.), *Cardiovascular Drugs and the Management of Heart Disease.* New York: Raven, 1982.

5. Adrenergic neuronal blocking agents
   Reserpine
   Guanethidine
6. Central depressants of sympathetic functions
   Alpha-methyldopa
   Clonidine
7. Ganglionic blocking agent
   Trimethaphan
8. Drugs that interfere with the renin-angiotensin system
   Saralasin
   Captopril

MAINTENANCE OF NORMAL BLOOD PRESSURE. Arterial blood pressure (BP) is proportional to the product of cardiac output (CO) multiplied by peripheral vascular resistance (PVR):

$$BP = CO \times PVR$$

The anatomic sites maintaining blood pressure are the heart, the kidney (regulating intravascular volume), the arterioles, and the capacitance vessels. The baroreceptors modulated by sympathomimetic amines in combination with renin-directed angiotensin also participate to maintain normal blood pressure (Fig. 18-2).

Antihypertensive medications (1) reduce the activities of peripheral and central sympathetic systems, (2) reduce peripheral vascular resistance, (3) interfere with renin-mediated angiotensin production, and (4) cause sodium and volume depletion [3, 5, 8, 9].

PHARMACOLOGY OF ANTIHYPERTENSIVE MEDICATIONS. Thiazide Diuretics. In addition to being safe antihypertensive medications themselves, thiazide diuretics potentiate the effects of other med-

ications used in essential hypertension. Furthermore, many antihypertensive medications retain Na^+ and water, and this side effect is reversed by diuretics. Consequently, thiazide diuretics are widely used in the treatment of hypertension, often as a first drug. The initial effect is diuresis, causing reduced blood volume, cardiac output, and blood pressure. The long-term effect is due to a direct action on the vascular wall, causing a reduction in total peripheral resistance and blood pressure. Because of loss of sodium, the vascular smooth muscle becomes less responsive to vasopressors such as angiotensin II and norepinephrine [2].

Thiazides have no effect on neurotransmission or central vasomotor reflexes and do not cause postural hypotension. The side effects are hyperglycemia, hyperuricemia, and hypokalemia.

Arteriolar and Venular Vasodilators. HYDRALAZINE (APRESOLINE). Hydralazine is the most often used drug in moderate to severe hypertension. The fall in total peripheral resistance causes reflex elevation of heart rate and an enhanced cardiac output. This cardiac acceleration, which may precipitate an anginal attack in susceptible individuals, can be blocked with beta-adrenergic blocking agents. Propranolol also has a synergistic effect in reducing blood pressure. The adverse effects of hydralazine include headache, palpitation, and gastrointestinal effects. Chronic administration of large doses causes a reversible lupus erythematosus–like syndrome. Hydralazine does not alter sympathetic functions.

DIAZOXIDE (HYPERSTAT). Diazoxide, which is administered intravenously, is used exclusively in malignant hypertension or hypertensive crisis. Diazoxide causes reflex cardiac acceleration and increased cardiac output. In addition, it results in hyperglycemia due to inhibition of insulin release from the beta cells. Since diazoxide causes sodium and water retention, it should be given with a diuretic such as furosemide or ethacrynic acid.

MINOXIDIL (LONITEN). Minoxidil, which is effective orally, is indicated in patients with severe hypertension who have become refractory or have not responded to other drugs. The side effects of minoxidil include sodium retention (controlled with a diuretic), tachycardia (controlled by a beta blocker), and pronounced hypertrichosis (may be used in alopecia).

NITROPRUSSIDE (NIPRIDE). Nitroprusside is used exclusively in malignant hypertension and hypertensive crisis. Like diazoxide, nitroprusside is a vasodilator and has been used effectively for acute myocardial infarction and in patients with chronic refractory heart failure. Nitroprusside is given by infusion, and its blood pressure–lowering effect is directly related to the rate of administration. On discontinuation, the blood pressure rises rapidly. In patients with rhodanase deficiency, lethal cyanide poisoning may occur, and in patients with renal failure, thiocyanate may accumulate, inhibiting iodine uptake and causing hypothyroidism.

PRAZOSIN (MINIPRESS). Prazosin is indicated in mild to severe hypertension. It is a direct vasodilator used

Fig. 18-1. *The structures of a few antihypertensive medications.*

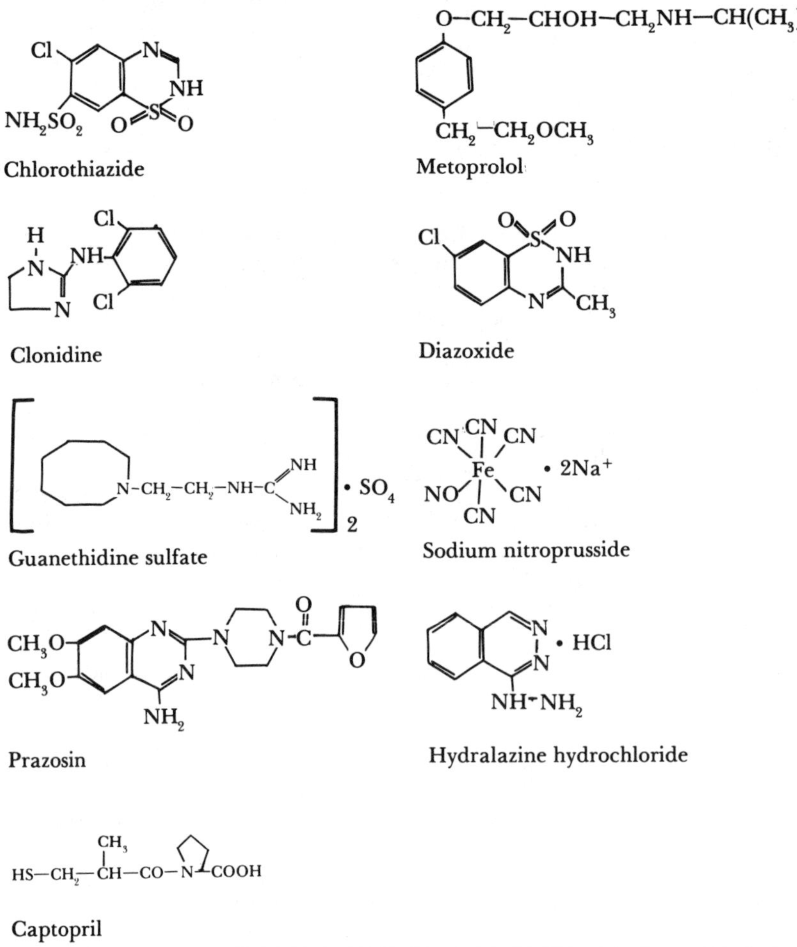

Chlorothiazide

Metoprolol

Clonidine

Diazoxide

Guanethidine sulfate

Sodium nitroprusside

Prazosin

Hydralazine hydrochloride

Captopril

in chronic therapy. The side effects are sedation, postural hypotension, and headache (due to vasodilatation). Prazosin is bound to plasma protein to the extent of 97 percent. When used for the first time or in larger than recommended doses, prazosin may cause pronounced hypotension, faintness, dizziness, and palpitation. These effects, which have been labeled "first-dose phenomenon," are seen especially in salt- and water-depleted patients. Therefore, the first dose of prazosin is given at bedtime and is small.

Alpha-Adrenergic Blocking Drugs. Alpha-adrenergic blocking drugs such as phenoxybenzamine cause too many side effects and relatively few beneficial effects to be useful in the routine treatment of hypertension. The alpha-adrenergic blocking drugs may be used during the removal of an adrenal medullary tumor, particularly when a beta blocker is employed to prevent cardiac arrhythmias. Manipulation of the tumor results in the release of norepinephrine and epinephrine, which produce excessive hypertension in the presence of a beta blocker, hence necessitating the administration of an alpha blocker.

Beta-Adrenergic Blocking Agents—Propranolol (Inderal) and Metoprolol (Lopressor). In the treat-ment of hypertension, a major use of the beta blockers is in combination with hydralazine. The direct vasodilators bring about reflex cardiac stimulation, and the beta blockers prevent these adverse effects. Beta blockers also reduce blood pressure by a central effect or a peripheral action (or both) to decrease renin activity. Metoprolol and atenolol are beta$_1$ selective, and they are safer agents in patients with asthma, diabetes mellitus, and low-renin hypertension. Some beta blocking agents such as pindolol have intrinsic sympathomimetic activity and may be used in pronounced bradycardia (sick sinus syndrome). Unlike propranolol, metoprolol is not a very lipid-soluble substance, does not enter the brain, and does not cause CNS toxicity.

Adrenergic Neuronal Blocking Drugs. RESERPINE (SERPASIL). Reserpine depletes catecholamine peripherally and centrally. Sympathetic reflexes are attenuated but not abolished. Reserpine is useful in mild to moderate hypertension. The onset of action is very slow (2–3 weeks) when it is given orally. Cholinergic hyperactivity such as diarrhea, bradycardia, and nasal stuffiness is a side effect of reserpine. Reserpine can activate peptic ulcer (cholinergic dominance) and cause depression (deplete norepinephrine). Reser-

Fig. 18-2. *Factors and drugs involved in maintaining and controlling blood pressure. (Modified and combined from N. L. Benowitz and H. R. Bourne, Antihypertensive Agents. In B. G. Katzung [ed.],* Basic and Clinical Pharmacology. *Los Altos, Calif.: Lange, 1982; and B. R. Rubin and M. J. Antonaccio, Captopril. In A. Scriabine [ed.],* Pharmacology of Antihypertensive Drugs. *New York: Raven, 1980.)*

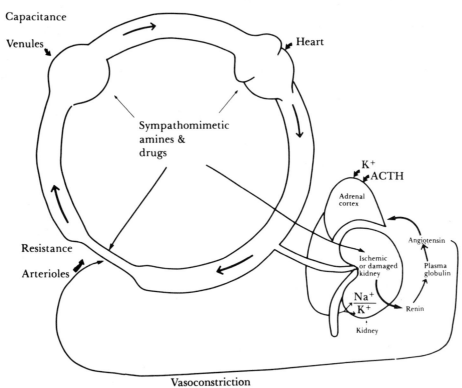

pine and propranolol have potential cardiac depressant activity and should not be used together.

GUANETHIDINE (ISMELIN). Guanethidine is the most potent drug in the management of moderate to severe hypertension. Its onset of action is slow. The effects of guanethidine on the adrenergic neuron include the following:

A transient rise in blood pressure (resembles amphetamine and tyramine)

Interference with conduction of nerve impulses and neurally mediated catecholamine release (resembles bretylium)

Catecholamine depletion (resembles reserpine)

Blockade of neuronal catecholamine uptake (resembles cocaine and tricyclic antidepressants)

Guanethidine abolishes sympathetic reflexes. Postural hypotension occurs frequently, as does impotence. Reserpine does not have this effect to so great an extent. Guanethidine and reserpine display the consequences of reduced sympathetic activity such as diarrhea, bradycardia, and nasal stuffiness (cholinergic predominance). Unlike reserpine, guanethidine does not cross the blood-brain barrier and does not cause sedation and depression. Reserpine does.

Central Depressants of Sympathetic Functions. AL-PHA-METHYLDOPA (ALDOMET). Alpha-methyldopa is used in mild to severe hypertension. It is converted to alpha-methylnorepinephrine, whose main hypotensive effect is due to stimulation of presynaptic alpha₂-adrenergic receptors, causing a reduction in release of norepinephrine. In addition, it reduces the peripheral vascular resistance without any alteration in the heart rate or cardiac output. Postural hypotension is mild and infrequent. The drug causes sedation, and tolerance develops to it. It causes a positive Coombs' test (25%). Alpha-methyldopa has a long onset and short duration of action. It is useful especially in hypertension complicated by renal dysfunction, since renal blood flow and glomerular filtration rate remain unaltered. It is contraindicated in liver disease and may produce hepatitislike symptoms.

CLONIDINE (CATAPRES). Clonidine is used in mild to severe hypertension. Like alpha-methyldopa, it reduces sympathetic outflow centrally, has a vagotonic effect, and enhances sensitivity to carotid sinus stimulation. Heart rate and cardiac output are lowered. Abrupt withdrawal causes a rapid rise in blood pressure (rebound hypertension), which may require treatment with alpha- and beta-adrenergic blocking agents, or by reinstatement of clonidine itself.

Ganglionic Blocking Agents. A ganglionic blocking agent such as trimethaphan reduces blood pressure, particularly in the standing position, causing orthostatic hypotension. In addition, it causes parasympathetic ganglionic blockade. Trimethaphan is used as an infusion in hypertensive crisis.

Captopril. Captopril (Capoten) is active in most forms of hypertension except aldosteronism. It inhibits the conversion of angiotensin I to angiotensin II, hence reducing the synthesis of a potent vasoconstrictor. It also inhibits the metabolism of bradykinin, enhancing the function of a vasodilating substance [7].

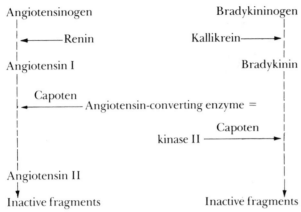

The pharmacology of antihypertensive agents most often used is summarized in Table 18-2.

HYPERTENSION IN THE ELDERLY. Treating hypertension in elderly patients requires different approaches from those appropriate for younger ones. Elderly patients, in general, have more advanced atherosclerosis, more evidence of ongoing cardiovascular abnormalities, increased alpha-adrenergic response to sympathetic stimulation, decreased beta-adrenergic response to sympathetic stimulation, increased total peripheral resistance, increased variability of blood pressure, and lower plasma renin activity [13].

The elderly patient may also manifest altered pharmacokinetic parameters such as altered drug distribution, impaired hepatic metabolism, decreased biliary excretion, decreased renal clearance and excretion, and increased susceptibility to drug interactions [13].

QUESTIONS ON ANTIHYPERTENSIVE MEDICATIONS

Answer questions 167 and 168 by using the following key: Select one answer to which *all* of the stated characteristics apply. No answer applies more than once.
    A. Reserpine.
    B. Alpha-methyldopa.
    C. Clonidine.
    D. Guanethidine.
    E. None of the above.
____ 167. Causes central alpha receptor stimulation; is contraindicated in liver and kidney diseases; should never be withdrawn abruptly.
____ 168. Depletes norepinephrine; has slow onset of action; has postural hypotension and impotence as prominent side effects.
Answer questions 169 and 170 by using the following key: Select one answer to which *all* of the stated characteristics

apply. No answer applies more than once.
    A. Hydralazine.
    B. Diazoxide.
    C. Nitroprusside.
    D. Trimethaphan.
    E. None of the above.
____ 169. Causes reflex cardiac stimulation; given by bolus injection; used with loop diuretic.
____ 170. Given by intravenous infusion; does not cause reflex increase in cardiac output; is light sensitive.
Answer questions 171–177 by selecting one answer that best completes the statement or answers the question.
____ 171. Which one of the following statements or indicated therapy is mismatched with drug or situation?
    A. Norepinephrine reduction in action and in level—occurs with clonidine, alpha-methyldopa, prazosin.
    B. Vasodilation—occurs with hydralazine, diazoxide, and nitroprusside.
    C. Diazoxide—may necessitate the use of furosemide.
    D. Propranolol and metoprolol—have essentially the same mechanism of action as guanethidine and reserpine.
____ 172. The reason thiazide diuretics such as hydrochlorothiazide or chlorthalidone are used extensively in the treatment of hypertension deals with the fact that they:
    A. Have antihypertensive action themselves.
    B. Potentiate the antihypertensive effects of other drugs.
    C. Negate the Na^+ retaining of vasodilators.
    D. All of the above.
____ 173. Which one of the following statements is *false*?
    A. Saralasin or captopril inhibits angiotensin synthesis or blocks its receptors.
    B. Minoxidil is used in refractory hypertension.
    C. Diazoxide and nitroprusside are used in hypertensive crisis.
    D. Methyldopa and hydralazine cause reduced renal blood flow.
____ 174. Which properties do thiazides and propranolol have in common when either is used chronically in hypertension?
    A. Both cause hypokalemia, hyperglycemia, and hyperuricemia.
    B. Both cause CNS lethargy and nightmares.
    C. Both down regulate ("reset") autoregulatory mechanisms, maintaining total peripheral resistance (TPR).
    D. Both are contraindicated in gout and asthma.
____ 175. In a chronic propranolol-treated patient, propranolol should be withdrawn slowly or gradually, because sudden propranolol withdrawal may:
    A. Precipitate angina pectoris.
    B. Cause myocardial infarction.
    C. Cause beta receptor up regulation.
    D. All of the above.
____ 176. Initially in managing a hypertensive patient with drugs using an "innovative" versus a "classic" approach:
    A. The older patients may be treated with a diuretic whereas the younger patients may be treated with a beta blocker.

Table 18-2. *Summary Pharmacology of Select Antihypertensive Medications*

	Indications	Mechanism of Action	Side Effects	Cautions or Contraindications	Comments
Thiazide diuretics	Alone—mild Combination—all forms except crisis	Volume depletion ↓ TPR	Hypokalemia Hyperglycemia Hyperuricemia	Acute gout	Potentiates other HBP medications No postural hypotension
Reserpine	Mild to moderate	NE depletion	Sedation Nasal congestion ↑ GI activity	Depression Peptic ulcer Propranolol R_x	Slow onset—weeks
Alpha-methyldopa (Aldomet)	Mild to severe	Reduces sympathetic outflow centrally (stimulating α_2)	Sedation Dry mouth Diarrhea	Liver disease	Short duration of action Wide dose range Maintains renal blood flow
Clonidine (Catapres)	Mild to severe	Reduces sympathetic outflow centrally	Sedation Dry mouth	Abrupt withdrawal Rebound hypertension	Tolerance Short duration of action
Prazosin (Minipress)	Mild to severe	Vasodilation	Sedation Postural hypotension	First-dose effect	Wide dose range Plasma protein binding
Propranolol (Inderal), metoprolol (Lopressor)	Mild to severe	β-blockade	Bronchospasm Cardiac depression Nightmares	Diabetes CHF Asthma	Slow withdrawal Wide dose range
Hydralazine (Apresoline)	Moderate to severe	Vasodilation	Cardiac stimulation Headache N and V	Angina	Short duration of action Maintains renal blood flow Lupus syndrome
Guanethidine (Ismelin)	Moderate to severe	NE depletion	Postural hypotension Impotence Diarrhea	Pheochromocytoma Cerebral or coronary insufficiency Propranolol R_x	Slow onset—days Drug interactions
Diazoxide (Hyperstat)	Crisis	Vasodilation	Salt retention Cardiac stimulation Hyperglycemia	Aortic aneurysm Cerebral or coronary insufficiency	IV push preferable Alkaline solution 3–12 hours duration Loop diuretic
Nitroprusside (Nipride)	Crisis	Vasodilation		Hypothyroidism Renal impairment	IV drip or infusion pump Constant BP monitoring Protect from light
Trimethaphan (Arfonad)	Crisis	Ganglionic blockade	Paralytic ileus Bladder atony	Renal impairment Preeclampsia	IV drip or infusion pump Postural changes helpful Supersensitivity

From F. Dalske, *Review of Concepts in Cardiovascular Pharmacology.* Omaha: University of Nebraska, 1979.

B. Treat all patients with a long-acting diuretic.
C. Treat all patients with a vasodilator that increases cardiac output so that left ventricle failure can be avoided.
D. None of the above.

____ 177. Metoprolol and atenolol are selective $beta_1$-adrenergic receptor blockers whereas propranolol is a nonselective $beta_1$- and $beta_2$-adrenergic receptor blocker. In using them, one should recall that:
A. The receptor selectivity is only relative in nature and in high doses $beta_1$ blockers also block $beta_2$ receptor sites.
B. The durations of action of propranolol and metoprolol are identical.
C. The CNS side effects of propranolol and metoprolol are identical.
D. The beta blockers are especially useful in digitalis-induced toxicity producing complete AV block.

ANSWERS ON ANTIHYPERTENSIVE MEDICATIONS

167. C.
168. D.
169. B.
170. C.
171. D.
172. D.
173. D.
174. C.
175. D.
176. A.
177. A.

REFERENCES

1. Benowitz, N. L., and Bourne, H. R. Antihypertensive Agents. In B. G. Katzung (ed.), *Basic and Clinical Pharmacology*. Los Altos, Calif.: Lange, 1982. P. 22.
2. Blaschke, T. F., and Melman, K. L. Antihypertensive Agents and the Drug Therapy of Hypertension. In A. G. Gilman, L. S. Goodman, and A. Gilman (eds.), *The Pharmacological Basis of Therapeutics* (6th ed.). New York: Macmillan, 1980. Pp. 793–818.
3. Buckley, J. P., and Ferrario, C. M. *Central Nervous System Mechanisms in Hypertension*. New York: Raven, 1981.
4. Dalske, R. *Review of Concepts in Cardiovascular Pharmacology*. Omaha: University of Nebraska, 1979.
5. Fregly, M. J., and Kare, M. R. *The Role of Salt in Cardiovascular Hypertension*. New York: Academic, 1982.
6. Onesti, G., and Kim, K. E. *Hypertension in the Young and the Old*. New York: Grune & Stratton, 1980.
7. Rubin, B. R., and Antonaccio, M. J. Captopril. In A. Scriabine (ed.), *Pharmacology of Antihypertensive Drugs*. New York: Raven, 1980. Pp. 21–42.
8. Scriabine, A. (ed.). *Pharmacology of Antihypertensive Drugs*. New York: Raven, 1980.
9. Scriabine, A., and Sweet, C. S. *New Antihypertensive Drugs*. New York: Spectrum, 1976.
10. Shepherd, J. T., and Vanhoutte, P. M. *The Human Cardiovascular System. Facts and Concepts*. New York: Raven, 1979.
11. Tuttle, E. P. Etiology and Pathogenesis of Systemic Hypertension. In J. W. Hurst et al. (eds.), *The Heart* (3rd ed.). New York: McGraw-Hill, 1974. Pp. 1164–1174.
12. Vanhoutte, P. M., and Leusen, I. *Vasodilatation*. New York: Raven, 1981.
13. Weber, M. A., and Drayer, J. I. M. Considerations in the Pharmacological Treatment of Hypertension. In G. A. Ewy and R. Bressler (eds.), *Cardiovascular Drugs and the Management of Heart Disease*. New York: Raven, 1982. Pp. 635–645.

19. Antianginal Drugs

Fame is the perfume of heroic deeds.

Socrates

Angina pectoris (strangulation, squeezing, and crushing of the chest) results primarily from coronary atherosclerosis, but also to a certain extent from coronary arthritis, fibromuscular hyperplasia of the coronary arteries, aortic valve disease (stenosis and regurgitation), idiopathic hypertrophic subaortic stenosis (obstructive cardiomyopathy), and mitral stenosis.

Myocardial ischemia may produce vasoactive substances, metabolic abnormalities, electrical instability, and ECG abnormalities (predisposing, but not necessarily leading, to ventricular arrhythmias), malfunctioning of the left ventricle, and always pain, which may be localized in the substernal area or become diffuse, radiating to the left shoulder and ulnar aspect of the left arm and hand. In addition to pain, anxiety, feeling of impending death, shortness of breath, diaphoresis, nausea and vomiting, and fainting may take place. Angina may occur during work and heavy physical exertion or during rest and sleep (angina decubitus). In either case, the signs and symptoms are identical [1, 4].

OXYGEN DEMAND OF THE HEART.
Unlike the skeletal muscle, in which anaerobic metabolism (conversion of pyruvic acid into lactic acid) usually accounts for 40 percent of the energy produced, the cardiac muscle predominantly employs aerobic metabolism (conversion of pyruvic acid to CO_2 and H_2O), and anaerobic metabolism is utilized only in extreme hypoxia. By adjustment of cardiac output, the heart constantly attempts to provide sufficient oxygen to the tissue to prevent hypoxia. The oxygen demand of the tissues changes from time to time and even from moment to moment. If the deficient supply of oxygen to a portion of the heart is permanent, necrosis will develop and myocardial infarction occurs. If the deficiency of oxygen is temporary, painful coronary insufficiency takes place and the patient is said to have suffered from an attack of angina pectoris. The factors (Fig. 19-1) that increase the oxygen demand of the heart are heart rate, contractile state, and wall tension.

The faster the heart beats, the more oxygen it utilizes. The larger the heart is, the more oxygen is required for its contraction. The greater the force of myocardial contraction, the higher the amount of oxygen consumed. Agents effective in the management of angina pectoris work by reducing oxygen demand and not by increasing oxygen supply. In order to increase the supply of oxygen, one must increase coronary blood flow and enhance AV oxygen difference. Since normally the heart extracts a great deal of oxygen from the blood, AV oxygen differences may not be augmented. Similarly, during myocardial ischemia, the blood vessels are dilated fully. Moreover, the atherosclerotic plaque may not allow further dilatation beyond that induced by ischemia. Useful pharmacologic agents therefore exert their beneficial effects in part by reducing oxygen consumption and largely by reducing the heart rate and relaxing vascular smooth muscles [3, 5].

ANTIANGINAL AGENTS. Nitrates and Nitrites.
The mechanism of therapeutic actions of nitrates and nitrites may be explained by their ability to relax vascular smooth muscle and consequently reduce cardiac preload and afterload.

CARDIAC HEMODYNAMICS. These agents cause arterial dilatation, reducing blood pressure and the work of the heart. They also cause venous dilatation, decreasing the venous return and ventricular volume, which in turn diminishes wall tension. The consequence of these events is a reduction in the work of the heart. Decreasing the blood pressure increases the heart rate by activation of carotid sinus reflexes. However, the extent of the reduction in wall tension is a greater beneficial factor than the elevated heart rate. The net effect is a reduction in the work of the heart. Furthermore, the nitrate-induced tachycardia may be blocked by administration of propranolol, a beta-adrenergic receptor blocking agent.

CORONARY CIRCULATION. Collateral vessels are silent blood vessels that become functional in hypoxic emergencies. By dilating, they allow greater blood flow to the ischemic areas. This effect of nitrate, which is greater than that produced by dipyridamole, seems to be potentiated by propranolol when it is used in combination with nitrates.

SMOOTH MUSCLE. Nitrites and nitrates dilate all smooth muscles. By dilating the cutaneous blood vessels, they cause blushing. By dilating the cerebral vessels, they cause headache. The appearance of headache and blushing are indications of the efficacy of these medications.

PHARMACOKINETICS. These agents are best absorbed through the mucous membrane of the mouth and the nose. Therefore, they are usually administered sublingually or buccally. Similarly, they may be inhaled. By these routes of administration the active ingredient is absorbed into the venous circulation, and by way of the vena cava it reaches the heart, aorta, and coronary arteries. If these agents are given orally, they will be metabolized to inactive compounds by nitrate reductase in the liver.

Fig. 19-1. *Relation between factors increasing myocardial oxygen supply and demand. (Concept patterned after B. Pitt, Physiology and Pathophysiology of the Coronary Circulation and the Role of Nitroglycerin. In P. Needleman [ed.], Organic Nitrates. Berlin: Springer-Verlag, 1975.)*

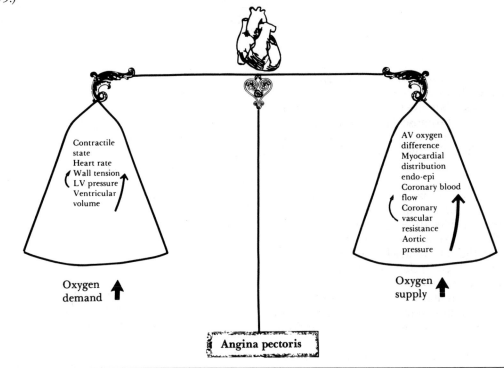

PHARMACOLOGIC PREPARATIONS. AMYL NITRITE.

$$CH_3 \diagdown$$
$$\diagup CH - CH_2 - CH_2 - NO_2$$
$$CH_3 \diagup$$

Amyl nitrite is a highly volatile liquid, sold in fragile glass ampules packaged in a protective cloth covering. The ampule can be crushed, resulting in rapid release of inhalable vapors. Amyl nitrite has a rapid onset of action and a duration of action of 8 to 10 minutes. The pronounced vasodilatation causes tachycardia, enhanced cardiac output, and vasoconstriction. Amyl nitrite is no longer used for angina.

NITROGLYCERIN.

$$CH_2 - O - NO_2$$
$$|$$
$$CH - O - NO_2$$
$$|$$
$$CH_2 - O - NO_2$$

Nitroglycerin dilates coronary arteries rapidly (1–2 minutes), but the duration of coronary dilatation is shorter than the duration of antianginal effects (30 minutes). In addition to coronary arteries, nitroglycerin dilates blood vessels in bronchi, the uterus, and the gastrointestinal tract. It has a pronounced effect on meningeal vessels. Flushing and headache are common.

Nitroglycerin may be provided continuously for 24 hours by a transdermal therapeutic system called Transderm-Nitro. This system releases 5 to 10 mg of nitroglycerin over 24 hours. Nitroglycerin is absorbed through the skin into the systemic circulation. The beneficial effect is apparent 30 minutes after the application of the pad and is terminated 30 minutes after its removal. Therefore, sublingual nitroglycerin should be used for an immediate effect followed by Transderm-Nitro as a prophylactic measure.

NITROGLYCERIN OINTMENT. Nitroglycerin may be applied topically (2% nitroglycerin ointment). Its hemodynamic and beneficial effects are apparent as early as 15 minutes and last up to 4 hours. Nitroglycerin ointment may be especially useful for angina decubitus, which may develop 3 hours after sleep.

ORAL NITRATES (ISOSORBIDE DINITRATES). Due to the first-pass effect, the orally administered nitrates such as isosorbide dinitrate will be effective only when given in large doses (30–40 mg q.i.d.). Isosorbide is effective in low doses (5 mg) when given sublingually.

Nonnitrate Coronary Vasodilators. DIPYRIDAMOLE (PERSANTINE). Dipyridamole, with a pharmacologic action similar to that of papaverine, is used only as a prophylactic measure and is not effective during an acute attack of angina. In contrast to nitroglycerin, dipyridamole dilates small resistance vessels (but not conducting or collateral vessels) by inhibiting the uptake and inactivation of adenosine, an effective coronary vasodilator. Dipyridamole also inhibits platelet aggregation [2].

Calcium Channel Blocking Agents. NIFEDIPINE (PROCARDIA). Nifedipine is absorbed orally or buccally. By

Table 19-1. *Synergistic Action of Propranolol and Nitrates in Angina Pectoris*

Physiologic Effect	Nitroglycerin	Propranolol	Combined Propranolol and Nitroglycerin
Heart rate	Increased	Decreased	No change
Blood pressure	Decreased	Decreased	Decreased
Left ventricle size	Decreased	Increased	No change
Myocardial oxygen consumption	Decreased	Decreased	Decreased substantially

its negative inotropic effect, by reducing afterload, and by dilating coronary arteries, nifedipine decreases oxygen consumption. Nifedipine is thought to be effective especially in angina caused by coronary artery spasm. In addition to the usual side effects associated with hypotension (headache and flushing), nifedipine may produce sedation and fatigue in some patients. On a rare occasion, by causing severe hypotension (coronary steal syndrome), nifedipine may exacerbate angina.

Beta-Adrenergic Blocking Agents. Beta-adrenergic receptor blocking agents such as propranolol may be used prophylactically in angina. By causing blockade of beta receptors in the heart, propranolol reduces blood pressure, cardiac contractility, cardiac output, and oxygen consumption. It should be recalled that propranolol is a cardiac depressant, and its injudicious use may lead to congestive heart failure. Propranolol is also frequently combined with nitrates to combat nitrate-induced reflex tachycardia. These synergistic effects are depicted in Table 19-1.

QUESTIONS ON ANTIANGINAL DRUGS

Select one answer that best completes the statement or answers the question.

____ 178. In long treatment of patients with angina pectoris, which of the following interventions may be necessary?
A. Correct hypertension.
B. Correct hyperthyroidism.
C. Correct hyperlipidemia.
D. Correct all of the above.

____ 179. Following administration of nitroglycerin, the change in cardiac hemodynamics is characterized by:
A. Venous dilation $->$ ↑ venous return $->$ ↑ ventricular volume $->$ ↑ wall tension
B. Constriction of collateral vessels.
C. Shifting the blood away from ischemic areas.
D. Arterial dilation $->$ ↓ BP $->$ ↓ work of the heart.

____ 180. One reason nitroglycerin and propranolol have low bioavailability following oral administration is that they are rapidly:
A. Protein bound.
B. Excreted unchanged.
C. Deposited in adipose tissue.
D. Metabolized.

____ 181. Transderm-Nitro is contraindicated in:
A. Stable angina.

B. Effort angina.
C. Variant angina.
D. Elevated ocular pressure and CSF pressure.

____ 182. Slow channel Ca^{2+} blocking agents may be used in all of the following *except* which one?
A. Hypertension.
B. Angina.
C. Arrhythmias.
D. Congestive heart failure.

____ 183. Propranolol (Inderal) is used in conjunction with nitroglycerin:
A. To block excess tachycardia.
B. To augment collateral circulation.
C. To reduce oxygen consumption.
D. All of the above.

ANSWERS AND EXPLANATION ON ANTIANGINAL DRUGS

178. D.
179. D.
180. D.
181. D.
Explanation: Substances causing vasodilatation such as nitrites and morphine increase the cerebrospinal fluid pressure. Therefore, they should be used cautiously in cases in which the cerebrospinal pressure is already high.
182. D.
183. D.

REFERENCES

1. Hurst, I. W., and Logue, R. B. The Clinical Recognition and Medical Management of Coronary Atherosclerotic Heart Disease. In I. W. Hurst et al. (eds.), *The Heart* (3rd ed.). New York: McGraw-Hill, 1974. Pp. 1038–1132.
2. MacLeod, S. M., and Zsoter, T. T. Antianginal Drugs. In P. Seeman, E. M. Sellers, and W. H. E. Roschlau (eds.), *Principles of Medical Pharmacology* (3rd ed.). Toronto: University of Toronto, 1980. Pp. 343–349.
3. Pitt, B. Physiology and Pathophysiology of the Coronary Circulation and the Role of Nitroglycerin. In P. Needleman (ed.), *Organic Nitrates*. Berlin: Springer-Verlag, 1975. Pp. 115–130.
4. Rubin, I. L., Gross, H., and Arbeit, S. R. *The Treatment of Heart Disease in the Adult*. Philadelphia: Lea & Febiger, 1972. Pp. 1–52.
5. Sonnenblick, E. H., and Skelton, C. L. Oxygen consumption of the heart: Physiologic principles and clinical implications. *Mod. Concepts Cardiovasc. Dis.* 40:9, 1971.

20. Anticoagulants

> The creation of a thousand forests is in one acorn.
> *Ralph Waldo Emerson*

The clotting of blood, which protects against hemorrhage, involves the sequential initiation, interaction, and completion of several stages in hemostasis. These are listed in Table 20-1. The adhesion and aggregation of platelets is mediated through release of ADP. Extensive numbers of pharmacologic agents such as acetylsalicylic acid, indomethacin, phenylbutazone, sulfinpyrazone, and dipyridamole inhibit platelet aggregation, inhibit thrombus formation, and may be of value in thrombotic disorders [3, 4]. The formation of fibrin itself takes place via a cascading group of reactions [2] involving numerous blood-clotting factors and taking place in several stages (Table 20-2).

Hemorrhage may result from (1) abnormalities or deficiency of platelets (thrombocytopenic purpuras), (2) deficiency of clotting factors (factors II, VII, IX, and X), (3) vitamin K deficiency (necessary to synthesize clotting factors), and (4) liver diseases in which clotting factors are synthesized. Increased clotting may take place in (1) thrombosis (enhanced formation of fibrin), (2) stasis and phlebitis (diminished circulation), and (3) embolism (dislocation and lodging of blood clots).

AGENTS USED IN AN IN VITRO SYSTEM.

The anticoagulants used in an in vitro system are oxalate, citrate, fluoride, and Ca^{2+} chelating agents such as EDTA. They chelate the ionic Ca^{2+} and interfere with the clotting mechanism.

HEPARIN. Commercial heparin is a sulfated mucopolysaccharide of repeating units of D-glucosamine, D-glucuronic acid, and L-iduronic acid (Fig. 20-1).

ORAL ANTICOAGULANTS. Coumarin. The coumarin anticoagulants include dicumarol, warfarin sodium (coumadin sodium), warfarin potassium (Athrombin-K), acenocoumarol (Sintrom), and phenprocoumon (Liquamar).

Indandione. The indandione derivatives are phenindione (Danilone, Hedulin, Indone), diphenadione (Dipaxin), and anisindione (Miradon). The pharmacologic properties of oral anticoagulants are identical qualitatively, but they are varied in their pharmacokinetic parameters and in their toxicities. The racemic warfarin sodium is the most widely used anticoagulant.

The comparative pharmacology of heparin and coumarin is shown in Table 20-3.

CAUTIONS AND CONTRAINDICATIONS.

Bleeding. The use of anticoagulants should be contraindicated in the presence of an active hemorrhage, in potential hemorrhage (acid-pepsin disease), and in hemorrhagic disorders (hemophilia).

Trauma. In traumatic injuries to the central nervous system and to the eyes, anticoagulants should be used with extreme caution. It is very difficult to control hemorrhage in these areas.

Table 20-1. *Stages in Hemostasis*

Stage	Initiator	Response or Outcome
Vascular	Tissue injury	Vasoconstriction
Platelet	Adhesion and aggregation	Plug formation
Plasma	Fibrin generation	Coagulation

Table 20-2. *Formation of Fibrin*

Stage	Formation	Needed Factors or Precursors
One	Plasma thromboplastin	Hageman factor (XII), antihemophilic globulin (VIII), Christmas factor (IX), plasma thromboplastin antecedent (PTA [XI]), calcium (IV), and platelet phospholipid
Two	Activated thromboplastin	Tissue thromboplastin (III), Stuart factor (X), proconvertin (VII), and calcium (IV)
Three	Thrombin	Prothrombin (II), proaccelerin (V), calcium (IV), and platelet
Four	Fibrin	Thrombin

Fig. 20-1. *The structures of selected anticoagulants.*

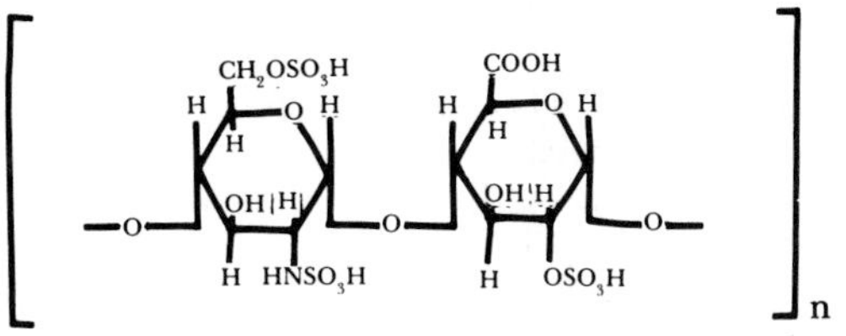

Heparin

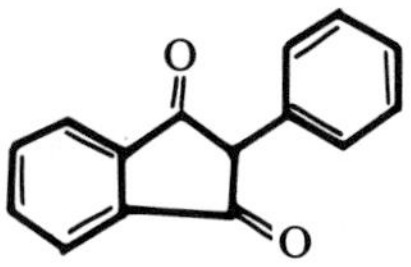

Phenindione

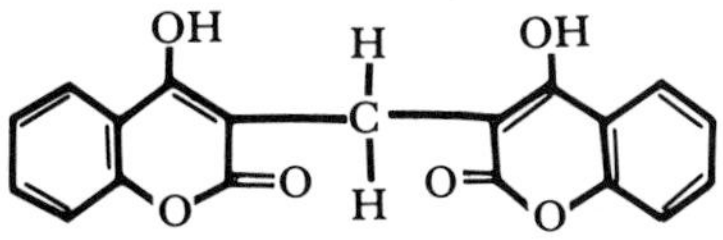

Dicumarol

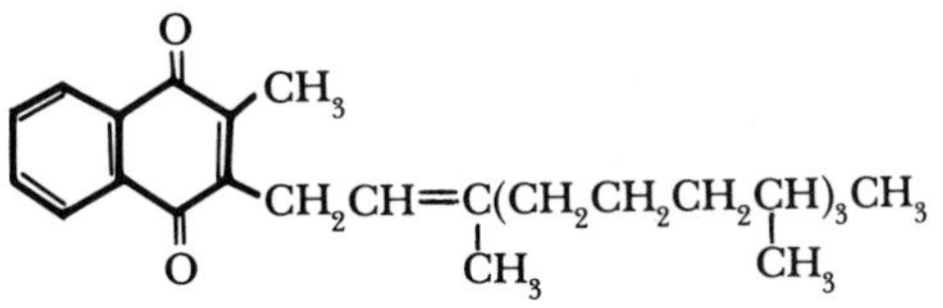

Vitamin K_1

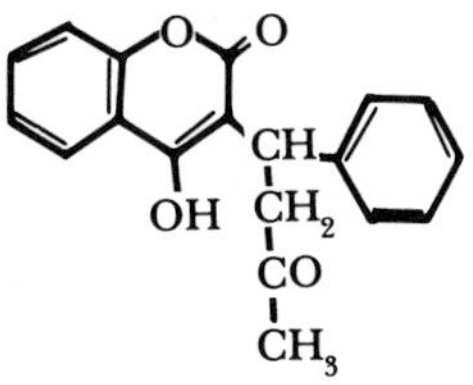

Warfarin

Table 20-3. *Pharmacology of Anticoagulants*

Properties Studied	Heparin	Coumarin
Chemistry	High negative charge	
Occurrence	Naturally occurring	Synthetic
Mechanism of action	Activates plasma antithrombin; blocks thromboplastin generation; neutralizes tissue thromboplastin	Inhibits the synthesis of factors II, VII, IX, and X, by blocking the action of vitamin K
PHARMACOKINETICS		
Route of administration	Subcutaneously Intravenously	Orally
Onset	Minutes (10–20)	48 hours
Duration	4 hours (subcutaneously)	2–10 days
Protein binding and metabolism	In liver by heparinase; inactive metabolite is excreted by the kidney	Bound to albumin (99%) side-chain reduction to alcohol (dextrowarfarin), oxidation to 7-hydroxywarfarin (levowarfarin)
Antagonists	Protamine sulfate, a strongly basic protein, forms complex with heparin to an inactive compound: 1 mg protamine for 100 units of heparin	Vitamin K, whole blood, fresh plasma

From F. Dalske, *Review of Concepts in Cardiovascular Pharmacology.* Omaha: University of Nebraska, 1979.

Pregnancy. Heparin may be used cautiously in pregnancy. Coumarin passes the placental barrier and is teratogenic in nature.

Hypertension. The presence of an aneurysm must be considered in an untreated hypertensive patient.

Hepatic and Renal Failure. Anticoagulants should be monitored carefully in severe hepatic and renal failure, vitamin K deficiency, alcoholism, and arthritis patients taking acetylsalicylic acid in large quantities. Furthermore, it should be recalled that anticoagulants are extensively metabolized and their metabolites excreted.

DRUG-DRUG INTERACTIONS. Interactions of oral anticoagulants with drugs, especially with barbiturates, salicylates, and phenylbutazone, are numerous and at times may become life threatening. All aspects of pharmacokinetics may be involved [4]. A few examples will be cited.

Drugs That Enhance the Response to Oral Anticoagulants.
By displacement of extensively bound anticoagulant from plasma albumin (e.g., chloral hydrate, clofibrate, phenylbutazone)
By inhibition of hepatic microsomal enzymes (e.g., chloramphenicol, clofibrate)
By reduction in the availability of vitamin K (e.g., anabolic steroids, broad-spectrum antibiotics)
By inhibition of clotting factor synthesis (e.g., anabolic steroids, salicylates)

Drugs That Diminish the Response to Oral Anticoagulants.
By inhibition of absorption of anticoagulants (e.g., griseofulvin, clofibrate)
By induction of hepatic microsomal enzymes (e.g., barbiturates, ethchlorvynol, glutethimide)
By stimulation of clotting factor synthesis (e.g., vitamin K)

The aforementioned interactions have not been reported with heparin [4].

USES OF ANTICOAGULANTS. Venous Thrombosis. An embolism may travel through the inferior vena cava and through the right heart to lodge eventually in the lung, producing pulmonary embolism. Susceptible patients may be treated prophylactically to diminish venous thrombosis.

Artificial Heart Valve. Foreign surfaces are more prone to clot formation. The newer techniques and materials used in surgery have reduced the use of anticoagulants. However, they may be employed effectively to prevent postsurgical clot formation.

Atrial Fibrillation. In cardiac arrhythmias, when the heart is beating rapidly but inefficiently, the formation of clots in atrial appendages is common. Conversion to normal sinus rhythm may cause the clots to be freed and to lodge in vital organs. Consequently, patients with arrhythmias may be treated with anticoagulants before and after conversion of the arrhythmia to a sinus rhythm.

Prophylaxis. Elderly persons leading a sedentary life or patients confined to bed are more prone to thrombus formation. Other superimposing factors are reduced muscular mass and increased venous tortuosity. Anticoagulant therapy may be used in selected patients.

Certain Elective Surgery. In certain elective surgery of the lower legs and abdomen, heparin may be administered a few hours before surgery and continued for several days postoperatively.

Myocardial Infarction. Minidose heparin (1,500 U subcutaneously) may be indicated in some but not all patients with myocardial infarction.

Fig. 20-2. *Stages of fibrinolysis and the action of epsilon-aminocaproic acid.*

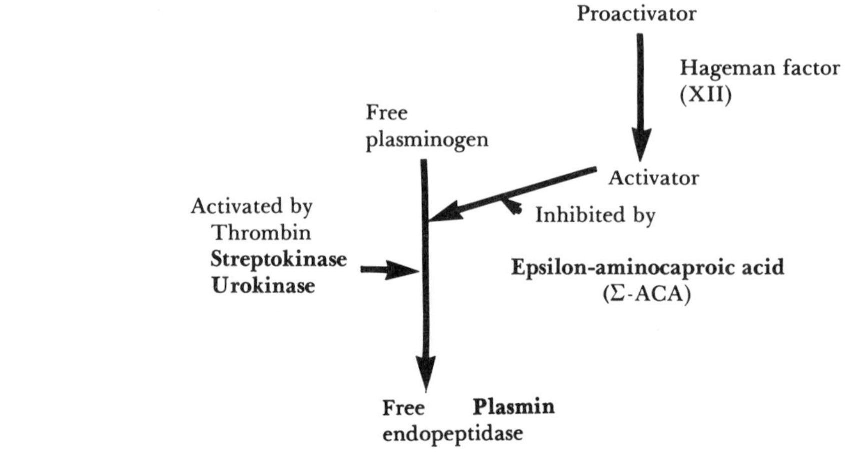

Therapeutic Fibrinolysis. Fibrinolysis takes place according to the scheme depicted in Figure 20-2.

Plasmin, an endopeptidase, hydrolyzes fibrin, fibrinogen, factor V, and factor VIII to their inactive products. Plasminogen is converted to plasmin by an activator. Hageman factor (XII) converts a proactivator to the active activator. Agents such as thrombin, streptokinase, and urokinase enhance the formation of plasmin and hence have fibrinolytic properties. Epsilon-aminocaproic acid (ε-ACA) inhibits the action of activator-mediated formation of plasmin and hence may be used as an antidote to streptokinase-urokinase, or in a defibrination syndrome, where bleeding from mucous membrane occurs (Fig. 20-2).

Streptokinase (Streptase) and Urokinase (Abbokinase). Streptokinase is obtained from group C beta-hemolytic streptococci. Urokinase is obtained from urine. When these agents are used, the degradation of fibrin, fibrinogen, factors V and VII, and hemostatic plugs may cause hemorrhage, especially from sites of trauma and injury. Consequently, anticoagulants should not be concomitantly used with these agents. The effects of streptokinase or urokinase may be antidoted by epsilon-aminocaproic acid.

QUESTIONS ON ANTICOAGULANTS

Select one answer that completes the statement or answers the question.

____ 184. With reference to fibrinolysis, which one of the following pairs have no relationship to each other in therapy?
  A. Streptokinase—plasmin synthesis.
  B. Streptokinase—epsilon-aminocaproic acid.
  C. Plasmin—defibrination syndrome.
  D. Urokinase—heparin.

____ 185. Streptokinase or urokinase is contraindicated in:
  A. Pulmonary embolism.
  B. Thrombophlebitis.
  C. Maintenance of arteriovenous shunt.
  D. Malignancy.

____ 186. Heparin and coumarin differ in each of the following aspects *except* which one?
  A. Onset of action and duration of action.
  B. Mechanism of action.
  C. Antidote required for an overdose.
  D. Use in severe untreated hypertension.

____ 187. As an anticoagulant, aspirin differs from coumarin only in which one of the following aspects?
  A. Mechanism of action.
  B. Being synthetic in nature.
  C. Usage.
  D. Route of administration.

____ 188. The coumarin anticoagulants:
  A. Are frequently involved in drug interactions.
  B. May be used during pregnancy.
  C. Should be monitored closely to detect changes in prothrombin time.
  D. A and B.
  E. A and C.

____ 189. Heparin:
  A. May be used subcutaneously.
  B. May be used during pregnancy.
  C. May be used along with a coumarin anticoagulant.
  D. Can have its toxicity antagonized by protamine.
  E. All of the above.

ANSWERS ON ANTICOAGULANTS

184. D.
185. D.
186. D.
187. A.
188. E.
189. E.

REFERENCES

1. Dalske, F. *Review of Concepts in Cardiovascular Pharmacology.* Omaha: University of Nebraska, 1979.
2. Loomis, T. A. Anticoagulant and Coagulant Drugs. In J. R. DiPalma (ed.), *Drill's Pharmacology in Medicine* (4th ed.). New York: McGraw-Hill, 1971. Pp. 1083–1098.
3. O'Reilly, R. A. Anticoagulant, Antithrombotic, and Thrombolytic Drugs. In A. G. Gilman, L. S. Goodman, and A. Gilman (eds.), *The Pharmacological Basis of Therapeutics* (6th ed.). New York: Macmillan, 1980. Pp. 1347–1366.
4. Roschlau, W. H. E., and Sellers, E. M. Anticoagulants. In P. Seeman, E. M. Sellers, and W. H. E. Roschlau (eds.), *Principles of Medical Pharmacology* (3rd ed.). Toronto: University of Toronto, 1980. Pp. 351–362.

21. Hematinic Drugs

A person who dares to waste one hour of time has not discovered the value of life.

Charles Darwin

Anemia is defined as a reduction in the circulating blood cell mass, which may be expressed as

A reduction in the volume of packed red blood cells per 100 ml (VPRC)
A reduction of blood hemoglobin concentration (BHGC)
A reduction of the red blood cell count (RBC)

The stages of granulocyte development, from differentiation of the hemocytoblast, are basophil erythroblast, polychromatophil erythroblast, normoblast, and erythrocyte. The principal process in differentiation of an erythrocyte is reduction in its size, loss of nucleus and cellular organelles, and acquisition of hemoglobin. The normal development of erythrocytes is dependent upon numerous factors such as hemoglobin (globin, heme, and iron), minerals (iron and cobalt), and vitamins (vitamin B_{12} and folic acid).

CAUSES OF ANEMIA. Anemia may result from excess destruction of erythrocytes, such as those seen in hereditary spherocytosis or congenital hemolytic jaundice, hereditary elliptocytosis, or acanthocytosis—a congenital absence of beta-lipoprotein. In addition, anemia may be caused by deficiencies of key enzymes, such as glucose 6-phosphate dehydrogenase or pyruvate kinase, or by nutritional deficiencies other than those of iron, cobalt, vitamin B_{12}, and folic acid. These anemias may be associated with the following:

Ascorbic acid deficiency (anemia associated with scurvy)
Pyridoxine deficiency (vitamin B_6 is involved in the synthesis of delta-aminolevulinic acid, an intermediate in the biosynthesis of heme
Riboflavin deficiency (glutathione reductase requires riboflavin)
Pantothenic acid (causes normocytic anemia)
Niacin deficiency (normocytic anemia)
Copper deficiency (copper is a cofactor for polyphenol oxidase, tyrosinase, cytochrome oxidase, lactase, and monoamine oxidase; in addition to ceruloplasmin, copper is bound to erythrocuprein)
Zinc deficiency (carbonic anhydrase)

Finally, anemia may result from chronic infection, inflammation, neoplastic disease, and numerous unknown causes (aregenerative anemia) [5].

Part One: Iron-Deficiency Anemia

Iron-deficiency anemias are caused by excessive loss or inadequate intake of iron. In women, menstruation and pregnancy (bleeding and breeding) may increase the requirement for iron. Iron deficiency in men may be due to blood loss secondary to hemorrhage associated with gastric ulcer or neoplasm. In children, iron deficiency is due to nutritionally inadequate diet.

METABOLISM OF IRON. The metabolism of iron is shown in Figure 21-1. In the body, the total content of iron in men and women is 50 and 35 mg per kilogram of body weight, respectively. Of this iron content, approximately 60 percent is associated with the hemoglobin, 13 percent is associated with myoglobin and iron-containing enzymes, and the remaining 27 percent is located in the storage sites. Men and women are different primarily in their storage of iron, which is substantially lower in women because of menstruation. Menstrual losses are increased by the use of intrauterine devices and are decreased when estrogen-containing oral contraceptive medications are used.

Iron is obtained mainly from diet at approximately 12 to 15 mg per day. Under normal circumstances, only 10 percent (1 mg) of ingested iron is absorbed. However, in iron-deficiency anemia, this is increased to about 40 percent. Naturally, the requirement of iron is increased in growth and development, in menstruation, pregnancy, blood donation, and in an extensive number of pathologic conditions causing anemia. Moreover, the chronic ingestion of certain drugs (e.g., aspirin) may alter the daily requirement.

Iron is absorbed better in ferrous Fe^{2+} than in ferric Fe^{3+} form. The extent of absorption of iron from the duodenum is thought to be regulated by mucosal proteins referred to as *mucosal block*. The absorbed iron is stored in mucosal *ferritin* or transported to plasma and bound to *transferrin*. Ordinarily, iron excretion and elimination are regulated to equal the amount of iron absorption. A major portion of iron (> 60%) in the body is collected by bone marrow and incorporated into hemoglobin in erythrocytes (Fig. 21-1). In general, four atoms of iron are incorporated into one molecule of hemoglobin. After the destruction of erythrocytes in 120 days by the reticuloendothelium (RE), the released iron is returned to transferrin and ferritin [1].

Fig. 21-1. *The pharmacokinetics of iron.*

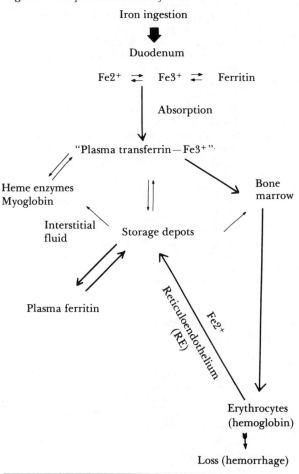

Iron ingestion

Duodenum

$Fe^{2+} \rightleftarrows Fe^{3+} \rightleftarrows$ Ferritin

Absorption

"Plasma transferrin — Fe^{3+}"

Heme enzymes
Myoglobin

Interstitial
fluid

Storage depots

Bone
marrow

Plasma ferritin

Fe^{2+}

Reticuloendothelium
(RE)

Erythrocytes
(hemoglobin)

Loss (hemorrhage)

Fig. 21-2. *The structure of deferoxamine, an iron-chelating agent.*

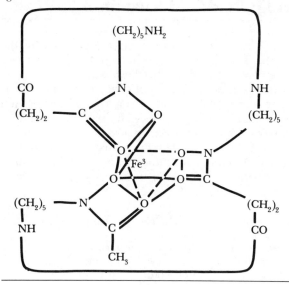

THERAPEUTIC PREPARATIONS OF IRON.

Oral Iron Preparations. Many oral preparations are available. In general, the ferrous salts (ferrous sulfate, ferrous gluconate, ferrous fumarate) are better absorbed than the ferric salts (ferric sulfate). Ferrous calcium citrate is mostly used during pregnancy to provide iron as well as calcium [4].

Parenteral Iron Preparations. The available medications include iron dextran (ferric hydroxide and high-molecular-weight dextran) for intramuscular uses, dextriferron (complex of ferric hydroxide and partially hydrolyzed dextran) for intravenous uses, and saccharated iron oxide (complex of ferric hydroxide and sucrose) for intravenous uses. These preparations are reserved for cases in which oral preparations are not tolerated, are not absorbed, are not rapid in their onset of action as desired for some patients, or are not suitable for unreliable patients.

Iron Toxicity. The lethal dose of iron is 12 gm of iron preparation containing 1 to 2 gm of elemental iron. Therefore, iron toxicity occurs rarely in adults but frequently in children. The mortality among untreated children is high (45%). The initial signs and symptoms of iron poisoning are those of gastrointes-

tinal origin—usually nausea, vomiting, and diarrhea. If the person is untreated, acidosis, cyanosis, and circulatory collapse may ensue. If death does not occur, gastric scarring and pyloric stenosis may result from the corrosive action of iron preparations. Treatment should include vomiting and lavage if the poisoning is discovered early, catharsis to hasten evacuation, $NaHCO_3$ to combat acidosis, and the administration of deferoxamine (Desferal), a specific iron-chelating agent (Fig. 21-2).

A dose of 100 mg of deferoxamine is able to bind 8.5 mg iron. The chelating effects of deferoxamine are maximum at acidic pH. Therefore, when given orally, the administration of deferoxamine must precede the application of $NaHCO_3$. In iron poisoning, deferoxamine may also be administered intramuscularly. In addition to being useful in iron poisoning, deferoxamine has been employed in iron overload such as ocular hemosiderosis or in hemochromatosis.

Part Two: Megaloblastic Anemia, Folic Acid, and Vitamin B$_{12}$

Both vitamin B$_{12}$ and folic acid are essential for the synthesis of DNA, which is impaired in patients with megaloblastic anemia. In the absence of adequate DNA synthesis, cells will not divide but will continue to grow. Megaloblastic anemia may also be associated with neurologic disturbances (paresthesias, diminution of sensation of vibration, loss of memory, confusion, irritability, and psychosis) that are due to deficiency of vitamin B$_{12}$ rather than folic acid. Vitamin B$_{12}$ deficiency may result from many factors including the following:

Failure of secretion of the glycoprotein intrinsic factor of Castle (pernicious anemia)
Absence of intestinal receptor for intrinsic factor
Gastrectomy (achlorhydria and lack of intrinsic factor)
Malabsorption syndrome (idiopathic steatorrhea)
Intestinal parasites (fish tapeworms)
Lack of vitamin B$_{12}$ binding protein in plasma (transcobalamin II, alpha globulin, beta globulin)
Vitamin B$_{12}$ antagonist (antibody to intrinsic factors) [2]

Vitamin B$_{12}$ must be administered parenterally. Folic acid deficiency may result from the following:

Nutritional deficiency
Malabsorption syndrome
Reduced folate binding protein
Folic acid antagonists (e.g., methotrexate)
Drugs reducing the level of folic acid (anticonvulsants, pyrimethamine)
Agents blocking purine synthesis (e.g., mercaptopurine, thioguanine) or pyrimidine synthesis (5-fluorouracil)
Hemolytic diseases (accelerated hematopoiesis)
Proliferative diseases and other conditions [2]

Folic acid is administered orally. It should not be used in pernicious anemia.

QUESTIONS ON HEMATINIC DRUGS

Select one answer that best completes the statement or answers the question.

_____ 190. Which one of the following pairs of agent and drug is improperly matched?
  A. Deferoxamine—Fe^{2+}.
  B. Ceruloplasmin—Cu^{2+}.
  C. Vitamin B$_{12}$—Zn^{2+}.
  D. Isoniazid—pyridoxine.

_____ 191. Which one of the following statements is *not* true?
  A. Iron salts are best absorbed in ferrous form.
  B. Deferoxamine binds iron best in acidic media.
  C. Vitamin B$_{12}$ and folic acid are biochemically interdependent.
  D. For absorption of folic acid, intrinsic factor is required.

_____ 192. One reason pyridoxine (vitamin B$_6$) deficiency causes anemia is the fact that B$_6$ is a coenzyme for which one of the following enzymes?

  A. Glutathione reductase.
  B. Carbonic anhydrase.
  C. Delta-aminolevulinic acid synthetase.
  D. Cytochrome oxidase.

_____ 193. Which one of the following iron salts would be therapeutically most suitable for a pregnant patient?
  A. Ferric sulfate.
  B. Ferrous calcium citrate.
  C. Ferrous sulfate.
  D. Ferrous fumarate.

_____ 194. Which one of the following statements about iron toxicity is *not* correct?
  A. It causes gastric scarring and pyloric stenosis.
  B. It causes circulatory collapse.
  C. It could be antidoted with deferoxamine.
  D. It is disabling, but not fatal.

_____ 195. Vitamin B$_{12}$ deficiency may result from:
  A. Lack of intrinsic factor.
  B. Steatorrhea.
  C. Gastrectomy.
  D. Tapeworm infections.
  E. All of the above.

ANSWERS AND EXPLANATIONS ON HEMATINIC DRUGS

190. C.
  Explanation: Vitamin B$_{12}$ (cyanocobalamin) contains a corrin ring resembling the porphyrin system of hemoglobin (four pyrrole-type rings). Coordinated to the four inner nitrogen atoms of the corrin, one atom of cobalt exists. In addition to a corrin ring, cyanocobalamin also contains an unusual ribonucleotide (5,6-dimethylbenzimidazole in the alpha-*N*-glycosyl linkage with D-ribose) [3].
191. D.
192. C.
  Explanation: Vitamin B$_6$ is involved in the synthesis of delta-aminolevulinic acid, which in turn is a precursor for the synthesis of protoporphyrin.
193. B.
  Explanation: Ferrous calcium citrate provides both calcium and iron.
194. D.
195. E.

REFERENCES

1. Finch, C. A. Drugs Effective in Iron Deficiency and Other Hypochromic Anemias. In A. G. Gilman, L. S. Goodman, and A. Gilman (eds.), *The Pharmacological Basis of Therapeutics* (6th ed.). New York: Macmillan, 1980. Pp. 1315–1330.
2. Hillman, R. S. Vitamin B$_{12}$, Folic Acid, and the Treatment of Megaloblastic Anemias. In A. G. Gilman, L. S. Goodman, and A. Gilman (eds.), *The Pharmacological Basis of Therapeutics* (6th ed.). New York: Macmillan, 1980. Pp. 1347–1366.
3. Lehninger, A. L. *Biochemistry* (2nd ed.). New York: Worth, 1976.
4. Roschlau, W. H. E. Hematinic Drugs. In P. Seeman, E. M. Sellers, and W. H. E. Roschlau (eds.), *Principles of Medical Pharmacology* (3rd ed.). Toronto: University of Toronto, 1980. Pp. 521–526.
5. Wintrobe, M. M., et al. *Clinical Hematology* (8th ed.). Philadelphia: Lea & Febiger, 1981.

22. Lipid-Lowering Agents

Chance favors only the prepared mind.

Louis Pasteur

Lipids, ordinarily water-insoluble substances, may be solubilized by bile and other intestinal contents. In the plasma, lipids interact with proteins to form lipoproteins, in which form major plasma lipids such as cholesterol, triglyceride, and phospholipids are found.

Lipoproteins may be classified according to their physiochemical behaviors during analytical ultracentrifugation (flotation class), preparative ultracentrifugation (density class), or electrophoretic preparation (electrophoretic mobility).

In terms of density as an index for classification of lipoproteins, the following lipoproteins are recognized [2]:

Class	Density
Chylomicrons, very-low-density lipoproteins (VLDL)	< 0.95
Low-density lipoproteins (LDL)	0.95–1.006
High-density lipoproteins (HDL)	1.063–1.21

The lipoprotein composition of each class varies dramatically. For example, the major lipoprotein of the chylomicron is triglyceride whereas the major lipoprotein of LDL is cholesterol (Fig. 22-1).

The dietary triglyceride, cholesterol, and phospholipids (involved in the assemblage of chylomicron particles) enter the plasma via the thoracic duct lymph. The triglyceride is removed by lipases, and cholesterol-rich remnants are then removed by the liver.

In addition to chylomicrons, VLDL also transports triglyceride, which has been synthesized from glucose and short-chain free fatty acids. Lipases remove triglyceride from VLDL, which, after loss of its apoproteins, is transformed into an intermediate lipoprotein form. Further degradation of this intermediate form, largely involving the removal of much of the remaining triglyceride, then leads to the formation of the ultimate remnants of VLDL, low-density lipoprotein. Low-density lipoprotein is probably, perhaps totally, a product of VLDL catabolism [2]. It too is probably ultimately removed by the liver (Fig. 22-2).

Each family of lipoproteins contains apoprotein possessing the following proposed functions:

To interact with lipoprotein receptor sites located on the cell surface

To activate enzymes (lipoprotein lipase) capable of catabolizing lipoproteins [4]

HYPERLIPOPROTEINEMIC STATES. Hyperlipoproteinemic states consist of heterogeneous

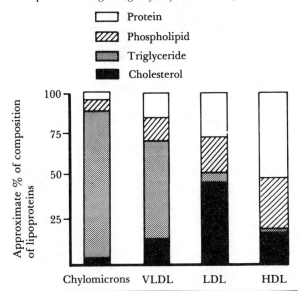

Fig. 22-1. *The composition of plasma lipoprotein. (From R. I. Levy and B. K. Rifkind, Lipid Lowering Drugs and Hyperlipidemia. In G. A. Avery [ed.], Antiarrhythmic, Antihypertensive and Lipid Lowering Drugs. Sydney: Adis, 1977.)*

groups of disorders in which the various lipoproteins exist in excess, resulting from either excess production or reduced destruction according to a classification shown in Table 22-1 [1].

LIPID-LOWERING DRUGS. Cholesterol, essential for the synthesis of adrenal, ovarian, and testicular steroid hormones, originates from two sources. The body synthesizes approximately 2 gm of cholesterol per day. In addition, between 300 and 800 mg of cholesterol is ingested in various diets. Cholesterol is excreted at amounts between 300 and 1,500 mg per day. The treatment of a hyperlipoid state may include (1) reduction in intake of cholesterol, (2) increase in excretion of cholesterol, and (3) reduction in the synthesis of cholesterol [3].

Clofibrate (Atromid S). Clofibrate reduces VLDL, triglyceride, and cholesterol. Clofibrate is thought to inhibit the synthesis of cholesterol by inhibiting the conversion of hydroxymethylglutarate to mevalonic acid, a precursor of cholesterol. The effect is apparent within 2 to 5 days following treatment. The drug is thought to be effective in patients with elevated VLDL, especially those who do not respond to dietary restriction. Clofibrate displaces coumarin and phenytoin from binding sites. Therefore, the pro-

Fig. 22-2. *The metabolism of chylomicrons* (top) *and normal lipoprotein metabolism* (bottom). *(From R. I. Levy and B. K. Rifkind, Lipid Lowering Drugs and Hyperlipidemia. In G. A. Avery* [ed.], Antiarrhythmic, Antihypertensive and Lipid Lowering Drugs. *Sydney: Adis, 1977.)*

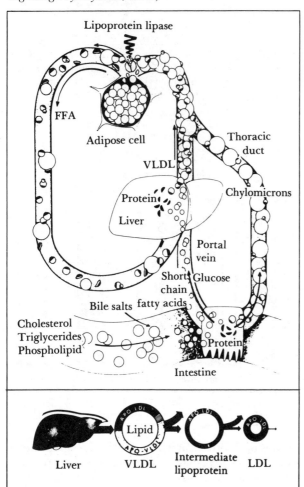

Table 22-1. *Types and Treatment of Hyperlipoproteinemia*

Type	Lipoprotein Increased	Treatment Indicated
I	Chylomicrons	Reduction of dietary fat
IIa	LDL	Cholestyramine, low-cholesterol diet, D-thyroxine
IIb	LDL and VLDL	Reduction of dietary fat, low-cholesterol diet, para-aminosalicylic acid, clofibrate, nicotinic acid
III	Abnormal IDL	Clofibrate, cholestyramine, D-thyroxine, low-cholesterol diet
IV	VLDL	Carbohydrate restriction, low-cholesterol diet, clofibrate
V	Chylomicrons and VLDL	Reduction of dietary fat, carbohydrate restriction, low-cholesterol diet, clofibrate, nicotinic acid

thrombin time should be checked on a regular basis in patients who are taking both clofibrate and coumarin. A flulike syndrome characterized by muscular cramps, tenderness, stiffness, and weakness may occur in some patients.

Cholestyramine (Questran). Cholestyramine is not absorbed. It exerts its effect by binding to bile acids in the intestine and hence eliminating them. In order to replenish the lost bile acid, cholesterol becomes converted to bile acid, and consequently the level of cholesterol is reduced. Cholestyramine has also been used in cholestasis to control intense pruritus. Cholestyramine reduces the level of LDL in 4 to 7 days, and the maximum effect is seen in 14 days.

In addition to binding to bile acid, cholestyramine binds numerous other drugs used for cardiovascular diseases that may be taken concomitantly with cholestyramine. The list includes chlorothiazide, phenylbutazone, phenobarbital, anticoagulants, digitalis, and fat-soluble vitamins (A, D, E, and K). Consequently, these and similar agents should be taken 1 hour before or 4 hours after administration of cholestyramine. Cholestyramine, which is given in large doses of 16 to 30 gm per day, causes severe constipation.

Nicotinic Acid. Nicotinic acid inhibits the release of free fatty acid, resulting in a fall in VLDL and then LDL. Nicotinic acid may cause intense flushing and itching (histamine release and vasodilatation). Tolerance to this effect develops.

Thyroxine (Choloxin). Hypothyroidism is associated with elevated levels of plasma lipids, and the reverse is the case with hyperthyroidism. D-Thyroxine increases the synthesis of cholesterol in the liver but also increases the fecal excretion of cholesterol and the rate of conversion of cholesterol to bile acid. Consequently, the level of LDL is reduced. It should be recalled that the dose of D-thyroxine is 2 to 6 mg. In higher than therapeutic doses, D-thyroxine may produce nervousness and insomnia, precipitate anginal attack, and cause cardiac dysrhythmias.

Probucol (Lorelco). Probucol lowers cholesterol and hence LDL following 1 to 3 months of treatment. It is then indicated in type II hyperlipoproteinemia. The few side effects reported for probucol are transient flatulence and diarrhea.

Beta-Sitosterol (Cytellin). Sitosterol is a plant steroid with a structure similar to that of cholesterol. It is not absorbed and interferes with absorption of cholesterol. Consequently, the level of LDL is reduced.

Another agent with reported hypolipidemic effects is neomycin. Since neomycin is not absorbed, it binds and forms an insoluble complex with bile acids and hence exerts a cholestyraminelike effect.

Para-aminosalicylic acid, an antituberculosis medication, has been reported to reduce both cholesterol and triglyceride. Therefore, by reducing LDL and VLDL, it is thought to be effective in type IIb hyperlipoproteinemia (Table 22-1).

QUESTIONS ON LIPID-LOWERING AGENTS

Select one answer that best completes the statement or answers the question.

_____ 196. Which one of the following is a mismatch between the drug and its properties or use?
   A. Clofibrate—inhibits cholesterol synthesis at a step prior to formation of mevalonic acid.
   B. Cholestyramine—not absorbed, enhances elimination of bile acid, may cause vitamin (A, D, E, K) deficiency.
   C. Nicotinic acid—causes vasodilatation, histamine release.
   D. Sitosterol—inhibits cholesterol synthesis.

_____ 197. Para-aminosalicylic acid is characterized by all the following properties except which one?
   A. It reduces both cholesterol and triglyceride.
   B. It is used by bacteria to synthesize folic acid.
   C. It has antituberculosis properties.
   D. It is contraindicated in patients with impaired renal function.

_____ 198. Which one of the following statements is not true about probucol?
   A. It reduces cholesterol level by inhibiting its synthesis.
   B. It increases the excretion of bile acids in the feces.
   C. It is effective in patients with primary hypercholesterolemia.
   D. It reduces triglyceride level.

_____ 199. Which one of the following statements about clofibrate is not true?
   A. When treating patients with clofibrate and anticoagulants, one should increase the doses of the latter.
   B. It inhibits the synthesis of cholesterol.
   C. It exerts its effect in 2 to 3 days.
   D. It is especially effective in patients with elevated LDL.

_____ 200. When thyroxine is used as a hypolipoproteinemic agent in a patient with coronary heart disease, the concomitant use of which one of the following drugs should concern the internist the least?
   A. Thioridazine (Mellaril).
   B. Amitriptyline (Elavil).
   C. Propranolol (Inderal).
   D. Isoproterenol (Isuprel).
   E. None of the above.

ANSWERS AND EXPLANATIONS ON LIPID-LOWERING AGENTS

196. D (see Adrenal Steroids).
197. B.
   Explanation: Para-aminobenzoic acid is used by bacteria to synthesize folic acid.
198. B.
199. A.
   Explanation: Clofibrate interacts with many drugs and especially anticoagulants. It is advisable to halve the dosage of anticoagulants when starting treatment with clofibrate.
200. C.
   Explanation: Thyroxine, especially in higher than 2- to 6-mg doses and in susceptible patients, may produce angina attack and cardiac dysrhythmias. Thioridazine (a neuroleptic) and amitriptyline (an antidepressant) have strong anticholinergic actions predisposing the heart to tachycardia. Isoproterenol, a beta-adrenergic agonist, has a similar action. Propranolol, a beta receptor antagonist, may have two beneficial effects: It may block the thyroxine-induced adrenergic hyperactivity and the thyroxine-induced nervousness. Indeed, propranolol has been shown to be useful in managing certain symptoms of thyrotoxicosis.

REFERENCES

1. Levy, R. I. Drugs Used in the Treatment of Hyperlipoproteinemia. In A. G. Gilman, L. S. Goodman, and A. Gilman (eds.), *The Pharmacological Basis of Therapeutics* (6th ed.). New York: Macmillan, 1980. Pp. 834–847.
2. Levy, R. I., and Rifkind, B. K. Lipid Lowering Drugs and Hyperlipidemia. In G. A. Avery (ed.), *Antiarrhythmic, Antihypertensive and Lipid Lowering Drugs*. Baltimore: University Park, 1977. Pp. 1–34.
3. Noseda, G., Lewis, B., and Paoletti, R. *Diet and Drugs in Atherosclerosis*. New York: Raven, 1980.
4. Posner, I. Mechanisms of Enzyme Activation in the Lipoprotein Lipase System. In A. M. Gotto, Jr., and R. Paoletti (eds.), *Atherosclerosis Reviews*, Vol. 9. New York: Raven, 1982. Pp. 123–156.

VII. Endocrine Pharmacology, Gastrointestinal Pharmacology, Pulmonary Pharmacology, Histaminics and Antihistaminics

23. Antidiabetic Agents

It is chance that makes brothers, but hearts that makes friends.

Von Geibel

Diabetes mellitus results in disturbances in the metabolism of carbohydrates, lipids, and proteins. The blood glucose is maintained usually within a range of 80 to 130 mg per 100 milliliters. When the level of glucose rises above 180 mg per 100 milliliters, glucose spills into the urine (glucosuria). The utilization of glucose by most tissues, including muscle and adipose tissue, is insulin dependent whereas the utilization of glucose by brain is insulin independent. In the absence of insulin, the organs other than brain are able to utilize amino acids and fatty acids as alternative sources of energy.

The release of insulin is closely coupled with the level of glucose. Hypoglycemia results in a low level of insulin and a high level of glucagon. Hypoglycemia then favors the process of glycogenolysis and gluconeogenesis.

Following ingestion of a meal or administration of glucose (e.g., in glucose tolerance test), the level of glucose rises, causing the release of insulin and inhibiting the release of hyperglycemic glucagon. In addition, the excess glucose will be transformed into glycogen in the liver and in the muscles. The high levels of amino acids and free fatty acids foster the formation of proteins in the muscles and triglyceride in the adipose tissues.

In a nondiabetic fasting subject, the ensuing hypoglycemia not only discourages the release of insulin but also activates the homeostatic mechanisms to block the action of insulin and to convert the storage forms of fuel into utilizable glucose. Consequently, a number of hormones including glucagon, epinephrine, and glucocorticoid are released that convert glycogen into glucose, triglyceride into free fatty acid, and proteins into amino acids (gluconeogenesis). Furthermore, the uptake and utilization of glucose in the peripheral tissue decrease. The muscles and other tissues utilize amino acids and free fatty acid, providing the brain an adequate supply of glucose.

In a diabetic individual with a deficiency of insulin, all the aforementioned measures discussed for a fasting individual may take place. A meal or the administration of glucose now causes pronounced hyperglycemia due to lack of insulin-dependent utilization of glucose by muscles and adipose tissues. The elevated level of glucose surpasses the renal threshold, and glucose may appear continuously in the urine. The osmotic diuretic effects of glucose cause polyuria and polydipsia. Chronic glucosuria may lead to urinary tract infection. In the absence of conversion to triglyceride, free fatty acid now becomes metabolized to ketone bodies, causing ketonuria and ketoacidosis (acetone or fruity breath). The continuous destruction of muscular proteins may cause muscle wasting and weight loss [1, 5].

CLASSES OF DIABETES MELLITUS. Diabetes mellitus is divided into two types: type I—insulin dependent (IDDM); and type II—noninsulin dependent (NIDDM).

Type I diabetic patients may have islet-cell antibodies and human leukocyte antigens (HLA). They are dependent on insulin to prevent ketosis and hence have insulinopenia. They are mostly children or young adults.

Type II diabetic patients are noninsulin dependent and are not prone to ketosis. Type II diabetes is not autoimmune related or HLA associated. The patients are older (> 40) subjects who may or may not be obese, and who may or may not have been treated with insulin for hyperglycemia [4].

SYMPTOMS OF DIABETES. The symptoms of a diabetic patient are thirst, anorexia, nausea, vomiting, abdominal pain, headache, drowsiness, weakness, coma, severe acidosis, air hunger (Kussmaul's breathing), sweetish odor of breath, hyperglycemia, decreased blood bicarbonate, decreased blood pH, and plasma that is strongly positive for ketone bodies [5].

COMPLICATIONS OF DIABETES. There are a number of complications of poorly treated or unstabilized diabetes.

Vascular Complications. Vascular complications may be characterized by microangiopathy (thickening of capillary basement membrane), intracapillary glomerulosclerosis (thickening of glomerular capillary basement membrane), and microangiopathy of blood vessels supplying the retina (diabetic retinopathy). Diabetes is still the leading cause of blindness in the world. In addition, atherosclerosis of peripheral arteries may take place [5].

Neuropathy. Diabetic neuropathy may be characterized by neuropathic ulcer, ptosis, diplopia, strabismus, loss of deep tendon reflex, ankle drop, wrist drop, paresthesia, hyperalgesia, hyperesthesia, and orthostatic hypotension (autonomic dysfunction) [5].

Intercapillary Glomerulosclerosis. Nephrotic syndromes are characterized by edema, albuminuria, and renal failure [5].

TREATMENT OF DIABETES. The therapy consists in correcting obesity (obese individuals are resistant to both endogenous and exogenous insulin), ex-

Table 23-1. *Nature and Action of Insulin Preparations*

Classification	Preparation	Onset of Action in Hours	Duration of Action in Hours
Fast acting	Insulin Injection (regular insulin)	1	6
	Prompt Insulin Zinc Suspension (semilente insulin)	1	14
Intermediate acting	Isophane Insulin Suspension (NPH insulin, isophane insulin)	2	24
	Insulin Zinc Suspension (lente insulin)	2	24
	Globin Zinc Insulin Injection	2	18
Long acting	Protamine Zinc Insulin Suspension	7	36
	Extended Insulin Zinc Suspension (ultralente insulin)	7	36

Data from J. Larner, Insulin and Oral Hypoglycemic Drugs: Glucagon. In A. G. Gilman, L. S. Goodman, and A. Gilman (eds.), *The Pharmacological Basis of Therapeutics* (6th ed.). New York: Macmillan, 1980.

ercising (which promotes glucose utilization and reduces insulin requirement), dieting (restrict excess carbohydrates), and taking insulin (primarily for polyuric, polydipsic, and ketonuric patients) [4].

TYPES OF INSULIN PREPARATIONS. Insulin preparations are either fast acting, intermediate acting, or long acting, as depicted in Table 23-1.

INDICATION FOR CRYSTALLINE (REGULAR) INSULIN. Crystalline insulin may be used for supplemental injection or for instituting corrective measures in infection, trauma, postoperative stabilization, and rehabilitation of patients, in ketoacidosis and coma. NPH insulin contains regular insulin.

INDICATION FOR ULTRALENTE OR SEMILENTE INSULIN. Ultralente or semilente insulin is used to eliminate nocturnal and early morning hyperglycemia.

COMPLICATION OF INSULIN THERAPY—HYPOGLYCEMIA. Hypoglycemia may result from either excess insulin or lack of sufficient amount of glucose. Severe hypoglycemia may cause headache, confusion, double vision, drowsiness, and convulsions. The treatment may include glucose or glucagon. Complications of hypoglycemia include:

Lipodystrophy, characterized by atrophy of subcutaneous fat

Insulin edema, characterized by generalized retention of fluid

Insulin resistance, characterized by excess requirement of daily insulin (> 200 U) [3]

AGENTS THAT ALTER THE RELEASE OF INSULIN. The release of insulin is increased by physiologic substances (glucose, leucine, arginine, gastrin, secretin, and pancreozymin) and by pharmacologic substances (oral hypoglycemic agents). The release of insulin is also inhibited by physiologic substances (epinephrine and norepinephrine) and by pharmacologic substances (thiazide diuretics, diazoxide, and chlorpromazine).

PHARMACOLOGY OF ORAL HYPOGLYCEMIC AGENTS. Oral hypoglycemic agents are advantageous in comparison with insulin in that by releasing insulin and by decreasing the release of glucagon they mimic physiologic processes, and fewer allergic reactions are caused by them. Furthermore, they are orally effective, obviating the need of daily administration. These agents and their duration of action are listed in Table 23-2.

The two recently introduced sulfonylurea oral hypoglycemic agents are glyburide (Diabeta, Micronase) and glipzide (Glibenese). These agents are more potent than the older drugs but have identical mechanisms of action.

Table 23-2. *Characteristic Oral Hypoglycemic Agents*

Chemical Type	Name	Duration of Action (hours)
Sulfonylurea	Tolbutamide (Orinase)	6–12
	Acetohexamide (Dymelor)	12–24
	Chlorpropamide (Diabinese)	60
	Tolazamide (Tolinase)	10–14

Since oral hypoglycemic agents require a functioning pancreas, they are ineffective in type I diabetic patients. They promote the release of insulin from the pancreatic beta cells and increase the number of insulin receptor sites. They are used in type II non-ketogenic diabetic patients who cannot be controlled by diet or weight loss alone and in whom the use of insulin has proved to be difficult.

TREATMENT OF DIABETIC KETOACIDOSIS.
Diabetic ketoacidosis may result from or be aggravated by infection, surgery, trauma, shock, emotional stress, and failure to take any or sufficient amounts of insulin. Treatment includes correcting hypokalemia by giving KCl, acidosis by providing bicarbonate, dehydration and electrolyte imbalance by instituting appropriate measures, and hyperglycemia by administering crystalline zinc insulin (CZI).

QUESTIONS ON ANTIDIABETIC AGENTS

Select one answer that best completes the statement or answers the question.

_____ 201. The treatment of ketoacidosis may include the administration of:
A. Potassium chloride.
B. Sodium bicarbonate.
C. Crystalline zinc insulin.
D. All of the above.

_____ 202. Which one of the following pairs of compounds have opposite effects on blood glucose?
A. Insulin—glucagon.
B. Insulin—chlorthiazide.
C. Insulin—cortisol.
D. A and C.
E. A, B, and C.

_____ 203. Agent(s) known to release insulin include:
A. Isoproterenol.
B. Phentolamine.
C. Leucine.
D. Arginine.
E. All of the above.

_____ 204. A patient with type I diabetes mellitus:
A. May have islet-cell antibodies.
B. May be 10 years old.
C. Is insulin dependent.
D. May have ketosis.
E. All of the above.

_____ 205. Complication of insulin therapy includes all of the following *except* which one?
A. Lipodystrophy.
B. Hypoglycemia.
C. Insulin edema.
D. Time-dependent enhanced sensitivity to insulin, requiring smaller doses.

ANSWERS ON ANTIDIABETIC AGENTS

201. D.
202. E.
203. E.
204. E.
205. D.

REFERENCES

1. Ensinck, J. W., and Williams, R. H. Disorders Causing Hypoglycemia. In R. H. Williams (ed.), *Textbook of Endocrinology* (6th ed.). Philadelphia: Saunders, 1981. Pp. 844–875.
2. Larner, J. Insulin and Oral Hypoglycemic Drugs: Glucagon. In A. G. Gilman, L. S. Goodman, and A. Gilman (eds.), *The Pharmacological Basis of Therapeutics* (6th ed.). New York: Macmillan, 1980. Pp. 1497–1523.
3. Martin, J. M., Ehrlich, R. M., and Holland, F. J. *Etiology and Pathogenesis of Insulin-Dependent Diabetes Mellitus.* New York: Raven, 1981.
4. Olson, O. C. *Diagnosis and Management of Diabetes Mellitus.* Philadelphia: Lea & Febiger, 1981. Pp. 1–8.
5. Porte, D., and Halter, J. B. The Endocrine Pancreas and Diabetes Mellitus. In R. H. Williams (ed.), *Textbook of Endocrinology* (6th ed.). Philadelphia: Saunders, 1981. Pp. 716–843.

24. Adrenal Steroids

The adrenal gland (cap of the kidney) is divided histologically into three zones:

Outer zone or zona glomerulosa
Middle zone or zona fasciculata
Inner zone or zona reticularis

The adrenal cortex synthesizes cholesterol and pregnenolone by a group of enzymatic reactions and according to the following steps [1, 6]:

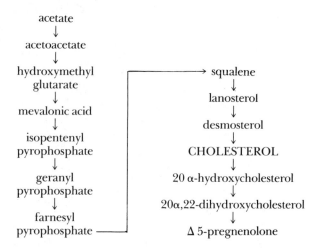

Pregnenolone is an important precursor for the synthesis of all steroids in the adrenal glands. Adrenal steroids are divided into three major categories: glucocorticoids, mineralocorticoids, and sex hormones.

THE GLUCOCORTICOIDS. The glucocorticoids influence mainly carbohydrate metabolism and to a certain extent protein and lipid metabolism. The main glucocorticoid is cortisol, with a daily secretion of 15 mg. Cortisol is synthesized by 11-beta-hydroxylation of 11-deoxycortisol. In addition to cortisol, the adrenal gland synthesizes and releases small amounts of corticosterone, which is synthesized from 11-deoxycorticosterone under the catalytic activity of 11-beta-hydroxylase. A deficiency of 11-beta-hydroxylase causes

Diminished secretion of cortisol
Diminished secretion of corticosterone
Enhanced compensatory secretion of ACTH
Enhanced secretion of 11-deoxycortisol and 11-deoxycorticosterone
Enhanced secretion of androgens

The clinical manifestations of 11-beta-hydroxylase deficiency are virilization (overproduction of androgen) and hypertension (overproduction of deoxycorticosteroids).

THE MINERALOCORTICOIDS. The mineralocorticoids influence salt and water metabolism and in general conserve sodium. The main mineralocorticoid is aldosterone, with a daily secretion of 100 μg. Aldosterone is synthesized from 18-hydroxycorticosterone by a dehydrogenase. The deficiency of 18-hydroxycorticosterone dehydrogenase results in diminished secretion of aldosterone. The clinical manifestations of dehydrogenase deficiency are as follows:

Sodium depletion
Dehydration
Hypotension
Potassium retention
Enhanced plasma renin

THE SEX HORMONES. Small quantities of progesterone, testosterone, and estradiol are also produced by the adrenal gland. However, in comparison to testicular and ovarian hormones, they play a minor role. Progesterone, which is the precursor of cortisol, aldosterone, testosterone, and estradiol, is synthesized from delta-5-pregnenolone by 3-beta-ol-dehydrogenase. Deficiency of this enzyme results in deficiency of cortisol and aldosterone. The patients require replacement therapy with both glucocorticoids and mineralocorticoids.

ADRENOCORTICOTROPIC HORMONE. Adrenocorticotropic hormone (ACTH) stimulates the synthesis of all adrenal steroids, but especially the glucocorticoids (Fig. 24-1).

The administration of psychoactive agents and emotional arousal originating from the limbic system are able to modify the functions of the pituitary-adrenal axis and to stimulate the synthesis of cortisol [2, 5]. Corticotropin, elaborated from anterior pituitary gland, is able to stimulate the synthesis of steroids including cortisol. The release of corticotropin is stimulated by hypothalamic corticotropin-releasing factor. Corticotropin (ACTH) produces the following effects:

It enhances the synthesis of pregnenolone.
It activates adenylate cyclase and enhances cyclic AMP level.
It enhances the level of adrenal steroids, and especially cortisol.
It reduces the level of ascorbic acid.

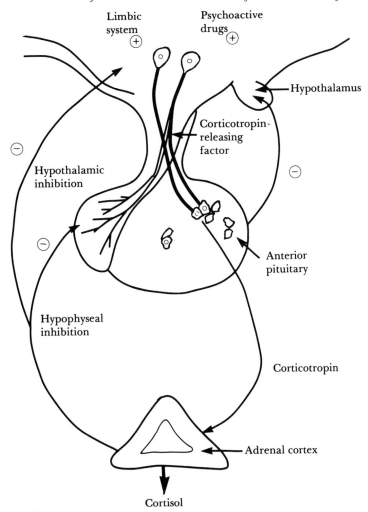

The level of cortisol is thought to control directly the secretion of ACTH through a negative feedback (−), which may be directed to both hypothalamus and anterior pituitary gland. Conversely, a reduction in the concentration of cortisol or cortisollike substance removes the negative effect and enhances the release of ACTH (Fig. 24-1).

The metyrapone test may be used diagnostically to evaluate the proper functioning of the anterior pituitary gland. The oral administration of metyrapone

Inhibits the activity of the enzyme 11-beta-hydroxylase, which is necessary for the synthesis of cortisol, corticosterone, and aldosterone

Enhances the release of corticotropin, which in turn increases the production of precursors (11-deoxycortisol and 11-deoxycorticosterone)

Enhances the appearance of 17-hydroxycorticosteroids and 17-ketogenic steroids

In the event the pituitary gland is nonfunctional and is unable to stimulate ACTH, these urinary metabolites will not increase [3, 6].

PHARMACOLOGY OF CORTISOL. Carbohydrate Metabolism. Cortisol (Fig. 24-2) has an antiinsulin effect and aggravates diabetes mellitus. It increases gluconeogenesis, inhibits the peripheral utilization of glucose, and causes hyperglycemia and glucosuria.

Protein Metabolism. Cortisol promotes the breakdown of proteins and inhibits protein synthesis. This effect causes muscle wasting in quadriceps femoris groups. Muscular activities may become difficult. The effect is opposite to that produced by insulin.

Lipid Metabolism. Cortisol causes abnormal deposition of fat pad called buffalo hump.

Electrolytes and Water Metabolism. Cortisol causes hypernatremia, hypokalemia, and hypercalciuria.

Uric Acid. Cortisol causes hyperuricemia by decreasing renal tubular resorption of uric acid.

Gastric HCl. Cortisol enhances the production of gastric hydrochloric acid.

Fig. 24-2. *The structures of selected corticosteroids.*

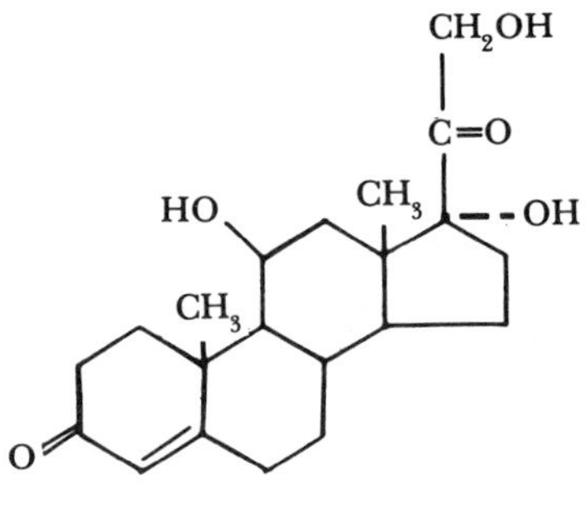

Cortisol

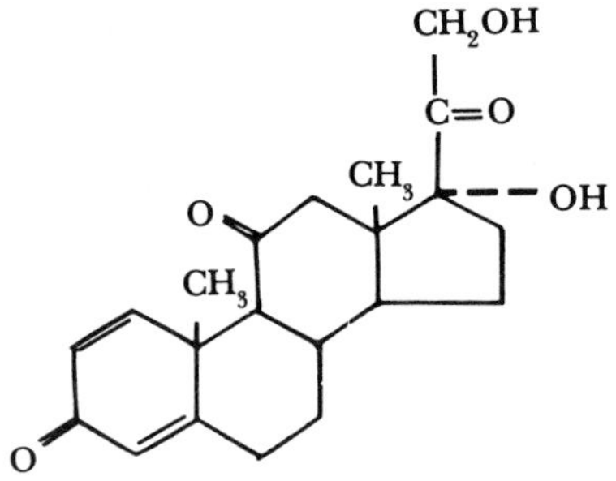

Prednisone

Blood Coagulation. Cortisol, like epinephrine, enhances the coagulability of blood.

Antiinflammatory Action. Cortisol exerts its antiinflammatory effect in part by blocking the release and action of histamine. In addition, it decreases the migration of polymorphonuclear leukocytes.

Hematologic Effects. Cortisol produces eosinophilia and causes involution of lymphoid tissues.

CUSHING'S SYNDROME. Cushing's syndrome is a rare condition (1/10,000) occurring primarily in the female population in the third or fourth decade of life. The basophilic adenoma of the anterior pituitary gland, hyperplasia, adenoma, and carcinoma of adrenal cortex may all lead to Cushing's syndrome. It is characterized by red cheeks, moon face, buffalo hump, thin skin, high blood pressure, pendulous abdomen with red striae, poor wound healing, osteoporosis, and some signs of virilism (enlarged clitoris) [6].

Treatment of Cushing's syndrome may include the following:

Removal of microadenoma by approaching the pituitary gland via the transsphenoidal route
Removal of the entire adenohypophysis and lifelong treatment with cortisol, thyroxine, and sex hormones
Bilateral adrenalectomy [6]

ECTOPIC ACTH SYNDROME. Hypercortisolism may be caused by production of ACTH by a nonpituitary neoplasm. The most common sources of ectopic ACTH are carcinoma of lung and pancreas.

ADDISON'S DISEASE. Addison's disease, also known as primary chronic adrenal cortical insufficiency syndrome, involves both male and female populations. It results primarily from atrophy of cortices and tuberculosis of adrenal gland. Addison's disease is characterized by mental apathy, confusion, hypotension, insensitivity to sympathomimetic pressor amines, impaired excretion of free water, hypersecretion of ACTH and melanocyte-stimulating hormone causing skin and mucous membrane pigmentation, fasting hypoglycemia (depleted liver glycogen), anorexia, and weight loss [6].

Addisonian crisis may result from combined cortisol and aldosterone deficiency along with extracellular volume depletion. The treatment includes intravenous administration of saline and parenteral administration of glucocorticoids. After crisis, glucocorticoid and fludrocortisone must be taken daily. Dexamethasone phosphate should be available to meet emergencies. The dose of fludrocortisone should be adjusted downward if edema, hypertension, or hypokalemia is present. Conversely, the doses of fludrocortisone should be increased if hypotension and hyperkalemia are evident. The administration of glucocorticoids in children should be monitored carefully to avoid growth retardation or adrenal insufficiency. Alternate-day therapy may be indicated in children [6].

PHARMACOLOGIC USAGE OF GLUCOCORTICOIDS. Glucocorticoids are vital in the treatment of adrenal insufficiency. In addition, they are used extensively in large pharmacologic doses as antiinflammatory and immunosuppressive agents. These nonendocrine uses are listed in Table 24-1.

PHARMACOLOGIC PREPARATIONS. Examples of antiinflammatory glucocorticoids are listed in Table 24-2.

Chronic use of glucocorticoids produces Cushing's syndrome, including acne, adrenal atrophy, aggravation of diabetes mellitus, aggravation of peptic ulcer, amenorrhea, hirsutism, hypernatremia and hypokalemia, hypertension, moon face, muscle wasting, necrotizing arthritis in rheumatoid patients, osteoporosis, and psychosis.

Table 24-1. *Nonendocrine Uses of Glucocorticoids*

Rheumatoid arthritis	Löffler's syndrome
Psoriatic arthritis	Berylliosis
Gouty arthritis	Idiopathic thrombocytopenic purpura
Bursitis and tenosynovitis	Autoimmune hemolytic anemia
Systemic lupus erythematosus	Lymphomas
Acute rheumatic carditis	Tuberculous meningitis
Pemphigus	Urticaria
Erythema multiforme	Chronic active hepatitis
Exfoliative dermatitis	Ulcerative colitis
Mycosis fungoides	Regional enteritis
Allergic rhinitis	Nontropical sprue
Bronchial asthma	Dental postoperative inflammation
Atopic dermatitis	Cerebral edema
Serum sickness	Subacute nonsuppurative thyroiditis
Allergic conjunctivitis	Malignant exophthalmos
Uveitis	Hypercalcemia
Retrobulbar neuritis	Trichinosis
Sarcoidosis	Myasthenia gravis
Organ transplantation	Alopecia areata

From G. W. Liddle, The Adrenals. In R. H. Williams (ed.), *Textbook of Endocrinology* (6th ed.). Philadelphia: Saunders, 1981. P. 289.

Table 24-2. *Glucocorticoids in Medicine*

Steroid	Antiinflammatory Potency	Sodium Retention
Betamethasone	20	0
Dexamethasone	20	0
Fludrocortisone	12	100
Paramethasone	6	0
Triamcinolone	5	0
Methylprednisolone	4	0
Prednisolone	3	0.8
Prednisone	2.5	0.8
Cortisol	1	1

Data from A. Goth, *Medical Pharmacology: Principles and Concepts* (11th ed.). St. Louis: Mosby, 1984.

Glucocorticoids are contraindicated in diabetes mellitus, digitalis therapy, glaucoma, hypertension, infection, osteoporosis, peptic ulcer, tuberculosis, and viral infection.

QUESTIONS ON ADRENAL STEROIDS

Select one answer that best completes the statement or answers the question.

___ 206. Examples of feedback regulation of hormone secretion are:
   A. Plasma cortisol and ACTH secretion.
   B. Plasma thyroxine and TSH secretion.
   C. Plasma glucose and insulin secretion.
   D. A, B, and C.

___ 207. Which one of the following substances is a precursor to both cholesterol and cortisol and whose synthesis is inhibited by clofibrate?
   A. Aspartic acid.
   B. Mevalonic acid.
   C. Glutamic acid.
   D. Myristic acid.

___ 208. Which one of the following enzymes and its product is a mismatch?
   A. Xanthine oxidase—uric acid.
   B. Glutamate decarboxylase—gamma-aminobutyric acid.
   C. 18-Hydroxycorticosterone dehydrogenase—delta-5-pregnenolone.
   D. Tyrosine hydroxylase—dopa.

___ 209. The oral administration of metyrapone does all of the following except which one?
   A. Stimulates the release of ACTH.
   B. Stimulates production of 11-deoxycortisol.
   C. Diminishes the production of 11-deoxycorticosterone.
   D. Enhances the appearance of 17-hydroxycorticosteroids.

___ 210. The action of cortisone is characterized by:
   A. Causing hyperglycemia.
   B. Enhancing the peripheral utilization of glucose.
   C. Having antiglucagon effect.
   D. Increasing gluconeogenesis.
   E. A and D.

___ 211. Cortisol causes all of the following except which one?
   A. Hypokalemia.
   B. Hypercalciuria.
   C. Hypouricemia.
   D. Hyperglycemia.

___ 212. The treatment of Cushing's syndrome may include:
   A. Removal of microadenoma.
   B. Removal of adenohypophysis.
   C. Bilateral adrenalectomy.
   D. All of the above.

___ 213. Hypercortisolism may be caused by:
   A. Carcinoma of the lung.
   B. Carcinoma of the pancreas.
   C. Neoplasm of pituitary gland.
   D. All of the above.

_____ 214. Addison's disease:
   A. May be characterized by cortisol and aldosterone deficiency.
   B. May manifest extracellular volume depletion.
   C. May be treated with saline and dexamethasone.
   D. All of the above.
_____ 215. Glucocorticoids are contraindicated in all of the following conditions *except* which one?
   A. Organ transplantation.
   B. Diabetes mellitus.
   C. Hypertension.
   D. Peptic ulcer.

ANSWERS AND EXPLANATIONS ON ADRENAL STEROIDS

206. D.
207. B.
   Explanation: Clofibrate inhibits cholesterol synthesis by preventing the conversion of hydroxymethylglutarate to mevalonic acid. Mevalonic acid is converted by numerous steps to cholesterol, to delta-5-pregnenolone, and finally to cortisol.
208. C.
   Explanation: The deficiency of 18-hydroxycorticosterone dehydrogenase results in diminished secretion of aldosterone.
209. C.
210. E.
211. C.
212. D.
213. D.
214. D.
215. A.

REFERENCES

1. Brooks, R. V. Biosynthesis and Metabolism of Adrenocortical Steroids. In V. H. T. James (ed.), *The Adrenal Gland: Comprehensive Endocrinology.* New York: Raven, 1979. Pp. 67–92.
2. Collu, R., et al. *Central Nervous System Effects of Hypothalamic Hormones and Other Peptides.* New York: Raven, 1979.
3. Federman, D. D. General Principles of Endocrinology. In R. H. Williams (ed.), *Textbook of Endocrinology* (6th ed.). Philadelphia: Saunders, 1981. Pp. 1–14.
4. Goth, A. *Medical Pharmacology: Principles and Concepts* (11th ed.). St. Louis: Mosby, 1984.
5. Jones, M. T., et al. *Interaction within the Brain-Pituitary-Adrenocortical System.* New York: Raven, 1979.
6. Liddle, G. W. The Adrenals. In R. H. Williams (ed.), *Textbook of Endocrinology* (6th ed.). Philadelphia: Saunders, 1981. Pp. 249–292.

25. Thyroid Hormones and Their Antagonists

Those bringing sunshine to the lives of others can not keep it from themselves.

Sir James Barrie

The thyroid gland synthesizes thyroxine and triiodothyronine, and these hormones are involved in the regulation of

Growth and development
Thermoregulation and calorigenesis
Metabolism of carbohydrate, proteins, and lipids
Hypophyseal thyrotropin secretion

The thyroid gland also synthesizes calcitonin, and this substance produces hypocalcemia by inhibiting bone resorption and by enhancing the urinary excretion of calcium and phosphate.

SYNTHESIS OF THYROID HORMONE. The steps involved in the synthesis of thyroid hormones are depicted in Figure 25-1. The ingested iodide (100–150 μg/day) is transported actively (iodide trapping) and then accumulated in the thyroid gland. The trapped iodide is oxidized by a peroxidase system to I^0 (active iodine), which iodinates the tyrosine residue of glycoprotein to yield monoiodotyrosine (MIT) and diiodotyrosine (DIT). This process is called iodide organification. The MIT and DIT combine to form triiodothyronine (T_3) whereas two molecules of DIT combine to form thyroxine (T_4). Thyroxine and triiodothyronine are released from thyroglobulin by pinocytosis and proteolysis of thyroglobulin by lysosomal enzymes. In circulation, 75 percent of thyroxine is bound to thyroxine-binding globulin (TBG), and the remainder is mostly bound to thyroxine-binding prealbumin (TBPA). Approximately 0.05 percent of thyroxine remains free. Triiodothyronine is similarly bound to TBG, only 0.5 percent of it remaining in the free form [1, 2].

Thyroxine may undergo deamination, decarboxylation, and glucuronic acid conjugation. However, it is mainly deiodinated in one of two ways. T_4 may be deiodinated to 3,5,3'-triiodothyronine, which is more efficacious than T_4. Alternatively, it may be deiodinated to pharmacologically inactive 3,3',5'-triiodothyronine (reverse T_3).

Calcitonin, a polypeptide of 32 amino acids, is produced by parafollicular cells (c cells) of the thyroid gland. The secretion of calcitonin is stimulated by

Calcium
Catecholamine and theophylline ($\uparrow$ cyclic AMP)
Glucagon
Cholecystokinin
Gastrin
Cerulein

The detailed metabolism of calcitonin has not been established.

THYROID-PITUITARY RELATIONSHIP. Thyrotropin-releasing hormone or factor (TRH), secreted by the hypothalamus, reaches the pituitary gland via the pituitary portal venous system and stimulates the release of thyroid-stimulating hormone (TSH), which in turn stimulates the synthesis of T_3 and T_4. The high level of thyroid hormones, mediated by a negative hypophyseal and hypothalamic feedback mechanism, inhibits the action of TRH in the hypothalamus (Fig. 25-2).

THYROTOXICOSIS. Thyrotoxicosis results when thyroid hormones are produced in excess, either by the thyroid gland (hyperthyroidism) or by tissues other than thyroid gland (e.g., choriocarcinoma in uterus or testis or pituitary tumor causing hypersecretion of TSH). Thyrotoxicosis may be due to overproduction of T_3, T_4, or T_3 and T_4. Excess TBG (occasionally) and excess TBPA (rarely) may also cause thyrotoxicosis. T_3 toxicosis may result from excess intake of liothyronine (T_3). T_4 toxicosis may result from the lack of conversion of T_4 to T_3 in elderly patients or in patients exposed to large quantities of iodine (as in x-ray contrast media). T_3 and T_4 toxicosis is seen in patients with Graves's disease, toxic multinodular goiter, and toxic adenoma [1, 2].

MANIFESTATION OF GRAVES'S DISEASE. Graves's disease (diffuse hyperthyroidism) occurs more frequently in women during childbearing years. It may be associated with thyrotoxicosis, exophthalmos, and goiter. In addition, it will manifest in tremor, excitability, emotional instability, rapid pulse, tachycardia, increased cardiac output, rapid respiration, facial flushing, warm and moist skin, increasing appetite, weight loss, muscle wasting, enlarged palpable lymph node, breast enlargement, and oligomenorrhea. The clinical manifestations of thyroid adenoma with nodular goiter vary dramatically from those produced by Graves's disease. Lymph enlargement, exophthalmos, and muscle

Fig. 25-1. *Trapping of the iodine and synthesis of triiodothyronine and thyroxine.*

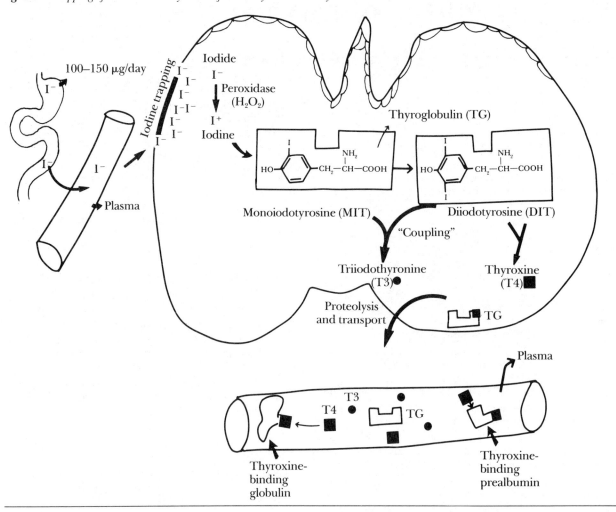

wasting and weakness are either absent or less pronounced. On the other hand, the cardiovascular manifestations (very rapid pulse, tachycardia, fibrillation, heart failure) are more prevalent [2].

THYROID HORMONE DEFICIENCY (HYPOTHYROIDISM). Hypothyroidism may result from

Atrophy of thyroid tissue
Failure of hypothalamic-pituitary axis to stimulate a normal thyroid gland (e.g., Sheehan's syndrome)
Goitrous hypothyroidism (e.g., Hashimoto's thyroiditis, iodine deficiency)

CLINICAL MANIFESTATION OF MYXEDEMA.
Myxedema may be characterized by coarse facial features (thick lips, puffy eyelids, sad expression), dry hair, slow speech, lethargy, memory impairment, cardiovascular abnormalities (slow pulse, hypotension, enlarged heart), cold skin, increased sensibility to cold, decreased sweating, dry wrinkled skin, and muscular weakness [2].

PHYSIOLOGIC EFFECTS OF THYROID HORMONES. Calorigenesis. Thyroid hormones stimulate calorigenesis and increase oxygen consumption through unknown mechanism(s). The basal metabolic rate is increased.

Protein Metabolism. Thyroid hormones increase protein synthesis. Growth is retarded by hypothyroidism and restored by replacement therapy.

Carbohydrate Metabolism. Thyroid hormones have antiinsulin effect and act synergistically with epinephrine to enhance glycogenolysis and hyperglycemia. Furthermore, they enhance the intestinal uptake of glucose and insulin degradation.

Lipid Metabolism. Thyroid hormones stimulate the synthesis, mobilization, and degradation of lipids. They lower cholesterol, and D-thyroxine is used in hyperlipoproteinemic states (see Chap. 22).

Vitamin Metabolism. The concentrations of thiamine, riboflavin, ascorbic acid, and vitamin B_{12} are reduced, and their requirements are increased in hyperthyroidism.

Fig. 25-2. *TSH-mediated increases in the synthesis of thyroxine and triiodothyronine and inhibition of their synthesis by negative hypothalamic-hypophyseal feedback mechanism(s).*

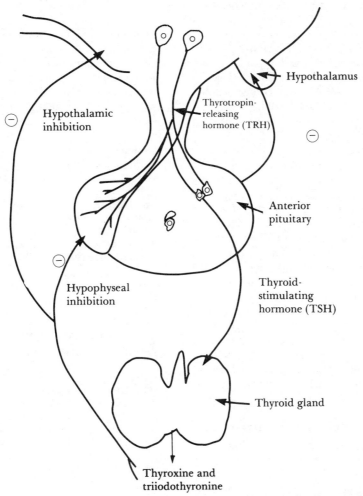

Catecholamine. Thyroid hormones enhance the tissue sensitivity to catecholamine through unknown mechanisms.

High-affinity binding sites (receptor sites) for thyroid hormones have been reported on the plasma membrane, mitochondria, and nucleus. The distribution of these receptor sites is nonuniform in the body (high in pituitary and heart), indicating diverse but organ-specific physiologic functions.

THYROID PREPARATIONS. Thyroglobulin (Proloid) is purified from hog thyroid gland and standardized to yield a T_4 to T_3 ratio of 2.5:1.0.

Levothyroxine sodium (Levothroid, Synthroid) is used for replacement therapy.

Liothyronine (Cytomel) has a short half-life and hence is used diagnostically in T_3 suppression test.

Liotrix (Euthroid, Thyrolar) is a combination of T_4 and T_3, standardized to yield a T_4 to T_3 ratio of 4:1.

ANTITHYROID AGENTS. The pharmacologic agents that interfere with and reduce the formation of thyroid hormones fall in the following categories.

Agents That Inhibit Iodide-Trapping Mechanism. Monovalent anions such as perchlorate (ClO_4^-), pertechnetate ($TcCO_4^-$), and thiocyanate (SCN^-) are able to inhibit competitively the active transport and accumulation of iodide. The effect is reversible with large concentrations of iodide. These agents are now obsolete and are no longer used. Goitrogenic vegetables (e.g., cabbage) contain thiocyanate.

Agents That Inhibit the Synthesis of Thyroid Hormones. Propylthiouracil, methimazole, and carbimazole exert their effects by inhibiting iodide organification and inhibiting the formation of diiodotyrosine (DIT).

These agents all possess a thiocarbamide moiety $(-N-\overset{\overset{\textstyle S}{\|}}{C}-R)$ that is essential for their antithyroid actions. The onset of their beneficial effects is slow, taking 3 to 4 weeks.

Agents That Inhibit the Release of Thyroid Hormones. Iodides (potassium iodide, Lugol's solution containing 5% iodine and 10% potassium iodide) exert their beneficial effects by inhibiting organification, inhibiting the release of thyroid hormones, and decreasing (inhibition of proteolysis) the size and vascularity of the gland, hence preparing the patient for surgery.

Agents That Cause Follicular Destruction. [131]I is given orally in the treatment of older patients with thyrotoxicosis. It accumulates in the storage follicles and emits beta rays with a half-life of 5 days. Radioactive iodine, which crosses the placental barrier, is contraindicated in pregnancy.

Treatment of Thyrotoxicosis. The treatment of thyrotoxicosis in younger patients may include the administration of antithyroid drug with propylthiouracil or methimazole. These agents are very slow in their onset of action, often taking years for remission to be apparent. The most serious reaction reported following administration of these drugs is agranulocytosis. In the event of multinodular goiters, subtotal thyroidectomy may be indicated. Patients are first treated with antithyroid drugs until they become euthyroid. This treatment is followed by potassium iodide to diminish vascularity as a preoperative measure. In addition to surgery, radioactive iodine is being used increasingly in treatment. The major complication following either surgery or treatment with radioactive iodine may be hypothyroidism requiring replacement therapy with levothyroxine.

TREATMENT OF THYROTOXIC CRISIS. Thyrotoxic crisis (thyroid storm) is precipitated by trauma, infection, surgery, and toxemia of pregnancy. The patient is feverish, and profuse sweating takes place. Tachycardia and tremors are present, and congestive heart failure may ensue. The supportive treatment includes any or all of the following measures:

1. The synthesis of thyroid hormone should be inhibited by using large doses of propylthiouracil (200 mg/4 hours). In addition to inhibiting synthesis, propylthiouracil inhibits the conversion of T_4 to T_3.
2. The release of thyroid hormone may be inhibited by sodium iodide given intravenously.
3. Large doses of dexamethasone should be given orally. This steroid inhibits the release of thyroid hormone and the conversion of T_4 to T_3.
4. Large doses of adrenergic antagonists such as propranolol, reserpine, or guanethidine may be tried.
5. Digitalis and diuretic may be required if congestive heart failure is present.
6. Antipyretics should be administered to reduce fever.
7. Any other supportive measures that may be indicated should be constituted to prevent the high mortality from thyrotoxic crisis [2].

TREATMENT OF NONTOXIC GOITER. Nontoxic goiter resulting from iodide deficiency is treated with an adequate amount of daily iodide. Hashimoto's thyroiditis is treated with thyroxine to suppress TSH secretion.

TREATMENT OF HYPOTHYROIDISM. Levothyroxine (2–25 µg/kg) is given for replacement therapy.

TREATMENT OF MYXEDEMA COMA. If hypothyroidism remains untreated, myxedema coma results. It is characterized by hypothermia (75°F), hypoglycemia, bradycardia, and hypotension. Alveolar hypotension may cause hypoxia, followed by lethargy, coma, and death. Treatment includes the following:

Administration of a loading dose of levothyroxine (300–400 µg given intravenously)
Administration of a daily dose of levothyroxine (50 µg)
Maintenance of respiration with mechanical ventilation and assisted oxygen administration
Evaluation of adrenocortical insufficiency and administration of corticosteroids
Hypertonic saline and glucose to alleviate hyponatremia and hypoglycemia

In addition, any other supportive therapy indicated should be instituted.

QUESTIONS ON THYROID HORMONES AND THEIR ANTAGONISTS

Select one answer that best completes the statement or answers the question.

_____ 216. Calcitonin causes hypocalcemia mostly by:
  A. Inhibiting bone resorption.
  B. Inhibiting osteolysis.
  C. Decreasing renal tubular resorption of calcium.
  D. All of the above.

_____ 217. The secretion of calcitonin is stimulated by:
  A. Calcium.
  B. Catecholamine.
  C. Glucagon.
  D. Cholecystokinin.
  E. All of the above.

_____ 218. Thyrotoxicosis may result from:
  A. Hyperthyroidism.
  B. Choriocarcinoma of uterus or testis.
  C. Hypersecretion of TSH.
  D. Pituitary tumor.
  E. All of the above.

_____ 219. Thyroxine in circulation is:
  A. Bound to thyroxine-binding globulin.
  B. Bound to thyroxine-binding prealbumin.
  C. Unbound to the extent of 95 percent.
  D. Bound to glutathione.
  E. Both A and B.

_____ 220. The physiologic actions of thyroid hormones are characterized by:
  A. Increased oxygen consumption.
  B. Enhanced basal metabolic rate.
  C. Antiinsulin effects.
  D. Hypolipoproteinemic effects.
  E. All of the above.

_____ 221. Methimazole exerts its effects by:
  A. Inhibiting iodide organification.
  B. Inhibiting the formation of diiodothyronine.
  C. Inhibiting iodide transport and accumulation.

D. A and B.
E. All of the above.

____ 222. One of the complications following treatment of thyrotoxicosis is:
A. Hypothyroidism.
B. Dysrhythmias and cardiac failure.
C. Orthostatic hypotension.
D. Insensitivity to sympathomimetic amines.

____ 223. The use of which one of the following substances should be contraindicated in thyroid storm?
A. Large dose of propylthiouracil.
B. Large dose of dexamethasone.
C. Large dose of isoproterenol.
D. Digitalis and diuretic.

ANSWERS AND EXPLANATIONS ON THYROID HORMONES AND THEIR ANTAGONISTS

216. A.
217. E.
218. E.
219. E.
220. E.
221. D.
222. A.

Explanation: The management of patients with thyrotoxicosis includes (a) antithyroid drugs to make them euthyroid, (b) potassium iodide to diminish vascularity, (c) surgery or radioactive iodide or both. Radioactive iodide may cause hypothyroidism requiring replacement therapy with levothyroxine.

223. C.

Explanation: Hyperthyroidism is associated with cardiac diseases. The cardiac output may be high and "high-output failure" may ensue. Consequently, during thyroid storm a beta-adrenergic blocking agent such as propranolol (and not the beta agonist such as isoproterenol) is indicated.

REFERENCES

1. Greenspan, F. S., and Dong, B. J. Thyroid and Antithyroid Drugs. In B. G. Katzung (ed.), *Basic and Clinical Pharmacology*. Los Altos, Calif.: Lange, 1982. Pp. 408–419.

2. Ingbar, S. H., and Woeber, K. A. The Thyroid Gland. In R. H. Williams (ed.), *Textbook of Endocrinology* (6th ed.). Philadelphia: Saunders, 1981. Pp. 117–242.

26. Vitamin D, Calcium Homeostasis, and Parathyroid Hormone

What would life be if we had no courage to attempt anything?

Vincent van Gogh

PARATHYROID DISORDERS. Four parathyroid glands are situated on the lateral lobes of the thyroid. The glands secrete parathyroid hormone in response to low serum calcium. This hormone increases the serum calcium levels by several mechanisms:

It stimulates bone resorption.
It increases intestinal absorption of calcium.
It increases the resorption of calcium by the renal tubules.
It acts on the kidney to decrease the tubular resorption of phosphate.

A reciprocal relationship exists between the level of calcium and phosphorus:

	Serum Ca	Serum Phosphate
Hyperparathyroidism	Elevated	Low
Hypoparathyroidism	Low	Elevated

In addition to parathyroid hormone, calcitonin is involved in calcium homeostasis. It (1) inhibits bone resorption and (2) prevents excess increase in the serum concentration of calcium by monitoring the action of parathyroid hormone [1].

HYPOPARATHYROIDISM. Hypoparathyroidism may result from any of the following:

Thyroidectomy for thyroid tumors (rare).
Congenital absence of parathyroid glands (rare).
Idiopathic hypoparathyroidism (rare). Since the patients also develop chronic mucocutaneous moniliasis, alopecia areata, and vitiligo, an autoimmune disease or a defect in cellular immunity has been suspected in these patients.
Surgical removal of the hyperplastic or neoplastic parathyroid glands.

Pathogenesis. In the absence of parathyroid hormones, the following events take place:

Serum calcium declines (reduced bone resorption).
Serum phosphorus increases (increased tubular resorption).
Neuromuscular irritability and tonic-clonic convulsions occur (low calcium tetany).
Laryngeal stridor, asthma, and other muscular spasms are apparent (irritability due to low calcium).
Ectopic calcifications take place in blood vessels, brain, sub-cutaneous tissue, muscles, and cartilage (calcium phosphate is an insoluble salt).

Other manifestations of hypoparathyroidism include lenticular cataracts, impaired dental structures, dry scaly skin, tendency to monilial infections, impaired mental acuity, and psychiatric disturbances.

Treatment. Hypocalcemic tetany is treated with intravenous administration of calcium gluconate or calcium chloride (5–10 ml of 10% solution). These agents exert their effects rapidly but transiently. It should be recalled too that 10-ml solutions of calcium chloride and calcium gluconate contain 270 mg and 70 mg of calcium, respectively. Moreover, since calcium chloride is a highly irritant substance, it should not be administered intramuscularly. Besides calcium salts, hypoparathyroidism is also treated with vitamin D_2 (ergocalciferol), which may be administered initially in large doses (400,000 IU), followed by maintenance doses of 50,000 to 100,000 IU per day (1 IU = 0.025 µg of cholecalciferol or vitamin D_3). Parathyroid hormone (100–300 U) is injected subcutaneously after the initial administration of calcium salt. The effect of parathyroid hormone is transient; it lasts only 3 to 4 weeks after its administration. It is thought that antibodies are formed against this polypeptide, which contains 87 residues of 17 amino acids.

PSEUDOHYPOPARATHYROIDISM. Pseudohypoparathyroidism is a rare condition in which the parathyroid glands are intact but the kidney tubules do not respond to parathyroid hormone. It is thought that parathyroid hormone exerts its effects by stimulating adenylate cyclase in the kidney, leading to the formation of cyclic AMP, which in turn inhibits the tubular resorption of phosphate. Patients suffering from pseudohypoparathyroidism lack renal adenylate cyclase. In the absence of an effective parathyroid action, the serum phosphorus is high, the serum calcium is low, and the parathyroid glands become hyperplastic. In addition, other signs of true hypoparathyroidism such as asthma, tetany, sparse hair, bone changes, abnormal dentition, poor eyesight, and neurologic and psychiatric abnormalities are evident.

Pseudohypoparathyroidism is diagnosed by clinical signs, by a high level of parathyroid hormone in the serum, and by low excretion of cyclic AMP in the urine. Treatment is the same as that described for hypoparathyroidism. The patients respond well to vitamin D.

HYPERPARATHYROIDISM.
Hyperparathyroidism results from parathyroid hyperplasia, parathyroid carcinoma, adenoma of parathyroid glands causing hypersecretion, and carcinoma of the lung and kidneys producing parathyroidlike hormones.

Pathogenesis. Hyperparathyroidism is associated with the following:

Stimulation of bone resorption and elevated serum level of calcium

Elevated urinary phosphate and decreased serum phosphate levels

Bone malformation in an untreated patient

Hypercalciuria, which may cause nephrolithiasis

Pancreatitis (calcification of pancreatic duct occurs but is rare)

Peptic ulcer (calcium stimulates gastric acid secretion)

Treatment. Hyperparathyroidism is surgically treated. Prior to surgery, the patients may be treated with corticosteroids, which antagonize vitamin D–induced intestinal absorption of calcium and also increase calcium excretion by the kidney.

QUESTIONS ON VITAMIN D, CALCIUM HOMEOSTASIS, AND PARATHYROID HORMONE

Select one answer that best completes the statement or answers the question.

_____ 224. Which one of the following agents may cause hypoparathyroidism in an epileptic patient?
   A. Sodium valproate.
   B. Phenobarbital.
   C. Ethosuximide.
   D. Carbamazepine.
_____ 225. The actions of glucocorticoids are characterized by their:
   A. Antagonizing vitamin D–stimulated intestinal calcium transport.
   B. Blocking collagen synthesis in bone.
   C. Reducing parathyroid hormone–stimulated bone resorption.
   D. All of the above.
_____ 226. Estrogens reduce the bone-resorbing action of parathyroid hormone by:
   A. Altering the renal response to parathyroid hormone.
   B. Altering vitamin D–binding protein.
   C. Enhancing the level of 1,25-dihydroxylated vitamin D.
   D. All of the above.
_____ 227. All of the following drugs alter calcium homeostasis *except* which one?
   A. Fluoride.
   B. Indomethacin.
   C. Thiazides.
   D. Mithramycin.

_____ 228. Osteoporosis may be caused by or from:
   A. Thyrotoxicosis.
   B. Hypogonadism.
   C. Glucocorticoid excess.
   D. All of the above.
_____ 229. Which one of the following unfortified food substances contains the highest amount of vitamin D?
   A. Milk.
   B. Egg yolk.
   C. Sardines.
   D. Shrimp.
_____ 230. Pseudohypoparathyroidism is characterized by deficiency of which one of the following enzymes?
   A. Na^+K^+ ATPase.
   B. Ca^+ ATPase.
   C. Adenylate cyclase.
   D. Phosphodiesterase.

Answer questions 231 to 234 by stating whether they are true or false statements.
_____ 231. Calcium chloride is a highly irritating substance and when injected subcutaneously it causes extreme pain.
_____ 232. Neonatal tetany may occur in the newborn of mothers with hyperparathyroidism.
_____ 233. Hypercalcemia causes muscle weakness, lethargy, and coma.
_____ 234. "Disuse" atrophy may lead to hypercalcemia.

ANSWERS AND EXPLANATIONS ON VITAMIN D, CALCIUM HOMEOSTASIS, AND PARATHYROID HORMONE

224. B.
225. D.
   Note: Glucocorticoids have been shown to be useful in the treatment of hypercalcemic states.
226. D.
   Note: Estrogens are effective in the treatment of postmenopausal osteoporosis.
227. B.
   Note: Fluoride increases bone formation.
      Thiazide reduces hypercalciuria.
      Mithramycin is used to treat Paget's disease.
228. D.
229. C.
230. C.
231. True.
232. True.
233. True.
234. True.

REFERENCE

1. Aurbach, G. D., Marx, S. J., and Spiegel, A. M. Parathyroid Hormone, Calcitonin, and the Calciferols. In R. H. Williams (ed.), *Textbook of Endocrinology* (6th ed.). Philadelphia: Saunders, 1981. Pp. 922–1032.

27. Posterior Pituitary Hormones: Oxytocin and Vasopressin

Part One: Oxytocin and Other Drugs Affecting Uterine Motility

The agents that stimulate the smooth muscles of the uterus, called oxytocics, are ergot alkaloids, prostaglandins, and oxytocin.

ERGOT ALKALOIDS. Ergonovine and methylergonovine have pronounced stimulating effects on the gravid uterus. These agents may be used to control postpartum uterine atony.

PROSTAGLANDINS. Prostaglandins of interest with respect to the reproductive system are carboprost tromethamine (Prostin M15), dinoprost tromethamine (Prostin F_2 Alpha), and dinoprostone (Prostin E_2).

Prostaglandins, by causing uterine contraction, are abortifacients. Prostin M15, Prostin F_2 Alpha, and Prostin E_2 are given intramuscularly, intraabdominally, or vaginally (suppositories), respectively. Agents that inhibit the synthesis of prostaglandins such as indomethacin are useful in preventing premature labor.

OXYTOCIN. Oxytocin is a single polypeptide with eight amino acids having the following sequence [5]:

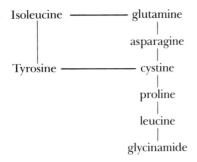

Isoleucine —————— glutamine
| |
| asparagine
| |
Tyrosine —————— cystine
|
proline
|
leucine
|
glycinamide

Oxytocin is synthesized in the cell bodies of supraoptic and paraventricular neurons and is then transported (complexed with neurophysin) in membrane-bound vesicles to the posterior lobe of the pituitary gland, where it may be released by reflex mechanism(s) initiated or amplified by genital stimulation, coitus, parturition, and suckling by one's infant. In addition to oxytocin, suckling releases prolactin. The action of oxytocin on uterus (muscular contraction and parturition) and mammary gland (contraction of myoepithelial cells and milk secretion) is a direct one without being influenced by the autonomic nervous system.

The uterus contains both alpha and beta$_2$ receptor sites. The stimulation of an alpha receptor site causes contraction whereas the stimulation of a beta$_2$ receptor site causes relaxation. Beta$_2$ receptor agonists such as ritodrine hydrochloride (Yutopar) or terbutaline sulfate (Brethine) are used to suppress premature labor [5].

For mammary development, lactation, and galactopoiesis, growth hormone, ovarian estrogen (duct formation), ovarian progesterone (lobule-alveolar development), adrenal corticoids, as well as prolactin and oxytocin, are required. The secretion of prolactin is modified by substances that stimulate or block dopamine receptor sites. Agents such as neuroleptics (chlorpromazine) may cause lactation in a nonpregnant woman [2]. On the other hand, dopamine receptor agonists such as bromocriptine (Parlodel) are used to prevent postpartum lactation.

The direct stimulatory effect of oxytocin is prominent in the gravid uterus during the late stage of pregnancy. The action of oxytocin is augmented by estrogen and inhibited by progesterone. The effect of oxytocin is specific for uterine muscle, since little effect is observed on intestinal muscle or coronary arteries. Oxytocin (Pitocin, Syntocinon) is used:

For induction of term labor. It may be contraindicated during the first and second stages of labor.

In controlling postpartum hemorrhage.

In preventing postpartum uterine atony.

In expulsion of the placenta.

In preventing postpartum breast engorgement in some cases by stimulating the milk letdown. The suckling stimulus initiates a neurogenic reflex transmitted through the spinal cord, midbrain, and hypothalamus, where it sponsors the release of oxytocin and finally lactation. Pain, stress, and adrenergic agonists are known to retard milk letdown [5].

Part Two: Vasopressin

The second hormone of the posterior pituitary gland is antidiuretic hormone (ADH or vasopressin). It has the following formula:

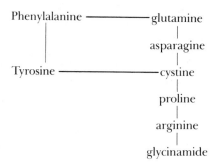

With the exception of two amino acids, vasopressin resembles oxytocin in structure. Oxytocin contains leucine and isoleucine whereas vasopressin contains phenylalanine and arginine. The site of synthesis, storage, and release of vasopressin is identical to that described for oxytocin [1]. The release of vasopressin is enhanced by stress and increased osmolarity of the blood. Furthermore, drugs such as nicotine, clofi-

Table 27-1. *Etiologies of Vasopressin-Sensitive Diabetes Insipidus*

A. Idiopathic form
  1. Nonfamilial form
  2. Familial form
B. Posthypophysectomy
C. Trauma
  1. Basilar skull fracture
D. Tumors
  1. Metastatic carcinoma
  2. Craniopharyngioma
  3. Suprasellar cysts
  4. Pinealoma
  5. Leukemia
E. Granuloma
  1. Sarcoid
  2. Tuberculosis
  3. Syphilis
F. Infections
  1. Meningitis
  2. Encephalitis
  3. Landry-Guillain-Barré syndrome
G. Vascular
  1. Cerebral thrombosis or hemorrhage
  2. Cerebral aneurysm
  3. Postpartum necrosis (Sheehan's syndrome)
H. Histiocytosis
  1. Eosinophilic granuloma
  2. Schüller-Christian disease

From R. W. Schrier and P. D. Miller, Water Metabolism in Diabetes Insipidus and the Syndrome of Inappropriate Antidiuretic Hormone Secretion. In N. A. Kurtzman and M. Martinez-Maldonado (eds.), *Pathophysiology of the Kidney.* Springfield, Ill.: Thomas, 1977. P. 969.

Table 27-2. *Acquired Causes of Nephrogenic Diabetes Insipidus*

A. Chronic renal disease
  1. Polycystic disease
  2. Medullary cystic disease
  3. Pyelonephritis
  4. Ureteral obstruction
  5. Far-advanced renal failure
B. Electrolyte disorders
  1. Hypokalemia
  2. Hypercalcemia
C. Drugs
  1. Lithium
  2. Demeclocycline
  3. Acetohexamide
  4. Tolazamide
  5. Glyburide
  6. Propoxyphene
  7. Amphotericin
  8. Methoxyflurane
  9. Vinblastine
  10. Colchicine
D. Sickle-cell disease
E. Dietary abnormalities
  1. Excessive water intake
  2. Decreased sodium chloride intake
  3. Decreased protein intake
F. Miscellaneous
  1. Multiple sclerosis
  2. Amyloidosis
  3. Sjögren's disease
  4. Sarcoidosis

From R. W. Schrier and A. Leaf, Effect of Hormones on Water, Sodium, Chloride, and Potassium Metabolism. In R. H. Williams (ed.), *Textbook of Endocrinology* (6th ed.). Philadelphia: Saunders, 1981. P. 1036.

brate, ether, barbiturate (not thiopental), morphine, and histamine stimulate the release of vasopressin whereas agents such as alcohol inhibit its release.

The primary physiologic role of vasopressin is to maintain the osmolarity of the blood by modulating the osmoreceptors in the anterior hypothalamus. The ADH-deficient diabetes insipidus (nonnephrogenic) may be treated with ADH. The nephrogenic diabetes insipidus may be controlled by thiazide diuretics. The etiologies of vasopressin-sensitive diabetes insipidus are shown in Table 27-1.

Lithium, when used chronically in a manic-depressive condition, causes ADH-unresponsive diabetes mellitus. In this case the kidney tubules become insensitive to ADH. Dose reduction obviates this syndrome with no residual effects. Chlorpropamide increases the sensitivity of the tubules to ADH. Inappropriate secretion of ADH seen in conditions such as bronchogenic carcinoma, head injury, and tuberculosis meningitis causes water retention. Lithium salts have been advocated in the management of inappropriate secretion of ADH.

PREPARATIONS. Vasopressin (Pitressin) may be administered subcutaneously or intramuscularly. It has a duration of action of 2 to 8 hours. Vasopressin tannate (Pitressin Tannate) is a suspension and should be injected intramuscularly only. It has a duration of action of 2 to 3 days. Desmopressin acetate (DDAVP) is used topically. Lypressin (Diapid) is used by intranasal spray. These agents may be employed in central diabetes insipidus (vasopressin sensitive), whose etiologies are shown in Tables 27-1 and 27-2.

QUESTIONS ON POSTERIOR PITUITARY HORMONES: OXYTOCIN AND VASOPRESSIN

Select one answer that best completes the statement or answers the question.

____ 235. For mammary development, lactation, and galactopoiesis, which agent(s) is (are) necessary?
A. Growth hormone.
B. Estrogen and progesterone.
C. Prolactin and oxytocin.
D. Glucocorticoids.
E. All of the above.

____ 236. Which pair of the following compounds have antagonistic effects on prolactin release?
A. Bromocriptine—chlorpromazine.
B. Reserpine—bromperidol.
C. Bromocriptine—levodopa.
D. None of the above.

____ 237. Oxytocin is used for:
A. Induction of labor.
B. Controlling postpartum hemorrhage.
C. Preventing postpartum lactation.
D. A and B.
E. A, B, and C.

____ 238. Pharmacologic agents causing nephrogenic diabetes insipidus include
A. Lithium.
B. Propoxyphene.
C. Amphotericin.
D. All of the above.

____ 239. The release of vasopressin is stimulated by the following substances *except* which one?
A. Clofibrate.
B. Thiopental.
C. Morphine.
D. Histamine.

____ 240. Vasopressin increases luminal water permeability of the collecting duct cells by stimulating which one of the following enzymes?
A. Adenylate cyclase.
B. Acetylcholinesterase.
C. Aconitase.
D. Adenosine kinase.

ANSWERS ON POSTERIOR PITUITARY HORMONES: OXYTOCIN AND VASOPRESSIN

235. E.
236. A.
237. D.
238. D.
239. B.
240. A.

REFERENCES

1. Baertschi, A. E., and Dreifuss, J. J. *Neuroendocrinology of Vasopressin, Corticoliberin and Opiomelanocortins*. New York: Academic, 1982.

2. Muller, E. E., et al. Drugs Affecting Prolactin Secretion. In G. Tolis et al. (eds.), *Prolactin and Prolactinomas*. New York: Raven, 1983. Pp. 83–103.

3. Schrier, R. W., and Leaf, A. Effect of Hormones on Water, Sodium, Chloride, and Potassium Metabolism. In R. H. Williams (ed.), *Textbook of Endocrinology* (6th ed.). Philadelphia: Saunders, 1981. Pp. 1032–1063.

4. Schrier, R. W., and Miller, P. D. Water Metabolism in Diabetes Insipidus and the Syndrome of Inappropriate Antidiuretic Hormone Secretion. In N. A. Kurtzman and M. Martinez-Maldonado (eds.), *Pathophysiology of the Kidney*. Springfield, Ill.: Thomas, 1977. Pp. 958–991.

5. Thomas, J. A., and Mawhinney, M. G. *Synopsis of Endocrine Pharmacology*. Baltimore: University Park, 1973. Pp. 44–57.

28. Reproductive Pharmacology

The larger the island of knowledge, the longer the shore-line of wonder.

Ralph Sockman

In the absence of pituitary gonadotropins, the gonads fail to develop properly and the removal of pituitary gland causes reproductory failure [2].

The hypothalamic releasing hormone (gonadoliberin, GnRH, LHRH, a single decapeptide) stimulates the release of both luteinizing hormone (LH, Luteropin) and follicle-stimulating hormone (FSH, Follitropin) from the anterior pituitary gland (Fig. 28-1). Follicle-stimulating hormone (FSH) induces development of ovarian follicles and maintains spermatogenesis. Luteinizing hormone (LH) induces development of ovarian follicles, causes ovulation, brings forth corpus luteal formation, and forms androgen in the male.

The activities of follicle-stimulating hormone and luteinizing hormone are in turn regulated by feedback inhibition:

Sertoli cells elaborate inhibin (a protein), which inhibits the release of FSH [3].
Testosterone from the Leydig cells as well as its metabolite, estradiol, are able to suppress the release of LH.
Inhibin inhibits the pituitary FSH response to luteinizing releasing hormone (LRH). Testosterone inhibits the action of LRH [7].

In addition to negative-feedback inhibition, positive-feedback regulation has been demonstrated. During the follicular phase, the elevated level of estradiol enhances the release of LRH and augments

Fig. 28-1. *Relationship and feedback regulation among the hypothalamic releasing factor (GnRH, LHRH), the pituitary hormones (FSH, LH), and the gonadal hormones (testosterone, estrogen, and progesterone).*

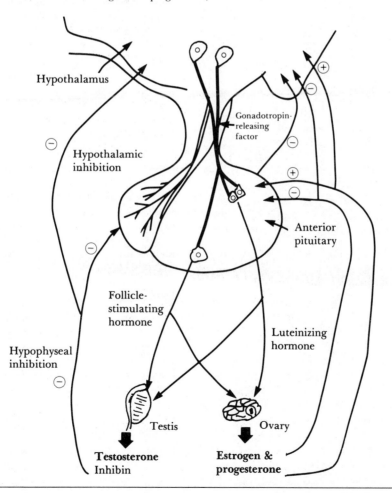

the responsiveness of the pituitary gland to LRH. Moreover, the elevated level of progesterone during ovulation imposes a positive-feedback role on FSH (Fig. 28-1). Indeed, the elevated level of estrogen and progesterone and the simultaneous surge of FSH and LH are the factors triggering ovulation [3].

THE NATURE OF HORMONE RECEPTORS.
Substances such as luteinizing hormone exert their effects by interacting with membrane-bound receptor sites. On the other hand, lipid-soluble hormones such as testosterone and 1,25-di-OH vitamin D enter the cell and bind to cytoplasmic receptors. After becoming activated, they are translocated to the nucleus and become bound to nuclear DNA and nuclear proteins, thereby stimulating the production of specific mRNA, which will sponsor the inherent physiologic function of the hormone (see Fig. 1-3B and C).

ACTION OF LUTEINIZING HORMONE IN TESTIS.
In the testicular Leydig cells, luteinizing hormone (LH) interacts with a specific membrane-bound receptor coupled to adenyl cyclase with the guanyl nucleotide subunit. This interaction converts ATP to cyclic AMP, which phosphorylates a cytoplasmic protein kinase destined to convert cholesterol to testosterone [1].

MECHANISM OF ACTION OF TESTOSTERONE.
Testosterone, a lipid-soluble substance, enters the cell and becomes enzymatically reduced to dihydrotestosterone by 5-alpha-reductase. Dihydrotestosterone becomes bound to a specific androgen receptor site located in the cytoplasm. The complex becomes activated and then is translocated to the nucleus, where it binds to chromatin acceptor site consisting of DNA and nonhistone chromosomal proteins (see Fig. 1-3C). This interaction results in the transcription of a specific mRNA, which is then relocated to the cytoplasm and is translated on cytoplasmic ribosomes, causing the synthesis of a new protein that sponsors the androgenic functions [4].

Part One: The Pharmacology of Estrogens

Estrogens are synthesized mainly in the ovaries, the placenta, and the adrenal glands. A minute amount of estradiol is synthesized in the testis. Estrogens are synthesized according to the following scheme [8]:

Cholesterol $\longrightarrow$ pregnenolone $\longrightarrow$ progesterone $\longrightarrow$

Androstenedione $\longrightarrow$ estradiol 17-beta $\longrightarrow$

Estrone $\longrightarrow$ estriol

PHYSIOLOGIC ACTIONS. Estrogen influences dramatically the growth and development of female reproductive organs (Table 28-1).

BIOCHEMICAL ACTIONS. The uterus and vagina are sensitive to the biochemical actions of estrogens, which are as follows [8]:

Early events—release of histamine, synthesis of cyclic AMP, stimulation of RNA polymerase, and increased excitability of myometrium
Intermediate events—synthesis of RNA and DNA, imbibition of water, and stimulation of certain enzymes
Late events—increased secretory activity, morphologic changes, increased protein synthesis, stimulation of lipid and carbohydrate metabolism, and increased gravimetric response

ESTROGEN PREPARATIONS. Estrogens are basically divided into three groups: natural steroids, semisynthetic steroids, and nonsteroid chemical compounds with estrogenic activities (Table 28-2).

THERAPEUTIC USES. Estrogens are used extensively in endocrine and nonendocrine diseases. A few of these indications are cited here:

Menopause	As replacement therapy
Atrophic vaginitis	To thicken epithelial cells and to proliferate mucosal cells
Hypopituitarism	To correct vaginal mucosal atrophy, maintain breast development, and minimize calcium loss from bone
Cancer	Used in postmenopausal mammary carcinoma
Primary hypogonadism	To correct ovarian failure
Osteoporosis	Estrogen by itself or with hypercalcemic steroid, used in osteoporosis
Primary amenorrhea	To cause proliferative endometrium
Uterine bleeding	To reverse estrogen deficiency if present (in this case, oral contraceptives containing 80–

Table 28-1. *Summary of Physiologic Actions of Estrogen*

Organ	Action
Uterus	Participate in growth and development of muscular and mucosal elements of uterus, oviducts, and fallopian tubes
Myometrium	Stimulate growth of myometrium at puberty and during pregnancy
Endometrium	Increase endothelium and "rebuild" endometrial lining in proliferative phase
Vagina	Increase epithelium layer in vaginal tract and enhance glandular secretion
Breast	Influence breast tissue at puberty, during each ovulatory cycle, and during pregnancy; participate in duct formation and, in conjunction with progesterone, oxytocin, and other hormones, prepare breasts for lactation

Table 28-2. *Naturally Occurring and Synthetic Estrogens*

Category	Drugs
Naturally occurring estrogen and derivatives	Estradiol (Estrace) Estradiol cypionate Estradiol valerate Ethinyl estradiol (Feminone) Micronized estradiol Piperazine estrone sulfate
Nonsteroidal synthetic estrogens	Chlorotrianisene (TACE) Dienestrol Diethylstilbestrol (Stilbestrol) Methallenestril Quinestrol (Estrovis)

	100 μg of estrogen are recommended)
Postpartum lactation	To relieve postpartum painful breast engorgement and to prevent postpartum lactation; bromocriptine is also effective
Control of height	To cause closure of epiphyses in unusually tall young girl
Dermatologic problems	Used with some success in acne

ADVERSE EFFECTS. Low-dose estrogens are safe only when taken for a limited period of time. The most often reported side effects are breakthrough bleeding, breast tenderness, and very infrequent gastrointestinal upset. When estrogens are used in large doses and injudiciously, they may cause thromboembolic disorders, hypertension in susceptible individuals, and cholestasis.

Estrogens are contraindicated in patients with estrogen-dependent neoplasm such as carcinoma of breast or endometrium. Vaginal adenocarcinoma has been reported in young women whose mothers were treated with diethylstilbestrol in an effort to prevent abortion.

ANTIESTROGENS. Clomiphene (Clomid) and tamoxifen (Nolvadex) modify or inhibit the actions of estrogens. These agents are able to bind to the cytoplasmic estrogen receptors, which are then translocated to the nucleus. By diminishing the number of estrogen-binding sites, they interfere with the physiologic actions of estrogens. Furthermore, by interfering with the normal hypothalamic and hypophyseal feedback inhibition of estrogen synthesis, these agents cause an increased secretion of LHRH, FSHRH, and gonadotropins. This leads to ovarian stimulation and ovulation. Clomiphene has been used successfully in some cases of infertility, causing multiple birth. Antiestrogens are able to arrest the growth of estrogen-dependent malignant mammary cells. Clomiphene has been used in certain cases of disseminated breast cancer.

Part Two: The Pharmacology of Progesterone

Progesterone is synthesized by the ovaries, the adrenal glands, and the placenta. In a nonpregnant person, it is produced by corpus luteum during the latter part of the menstrual cycle and under the influence of luteinizing and luteotropic hormones. In a pregnant person, it is produced initially by corpus luteum under the influence of chorionic gonadotropins, and after failure of corpus luteum it is synthesized by placenta.

Progesterone is not only an important progestin but an important precursor for androgen. It is synthesized according to the following reactions:

Acetate $\longrightarrow$ cholesterol $\longrightarrow$ pregnenolone $\longrightarrow$

Progesterone $\longrightarrow$ testosterone $\longrightarrow$ estradiol

Absorbed rapidly when given orally, progesterone has a plasma half-life of 5 minutes. It is completely metabolized in the liver and is cleared completely by "first passage" through the liver.

PHYSIOLOGIC ACTIONS. Progesterone initially prepares the uterus for implantation of the fertilized egg and prevents uterine contraction so that the fetus will not be expelled. Progesterone has been used in the past for threatened abortion. In addition, progesterone exerts effects on secretory cells of the mammary glands. It competes with aldosterone and causes a decrease in Na^+ resorption, and therefore antagonizes aldosterone-induced Na^+ retention. Progesterone increases the body temperature and decreases the plasma level of many amino acids.

PROGESTERONE AND PROGESTINS. Progesterone, which must be injected and has a short duration of action, has been replaced by progestins. The newer synthetic derivatives are effective orally and have longer duration of action. Unlike progesterone, some of these agents have androgenic, estrogenic, and even glucocorticoidlike effects (Table 28-3).

THERAPEUTIC USES OF PROGESTINS. Progestins are used (1) as antifertility agents and (2) in dysfunctional uterine bleeding, which may occur as a result of insufficient estrogen or continued secretion of estrogen in the absence of progesterone.

Amenorrhea. Progestins such as medroxyprogesterone are useful in the diagnosis and treatment of amenorrhea.

Dysmenorrhea. Since prostaglandin $F_{2\alpha}$ is capable of inducing contraction in the uterus, agents that are able to block the synthesis of prostaglandin such as aspirin or aspirinlike substances have been shown to be effective in dysmenorrheea (painful menstruation). For the sexually active woman, oral contraceptives have proved effective in relieving dysmenorrhea.

Endometriosis. Endometriosis, formerly treated with surgical removal of ovaries and uterus, is now treated with continuous administration of progestin, or progestin combined with estrogen. In addition, progestin may be useful in endometrial carcinoma.

Suppression of Postpartum Lactation. Estrogen, progesterone, and bromocriptine (a dopamine receptor agonist) all are effective in suppressing postpartum lactation.

ANTIFERTILITY AGENTS. Use of oral contraceptive medications has brought the pregnancy rate to approximately 1 to 2 percent. Antifertility agents may exert their effects by preventing ovulation, suppressing the actions of gonadotropins, interfering with implantation, and interfering with gestation.

The most commonly used antifertility medications are as follows [5]:

1. The combination preparation containing both progestin and estrogen. In general, a potent estrogen such as ethinyl estradiol or its methyl ether derivatives (mestranol) is combined with one of the several progestins such as norethindrone and its acetate ester: norgestrel, norethynodrel, and ethynodiol acetate. The combination preparations are taken for 20 to 21 days and then are not taken for 7 or 8 days (Table 28-4).

Table 28-3. *Progesterone and Selected Progestins*

Agent	Action
Progesterone (Progelan)	Must be given intramuscularly; brief duration of action
Ethisterone (17α-ethinyltestosterone)	Effective orally
Ethynodiol acetate	Potent progestin
Hydroxyprogesterone caproate (Delalutin)	Long acting; given intramuscularly
Medroxyprogesterone acetate (Provera)	Effective orally
Megestrol acetate (Megace)	Orally effective antifertility agent
Norethindrone (Norethisterone)	Potent oral progestin; mild androgenic effect
Norethynodrel	Used as an antifertility agent
Norgestrel (18-homonorethisterone)	Potent progestin

Table 28-4. *Antifertility Agents*

Trade Name	Mg—Estrogen	Mg—Progestin
Lo/Ovral	0.02 Ethinyl estradiol	0.3 Norgestrel
Loestrin 1/20, Zorane 1/20	0.02 Ethinyl estradiol	1 Norethindrone
Loestrin 1.5/30, Zorane 1.5/30	0.03 Ethinyl estradiol	1.5 Norethindrone
Ovcon-35	0.035 Ethinyl estradiol	0.4 Norethindrone
Brevicon, Modicon	0.035 Ethinyl estradiol	0.5 Norethindrone
Norinyl 1 + 50, Ortho-Novum 1/50	0.05 Mestranol	1 Norethindrone
Ovral	0.05 Ethinyl estradiol	0.5 Norgestrel
Demulen	0.05 Ethinyl estradiol	1 Ethynodiol diacetate
Ovcon-50, Zorane 1/50	0.05 Ethinyl estradiol	1 Norethindrone
Norlestrin, 1	0.05 Ethinyl estradiol	1 Norethindrone acetate
Norlestrin, 2.5	0.05 Ethinyl estradiol	2.5 Norethindrone acetate
Ortho-Novum, 10 mg	0.06 Mestranol	10 Norethindrone
Enovid, 5 mg	0.075 Mestranol	5 Norethynodrel
Norinyl 1 + 80, Ortho-Novum 1/80	0.08 Mestranol	1 Norethindrone
Ovulen	0.10 Mestranol	1 Ethynodiol diacetate
Norinyl, 2 mg, Ortho-Novum, 2 mg	0.10 Mestranol	2 Norethindrone
Enovid-E	0.10 Mestranol	2.5 Norethynodrel
Enovid, 10 mg	0.15 Mestranol	9.85 Norethynodrel

Data from F. Murad and R. C. Haynes, Jr., Estrogens and Progestins. In A. G. Gilman, L. S. Goodman, and A. Gilman (eds.), *The Pharmacological Basis of Therapeutics* (6th ed.). New York: Macmillan, 1980.

2. Sequential preparations, in which an estrogen is taken for 14 to 16 days and a combination of an estrogen and a progestin for 5 to 6 days. These preparations are no longer used.
3. Single-hormone preparations—either an estrogen alone (morning-after pill) or a progesterone alone (mini-pill).
4. Intrauterine device (IUD) containing a slow-releasing progestin preparation (Progestasert).

Mechanism of Action. The antifertility agents (Table 28-4) suppress ovulation by

1. Inhibiting the release of hypophyseal ovulation-regulating gonadotropin
2. Producing "thick" mucus from the cervical glands and hence impeding the penetration of sperm cells into the uterus to fertilize the ovum
3. Impeding the transfer of the ovum from oviduct to uterus
4. Preventing implantation of the fertilized ovum should fertilization take place

Side Effects. Oral contraceptive preparations have occasionally produced nausea, weight gain, edema, headache, dizziness, tenderness of breasts, depression, altered carbohydrate metabolism, altered thyroid function, altered blood coagulation, altered liver functions, and hypertension. Not all of these side effects occur in all patients at all times. Contraindications for oral contraceptive preparations are thromboembolic and cerebrovascular diseases, impaired liver function, estrogen-dependent carcinoma, undiagnosed bleeding, and pregnancy [7].

Part Three: The Pharmacology of Androgens

Testosterone, the male sex hormone, is responsible for the development and maintenance of male sex organs (penis, prostate gland, seminal vesicle, and vas deferens) and secondary sex characteristics. Testosterone also has anabolic effects. Like progesterone, testosterone is metabolized very rapidly by the liver by first-pass mechanism, hence requiring structural modifications. For example, the 17-OH group of testosterone may be modified by addition of propionic acid to yield testosterone propionate, cyclopentylpropionic acid to yield testosterone cypionate, or enanthate to yield testosterone enanthate. The 17 position may be methylated to yield methyltestosterone. Furthermore, a fluorine and a methyl group may be inserted to yield fluoxymesterone. In general, these agents are more effective when given orally and have longer duration of action (Table 28-5).

USES OF ANDROGENS. Testosterone and derivatives are used [6] in hypogonadism (eunuchoidism), hypopituitarism, accelerated growth, aging man, osteoporosis, anemia, endometriosis, promotion of anabolism, suppression of lactation, and carcinoma of breast.

SIDE EFFECTS. The side effects of these compounds are as follows:

Masculinization in women (such as hirsutism, acne, depression of menses, and clitoral enlargement) and of their female offspring. Therefore, androgens are contraindicated in pregnant women.

Prostatic hypertrophy in males, causing urinary retention. Therefore, androgens are contraindicated in patients with prostatic carcinoma.

Table 28-5. *Examples of Anabolic and Androgenic Steroids*

STEROIDS WITH ANABOLIC ACTIVITIES
Dromostanolone propionate (Drolban)
Ethylestrenol (Maxibolin)
Methandrostenolone (Dianabol)
Nandrolone decanoate (Deca-Durabolin)
Nandrolone phenpropionate (Durabolin)
Oxandrolone (Anavar)
Oxymetholone (Adroyd)
Stanozolol (Winstrol)
Testolactone (Teslac)

STEROIDS WITH ANDROGENIC PROPERTIES
Fluoxymesterone (Halotestin)
Methyltestosterone (Metandren)
Testosterone (Android-T)
Testosterone cypionate (Depo-Testosterone)
Testosterone enanthate (Delatestryl)

ANTIANDROGENS. Cyproterone inhibits the action of androgens. Gossypol is an experimental drug tested as a contraceptive for males. It prevents spermatogenesis without altering the other endocrine functions of the testis.

QUESTIONS ON REPRODUCTIVE PHARMACOLOGY

Select one answer that best completes the statement or answers the question.

_____ 241. Anabolic steroids:
   A. Reduce the negative nitrogen balance.
   B. Are used in postoperative recovery.
   C. Are used in debilitating diseases.
   D. All of the above.

_____ 242. Long-term therapy with androgens in large doses in women is restricted to:
   A. Premenopausal metastatic or advanced breast cancer.
   B. Anemia.
   C. Endometriosis.
   D. Osteoporosis.

_____ 243. Estrogens are used in all the following cases *except* which one?
   A. To enhance postpartum milk letdown.
   B. Osteoporosis.
   C. Atrophic vaginitis.
   D. Primary hypogonadism.

_____ 244. Which one of the following compounds has antiestrogenic properties?
   A. Clomiphene.
   B. Tamoxifen.
   C. Clofibrate.
   D. A and B.

_____ 245. The antifertility agents exert their effects by:
   A. Inhibiting the release of gonadotropin.
   B. Impeding the transfer of ovum to uterus.
   C. Impeding implantation of fertilized ovum.
   D. All of the above.

_____ 246. Which one of the following agents inhibits spermatogenesis?
   A. Gossypol.
   B. Gelusil.
   C. Gemcadiol.
   D. Gestodene.

ANSWERS ON REPRODUCTIVE PHARMACOLOGY

241. D.
242. D.
243. A.
244. D.
245. D.
246. A.

REFERENCES

1. Bardin, C. W., and Paulsen, C. A. The Testis. In R. H. Williams (ed.), *Textbook of Endocrinology* (6th ed.). Philadelphia: Saunders, 1981. Pp. 293–354.
2. Catt, K. J. *An ABC of Endocrinology.* Boston: Little, Brown, 1971.

3. Federman, D. D. General Principles of Endoerinology. In R. H. Williams (ed.), *Textbook of Endocrinology* (6th ed.). Philadelphia: Saunders, 1981. Pp. 1–14.

4. Grumbach, M. M., and Conte, F. A. Disorders of Sex Differentiation. In R. H. Williams (ed.), *Textbook of Endocrinology* (6th ed.). Philadelphia: Saunders, 1981. Pp. 423–514.

5. Murad, F., and Haynes, R. C., Jr. Estrogens and Progestins. In A. G. Gilman, L. S. Goodman, and A. Gilman (eds.), *The Pharmacological Basis of Therapeutics* (6th ed.). New York: Macmillan, 1980. Pp. 1420–1447.

6. Murad, F., and Haynes, R. C., Jr. Androgens and Anabolic Steroids. In A. G. Gilman, L. S. Goodman, and A. Gilman (eds.), *The Pharmacological Basis of Therapeutics* (6th ed.). New York: Macmillan, 1980. Pp. 1448–1465.

7. Sellers, E. A. Gonadal Hormones. In P. Seeman, E. M. Sellers, and W. H. E. Roschlau (eds.), *Principles of Medical Pharmacology* (3rd ed.). Toronto: University of Toronto, 1980. Pp. 399–409.

8. Thomas, J. A., and Mawhinney, M. G. *Synopsis of Endocrine Pharmacology.* Baltimore: University Park, 1973.

29. Gastrointestinal Pharmacology

It is high time that the ideal of success should be replaced by the ideal of service.

Albert Einstein

Part One: Antiemetics

The physiologic purpose of nausea is to prevent food intake; of vomiting, to expel the food or other toxic substances present in the upper part of the gastrointestinal tract. Protracted vomiting not only may cause electrolyte imbalance, dehydration, or malnutrition syndrome but also may result in mucosal laceration and upper gastrointestinal hemorrhage (Mallory-Weiss syndrome).

Nausea or vomiting or both may occur when the stomach is overly irritated, stimulated, or distended (overeating). In addition, nausea and vomiting may occur when the chemoreceptor trigger zone for emesis or the vomiting center is directly stimulated. The specific and rational use of antiemetic agents depends on the nature of the emesis-inducing problem. A few cases will be cited.

Pharmacologic agents such as aspirin and levodopa may cause vomiting by irritating the stomach directly. Furthermore, agents such as aminophylline, isoniazid, reserpine, antiinflammatory steroids, or caffeine may cause vomiting in susceptible individuals by releasing hydrochloric acid. Drug-induced emesis may be corrected by ingestion of the drugs with meals. The antiemetics are not effective in these conditions and their use is not justified.

Besides agents stimulating or irritating the stomach, many other factors may be responsible for inducing emesis centrally. The central control of vomiting is vested in two areas:

1. The vomiting center is located in the lateral reticular formation in the midst of a group of cells governing such activities as salivation and respiration.
2. The chemoreceptor trigger zone is a narrow strip along the floor of the fourth ventricle, located in close proximity to the vomiting center.

The functions of these two areas are distinct but interdependent.

The vomiting center is activated by impulses that originate from the gastrointestinal tract and other peripheral structures. In addition, there are unidentified tracts from the cerebral cortex to the vomiting center. Indeed, emotional trauma and unpleasant olfactory and visual stimuli may cause nausea and vomiting. Finally, the stimulation of the vestibular apparatus (movements of the head, neck, and eye muscles) may cause nausea and vomiting by stimulating the vomiting center. On the other hand, circulating chemicals, toxins, viruses, and ions may cause nausea and vomiting by first stimulating the chemoreceptor zone for emesis, which in turn stimulates the vomiting center. The oral administration of an irritant substance such as $CuSO_4$ causes nausea and vomiting by stimulating the vomiting center whereas the intravenous administration of $CuSO_4$ causes nausea and vomiting by stimulating the chemoreceptor zone for emesis. Apomorphine and morphine cause vomiting by stimulating the chemoreceptor. Nausea and vomiting may be precipitated by other factors too:

Emotional disturbances
Stimulation of vestibular apparatus
Radiation
Cancer chemotherapy
Pregnancy
Surgical operation
Many disease processes

SELECTION OF ANTIEMETIC AGENTS.

1. Psychogenically induced vomiting is best controlled by the use of sedatives and antianxiety agents such as

Phenobarbital
Buclizine (Softran), which also has antihistaminic property
Hydroxyzine (Atarax), which also has antihistaminic property

2. Nausea and vomiting of motion sickness is best treated with antihistaminic agents, which have a considerable amount of anticholinergic activity, e.g.,

Chlorpheniramine (Chlor-Trimeton)
Diphenhydramine (Benadryl)
Dimenhydrinate (Dramamine)
Cyclizine (Marezine)
Meclizine (Bonine)
Promethazine (Phenergan), a phenothiazine derivative lacking antipsychotic property and with predominantly antihistaminic property
Diphenidol (Vontrol)
Trimethobenzamide (Tigan)

3. Nausea and vomiting associated with chemico-physical agents that stimulate the chemoreceptor trigger zone for emesis is best treated with a member of the phenothiazine derivatives. With the exception of thioridazine (Mellaril), they all have antiemetic effects. The most often used are

Chlorpromazine (Thorazine)
Fluphenazine (Prolixin, Permitil)
Perphenazine (Trilafon)
Promazine (Sparine)

Promethazine (Phenergan)
Thiethylperazine (Torecan)
Triflupromazine (Vesprin)
Prochlorperazine (Compazine)

Phenothiazine derivatives depress the chemoreceptor trigger zone for emesis. Large doses inhibit the vomiting center. It has been reported that thiethylperazine (Torecan) depresses both the chemoreceptor and the vomiting center.

4. Radiation-induced emesis, or uncontrolled vomiting in patients undergoing radiation therapy, may necessitate either discontinuation of treatment or prophylactic treatment with phenothiazine antiemetics.

5. Antineoplastic agents such as nitrogen mustard or cisplatin may cause disabling nausea and severe vomiting. Triflupromazine has been shown to be more effective than chlorpromazine. Recent studies have suggested that naturally occurring cannabinoid (marijuana) or synthetic cannabinoids (Nabilone) are also effective in combating vomiting associated with cancer chemotherapeutic agents. In addition to antiemetic effects, cannabinoids increase appetite, cause euphoria, and are analgesics. These properties are useful in a patient with terminal stages of cancer.

6. Postoperative nausea and vomiting is directly related to the type and the dose of the anesthetic used. It has been shown that with the use of a muscle relaxant, which substantially reduces the amount of anesthetic to be used, the incidence of postoperative nausea and vomiting is lessened. However, most members of the phenothiazines may be used to control postoperative emesis.

7. Nausea and vomiting associated with the first trimester of pregnancy is benign and self-limiting. If at all possible, no medications should be used. If absolutely necessary, antihistaminics (meclizine, trimethobenzamide) may be effective. Pyridoxine (vitamin B_6) should not be used, since it may predispose to vitamin B_6–dependent syndrome in the infant.

Part Two: Laxatives and Cathartics

Constipation may be defined as the passage of excessively dry stools, infrequent stools, or stools of insufficient size. Constipation is a symptom and not a disease. It may be of brief duration (e.g., when one's living habits and diet change abruptly) or it may be a lifelong problem as seen in congenital aganglionosis of the colon (Hirschsprung's disease). The causes of constipation are listed in Table 29-1 [5].

In addition to these extensive categories, the following drugs may lead to constipation:

Anticholinergic drugs found in many of the over-the-counter (OTC) medications
Antiparkinsonian drugs with anticholinergic properties (e.g., trihexyphenidyl, ethopropazine)
Antihistaminic drugs with anticholinergic properties (e.g., diphenhydramine)
Neuroleptics with anticholinergic properties (e.g., thioridazine)
Antidepressants with anticholinergic properties (e.g., amitriptyline)
Anticonvulsants with anticholinergic properties (e.g., carbamazine)
Analgesics (e.g., morphine, codeine, and diphenoxylate)
Ganglionic blocking agents (e.g., mecamylamine hydrochloride, pempidine)
Antacids (calcium- or aluminum-containing compounds)

Constipation involves the subjective sensations of incomplete emptying of the rectum, bloating, passage of flatus, lower abdominal discomfort, anorexia, malaise, headache, weakness, and giddiness.

LAXATIVES AND CATHARTICS. Although often used interchangeably, the terms *laxative* and *cathartic* do have slightly different meanings. A laxative effect suggests the excretion of a soft, formed stool, while catharsis implies a more fluid and complete evacuation.

Irritants. These agents include cascara sagrada, castor oil, senna, rhubarb, phenolphthalein, and acetphenolisatin. Phenolphthalein is a constituent of many OTC preparations including Correctol, Ex-Lax, Feen-A-Mint. Most of these agents (exception, castor oil) are slow in their onset of action (24 hours).

Phenolphthalein is thought to exert its effect by inhibiting the movement of water and sodium from colon to blood, and by stimulating mucus secretion. When misused chronically, the loss of mucus by phenolphthalein may cause lower plasma proteins.

Castor oil becomes hydrolyzed to ricinoleic acid, the active cathartic. It has an onset of action of 2 to 6 hours.

The misuse of any of these agents has been shown to cause hypokalemia, dehydration, and cathartic colon (ulcerative colitislike). Phenolphthalein-containing products may make the color of alkaline urine red.

Table 29-1. *Major Causes of Constipation*

1. Functional causes
    Fiber-deficient diets
    Inadequate evacuatory habits
    Variants of "irritable bowel syndrome"
    Psychoses and mental deficiency
    Debilitation and extreme old age
2. Colonic diseases
    Chronic obstructive lesions (e.g., tumors, strictures)
    Ulcerative colitis
    Collagen vascular diseases with muscular abnormalities
3. Rectal diseases
    Stricture (e.g., ulcerative colitis, postsurgical)
    Painful conditions (fissure, abscess)
    Prolapsed rectal mucosa
    Rectocele
4. Neurologic diseases
    Hirschsprung's disease
    Ganglionneuromatosis
    Chagas' disease
    Intestinal pseudoobstruction
    Spinal cord injuries and disease
    Parkinson's disease
    Cerebral tumors and cerebrovascular disease
5. Metabolic diseases
    Porphyria
    Hypothyroidism
    Hypercalcemia
    Pheochromocytoma
    Uremia

From S. Philips, Disorders of Gastrointestinal Motility. In J. B. Wyngaarden and L. H. Smith, Jr. (eds.), *Cecil's Textbook of Medicine* (6th ed.). Philadelphia: Saunders, 1982. P. 668.

Bulk Saline Laxatives. These agents may be classified into inorganic salts (magnesium sulfate, magnesium citrate, milk of magnesia, sodium sulfate, sodium phosphate) and organic hydrophilic colloids (methylcellulose, carboxymethylcellulose [Metamucil], plantago seed, agar, psyllium, bran, and fruits). They exert their effects by absorbing and retaining water, by increasing bulk, by stimulating colonic peristaltic movements, and by lubricating and hydrating the desiccated fecal materials.

These agents are more effective when administered with water. The onset of action of inorganic salts is relatively fast (2–6 hours) whereas the onset of action of colloids is relatively slow (1–3 days). Though very effective and safe, these medications should not be used when the intestinal lumen has been narrowed. Chronic use of saline cathartics may pose problems for certain individuals. For example, magnesium salts have caused hypermagnesemia, coma, and death in patients with renal insufficiency. Sodium salts may cause congestive heart failure.

Lubricants. These agents are mineral oil and dioctyl sodium sulfosuccinate (Colace). Colace is used in the pharmaceutics industry as an emulsifying and dispersing substance. Both agents are taken orally. They do not influence peristalsis but soften desiccated stools or delay desiccation of fecal materials. They are especially useful in patients with painful bowel movement resulting from inspissated stools or inflammation of the anal sphincter such as that seen in hemorrhoids. Mineral oil, when used chronically, may interfere with absorption of fat-soluble vitamins and other essential nutrients. Lipid pneumonitis may occur if mineral oil is employed as a vehicle for drugs to be given nasally.

USES OF LAXATIVES. Poisoning. In this case, laxatives are used to hasten elimination and to reduce absorption of the poison.

Anthelmintics. Laxatives are used before and after treatment with anthelmintic drugs.

Radiology. Laxatives are used to clean the gastrointestinal tract prior to the application of radiographic techniques.

Problems Associated with Inflammation of Anal Sphincter. Laxatives may be used in patients with hemorrhoids or fissures.

Special Circumstances. Colace may be used in patients in whom "straining at the stool" may be harmful.

Part Three: Antidiarrheal Agents

Diarrhea and associated fecal urgency and incontinence may be defined as passage of liquefied stool with increased frequency. Diarrhea may result from the inhibition of ion transport or from stimulation of ion secretion in the intestine (Table 29-2).

In addition to impairment of ion transport and ion secretion, diarrhea may result from osmotic diarrhea, in which poorly absorbable solutes are present in the intestine. Finally, diarrhea may stem from deranged intestinal motility of numerous causes outlined in Table 29-3.

TREATMENT OF DIARRHEA. The treatment may include the following measures:

Fluid replenishment is achieved by ingestion of liquids and salty food.
Antiinflammatory agents, such as prednisone, may be effective in diarrhea associated with bowel disease.
Hypolipoproteinemic substances such as cholestyramine, which binds bile acid in the intestine, have been used in diarrhea associated with bile acid malabsorption.
Neuroleptics such as phenothiazine derivatives inhibit the intestinal ion secretion caused by cholera toxin and *E. coli* enterotoxins.
Bismuth subsalicylate prevents infection with enterotoxin-producing *E. coli*.

Table 29-2. *Some Causes of Secretory Diarrhea—Agents or Diseases That Produce Diarrhea by Virtue of Inhibition of Ion Absorption and/or Stimulation of Ion Secretion*

I. Agents that activate the adenylate cyclase–cyclic AMP system
    A. Cholera toxin
    B. Heat-labile toxin of *E. coli*
    C. *Salmonella* enterotoxin
    D. Vasoactive intestinal polypeptide (VIP)
    E. Prostaglandins
    F. Dihydroxy bile acids, long-chain fatty acids
II. Agents that probably do not activate the adenylate cyclase–cyclic AMP system
    A. Heat-stable toxin of *E. coli*
    B. Enterotoxins of *Clostridium perfringens, Pseudomonas aeruginosa*, and *Klebsiella pneumoniae*
    C. Calcitonin
    D. Serotonin
    E. Castor oil, phenolphthalein
III. Chronic secretory diarrhea
    A. Pancreatic cholera syndrome (VIP, calcitonin)
    B. Medullary carcinoma of thyroid (calcitonin, prostaglandins)
    C. Ganglioneuroma and ganglioneuroblastoma
    D. Malignant carcinoid syndrome (serotonin)
    E. Villous adenoma of the rectum
    F. Surreptitious laxative abuse
    G. Fatty acid and bile acid malabsorption

From J. S. Fordtran, Diarrhea. In J. B. Wyngaarden and L. H. Smith, Jr. (eds.), *Cecil's Textbook of Medicine* (6th ed.). Philadelphia: Saunders, 1982.

Table 29-3. *Some Causes of Diarrhea in Five Different Clinical Categories*

A. Acute diarrhea
    1. Viral, bacterial, and parasitic infections
    2. Food poisoning
    3. Drugs (acute or chronic)
    4. Heavy-metal poisoning (acute or chronic)
B. Traveler's diarrhea
    1. Bacterial infections
        a. Mediated by enterotoxins, e.g., heat-labile and/or heat-stable producing *E. coli*
        b. Mediated mainly by invasion of mucosa and inflammation, e.g., invasive *E. coli*, *Shigella*, *Campylobacter*
        c. Mediated by combination of invasion and enterotoxins, e.g., *Salmonella*
    2. Viral and parasitic infections
C. Chronic and recurrent diarrhea
    1. Irritable colon syndrome
    2. Inflammatory bowel disease
    3. Parasitic infections
    4. Malabsorption syndromes
    5. Drugs (acute or chronic)
    6. Heavy-metal poisoning (acute or chronic)
D. Chronic diarrhea of unknown origin (previous work had failed to reveal diagnosis)
    1. Surreptitious laxative abuse
    2. Irritable colon syndrome
    3. Unrecognized inflammatory bowel disease
    4. Other cause of chronic diarrhea that was previously overlooked
E. Incontinence
    1. Cause of sphincter dysfunction
        a. Anal surgery for fissure, fistulas, or hemorrhoids
        b. Episiotomy or tear during childbirth
        c. Anal Crohn's disease
        d. Diabetic neuropathy
        e. Idiopathic

From J. S. Fordtran, Diarrhea. In J. B. Wyngaarden and L. H. Smith, Jr. (eds.), *Cecil's Textbook of Medicine* (6th ed.). Philadelphia: Saunders, 1982.

Local anesthetic ointments may be helpful when used for a short period of time in symptomatic treatment of perianal discomfort.
Opiates may have a place in treatment.

The agents used are codeine, diphenoxylate and atropine (Lomotil), and loperamide. Since it causes less addiction than codeine, loperamide is now the most often used antidiarrheal agent. All these agents may reduce the propulsive activity of the gut, enhance contact time between intestinal mucosal and luminal contents, enhance active chloride absorption, and hence oppose the secretory effects of toxin. Opiate antidiarrheal agents should not be used in severe ulcerative colitis with impending toxic megacolon, and in shigellosis (prolongs duration).

Part Four: Treatment of Acid-Pepsin Disease

The medical treatment of esophageal, gastric, and duodenal ulcer includes (1) relief of symptoms, (2) increase in rate of healing, (3) prevention of complications, and (4) prevention of recurrence [4].

The treatment includes use of antacids, anticholinergic drugs, and histamine H_2 receptor antagonists.

ANTACIDS. Since acid-pepsin disease rarely occurs in the absence of gastric acid and pepsin, antacids are highly effective in the overall management of acid-pepsin diseases. Antacids consist of mixtures of magnesium, aluminum, and calcium compounds. Their efficacy is based on their inherent property to react and to neutralize gastric acid. The pharmacology of antacids is summarized in Table 29-4. Sodium bicarbonate, which may leave the stomach rapidly, has the potential risk of causing alkalosis and retaining sodium. Calcium salts may cause hypercalcemia, which may be detrimental in patients with impaired renal function. Aluminum salts may decrease the absorption of tetracyclines and anticholinergic drugs.

ANTICHOLINERGIC DRUGS. Vagal impulses release acetylcholine at the parietal cell and at gastric mucosal cells containing gastrin, a peptide hormone. Both the directly released acetylcholine and the indirectly released gastrin then stimulate the parietal cell to secrete H^+ into the gastric lumen.

The most useful anticholinergic drug is propantheline (Pro-Banthine). It depresses gastric motility and secretion. The production of pepsin is also reduced. Propantheline (Fig. 29-1) may be used as adjunct therapy in combination with antacids but not as a single agent [4]. The timing of medication is critical in ulcer therapy. Anticholinergic drugs should be given about 30 minutes before meals, and antacids about 1 hour after meals. The dose of antacid is often doubled just before bedtime. The side effects and contraindications for propantheline are identical to those described for atropine (prostatic hypertrophy, urinary retention, glaucoma, and cardiac arrhythmias).

HISTAMINE H_2 RECEPTOR ANTAGONISTS. The histamine receptors are classified as H_1, blocked by agents such as diphenhydramine and other antiallergic agents, and H_2, blocked by cimetidine (Tagamet) and ranitidine (Zantac). Cimetidine (Fig. 29-1) has no effect on most histamine (H_1)-mediated effects such as bronchoconstriction [1].

SUMMARY PHARMACOLOGY OF CIMETIDINE. Cimetidine, which is far more efficacious than anticholinergic drugs, is used in duodenal ulcers, in gastrinoma, and in gastroesophageal reflux. It is absorbed orally, has a plasma half-life of 2 hours, and is excreted mainly unchanged by the kidney. The doses of cimetidine must be reduced in impairment of renal functions. The few and seldom occurring adverse effects of cimetidine include gynecomastia (may bind to androgen receptor sites), galactorrhea (especially in patients with gastrinoma), granulocytopenia, agranulocytosis (very rare), mental confusion (especially in the elderly), restlessness, seizures, and reduced sperm count [4]. Ranitidine is more effective than cimetidine and allegedly has fewer side effects.

Table 29-4. *Summary Pharmacology of Antacids*

Antacid	Relative Potency	Onset	Advantages	Disadvantages
NaHCO₃ (OTC by lay public)	+ +	Immediate	Cheap	CO₂ distention, alkalosis, brief action, acid rebound (small), Na retention
Al(OH)₃	+	Slow	Demulcent astringent	Constipation, PO₄ depletion (rare), binds tetracycline and anticholinergics
CaCO₃	+ + +	Fast	Prolonged action, cheap, antipeptic	Constipation, chalky taste, acid rebound, hypercalcemia if used longer than 1 week
Mg(OH)₂ (milk of magnesia)	+ + +	Intermediate	Prolonged action	Laxative, Mg²⁺ absorption, care in renal dysfunction

+, + +, and + + + mean efficacious, moderately efficacious, and very efficacious.
From F. Dalske, *Review of Concepts in Gastrointestinal Pharmacology*. Omaha: University of Nebraska, 1979.

Fig. 29-1. *Structure of agents effective in acid-pepsin disease.*

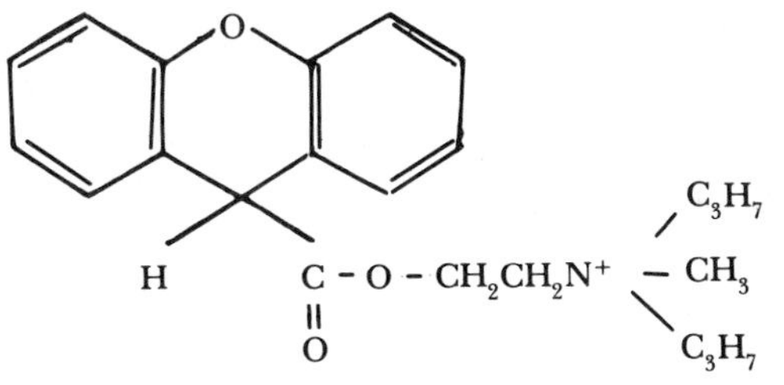

Propantheline

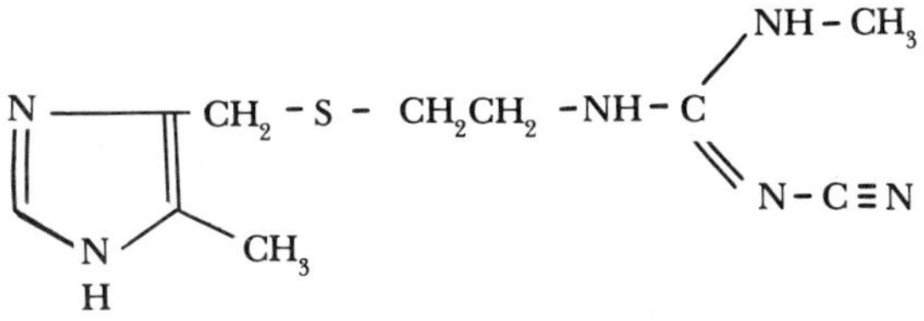

Cimetidine

QUESTIONS ON GASTROINTESTINAL PHARMACOLOGY

Select one answer that best completes the statement or answers the question.

_____ 247. All of the following statements about cimetidine are correct *except* which one?
   A. It inhibits histamine-evoked gastric secretion.
   B. It is a noncompetitive antagonist of H_2 receptors.
   C. It inhibits gastrin-evoked gastric secretion.
   D. It inhibits pentagastrin-evoked gastric secretion.

_____ 248. Which one of the following is *not* a reported side effect of cimetidine?
   A. Increased sperm count.
   B. Gynecomastia.
   C. Galactorrhea.
   D. Seizure.

_____ 249. Which one of the following phenothiazine derivatives is devoid of an antiemetic effect?
   A. Chlorpromazine.
   B. Prochlorperazine.
   C. Thioridazine.
   D. Trifluopromazine.

_____ 250. Which one of the following drug(s) is (are) able to cause constipation?
   A. Amitriptyline.
   B. Thioridazine.
   C. Trihexyphenidyl.
   D. All of the above.

ANSWERS AND EXPLANATION ON GASTROINTESTINAL PHARMACOLOGY

247. B.
248. A.
249. C.
250. D.
   Explanation: Amitriptyline (an antidepressant), thioridazine (a neuroleptic), and trihexyphenidyl (an antiparkinson's drug) are all potent anticholinergic drugs.

REFERENCES

1. Code, C. F. Histamine Receptors and Gastric Secretion. In C. R. Ganellin and M. E. Parsons (eds.), *Pharmacology of Histamine Receptor*. Bristol, Eng.: John Wright, 1982. Pp. 217–235.
2. Dalske, F. *Review of Concepts in Gastrointestinal Pharmacology*. Omaha: University of Nebraska, 1979.
3. Fordtran, J. S. Diarrhea. In J. B. Wyngaarden and L. H. Smith, Jr. (eds.), *Cecil's Textbook of Medicine* (6th ed.). Philadelphia: Saunders, 1982. Pp. 671–678.
4. Isenberg, J. I. Peptic Ulcer: Diagnosis and Medical Treatment. In J. B. Wyngaarden and L. H. Smith, Jr. (eds.), *Cecil's Textbook of Medicine* (6th ed.). Philadelphia: Saunders, 1982. Pp. 644–650.
5. Philips, S. Disorders of Gastrointestinal Motility. In J. B. Wyngaarden and L. H. Smith, Jr. (eds.), *Cecil's Textbook of Medicine* (6th ed.). Philadelphia: Saunders, 1982. Pp. 661–671.

30. Pulmonary Pharmacology

We work not only to produce but to give value to time.
Eugene Delacroix

The principal functions of the lungs are oxygenation of the blood and excretion of carbon dioxide and water. In accomplishing these tasks, the lungs and the heart are structurally and functionally interdependent, and the malfunctioning of one system will eventually compromise the function of the other. Pulmonary diseases often become manifested in the following ways:

Coughing and expectoration, frequently caused by inflammation of the bronchi, may be associated with viral infection, bacterial infection, pulmonary tuberculosis, carcinoma of the lung, and bronchial asthma.

Dyspnea (shortness of breath) may involve both the respiratory and the cardiovascular systems.

Pain (chest pain) may result from inflammation of pleura as seen in pneumonia, thromboembolism, myositis, and myocardial ischemia.

Hemoptysis (blood in the sputum) may result from bronchogenic carcinoma, bronchiectasis, bronchitis, and other inflammatory disorders [6].

Part One: Antitussives and Expectorants

Coughing may be transient and inconsequential or may linger on and be indicative of severe intrathoracic disease. Coughing may be "productive," having expectorant property to clear the airways of excess secretions, or "unproductive," occurring after innocuous stimuli and causing further irritation and mucosal trauma. Antitussive preparations should be used only in unproductive cough. The termination of a productive cough may result in accumulation of secretions and further impairment of oxygenation and gas exchange [6].

ANTITUSSIVE MEDICATIONS. These medications may be divided into narcotic (e.g., codeine) and nonnarcotic (e.g., dextromethorphan and levopropoxyphene) agents. Some smooth muscle relaxants and antihistaminics also have antitussive properties.

Codeine. Most narcotics (morphine, codeine, dihydrocodeinone, methadone, and levorphanol) have antitussive properties. Codeine is primarily used because it has a low addictive liability and is effective orally. Antitussive doses of narcotics are lower than analgesic doses.

Dextromethorphan (Romilar). Dextromethorphan, like codeine, exerts its antitussive property by elevating the cough threshold in the medulla. Unlike codeine, dextromethorphan has no respiratory depressant, analgesic, or addictive properties. Furthermore, it does not cause drowsiness, narcosis, or gastrointestinal irritation.

Levopropoxyphene Napsylate (Novrad). Unlike dextropropoxyphene (Darvon), levopropoxyphene has no analgesic or respiratory depressant properties.

Noscapine (narcotine, Nectadon). Noscapine is a naturally occurring opium alkaloid similar in structure and function to papaverine. It is antitussive and has no analgesic or addicting properties.

Diphenhydramine and chlorcyclizine are antihistaminic agents with antitussive properties. Dimethoxanate (Cothera) and pipazethate (Theratuss) are phenothiazine derivatives without analgesic, but with weak antitussive and local anesthetic properties.

MUCOLYTIC AGENTS. Acetylcysteine (Mucomyst) is an *N*-acetyl derivative of L-cysteine. It is given by aerosol and is able to liquefy excess mucus, especially in patients with pneumonia, chronic bronchitis, cystic fibrosis, bronchiectasis, and emphysema. Acetylcysteine exerts its effect by splitting the disulfide bond of mucin and reducing its viscosity. The respiratory fluid will be eliminated by drainage or expectoration. In a weakened debilitated patient, suctioning of excess fluid may become necessary.

MUCOKINETIC AGENTS (EXPECTORANTS). Ammonium chloride, ammonium carbonate, potassium citrate, potassium iodide, ipecac, creosotes, guaiacols, and volatile oils (oils of anise, eucalyptus, lemon, pine, and turpentine) are all expectorants. They increase the respiratory tract fluid and prevent the drying of secretions that when solidified form mucous plugs obstructing airway and preventing gas exchange.

Part Two: Pharmacology of Asthma

Bronchial asthma is a disorder characterized by paroxysmal and reversible bronchospasm manifested in cough, wheeze, and dyspnea resulting from hyperresponsivity of tracheobronchial smooth muscles to mechanical, chemical, environmental, allergic (extrinsic asthma), pharmacologic, or unknown stimuli. This awkward characterization should not be viewed as a definition but as a denotation that the pathophysiology of asthma is complex, defying oversimplification.

CLASSIFICATION OF ASTHMA. Asthmatic patients are divided into two major subgroups of extrinsic and intrinsic asthma [4].

Extrinsic Asthma. Extrinsic asthma, which shows seasonal variation, occurs in childhood and the adolescent period. It is caused by known and specific allergies such as danders, dusts, pollens, and foods. The asthmatic attacks are self-limiting, and responses to antiasthmatic drugs and hyposensitization procedures are favorable.

Intrinsic Asthma. Intrinsic asthma, which occurs in patients aged 30 and older, is more severe and is caused by no known allergies. The triggering factors are infection, pollution, cold, and exercise. The asthmatic attacks are more fulminant, and responses to antiasthmatic drugs and hyposensitization procedures are less favorable.

In extrinsic asthma, the proposed mechanisms leading to bronchoconstriction commence with sensitization of a patient by an allergen such as inhaled pollen, which is digested by mucosal lysozyme releasing water-soluble proteins. The absorption of these proteins results in release of a specific immune globulin E (IgE) by plasma cells of the lymphoid tissue in the respiratory tract. The formed IgE attaches to the surface of mast cells and basophils. The reexposure of the atopic patient to the same pollen causes an allergic reaction. The IgE-sensitized mast cells in the presence of the antigen release preformed pharmacologic substances (mediators) such as histamine, slow-reacting substance of anaphylaxis (SRS-A), eosinophil chemotactic factor of anaphylaxis (ECF-A), serotonin, kinins, and prostaglandins [5]. These substances cause vasodilatation, secretion of thick mucus, mucosal edema (vasodilatation) and inflammation, and bronchoconstriction. The bronchial obstruction produced by these factors is followed by typical symptoms of bronchial asthma. Infections are able to cause bronchoconstriction by causing mucosal edema and inflammation. Substances such as cromolyn sodium that prevent the release of mediators are very useful prophylactic agents in the management of asthma.

In addition to the immunologic mechanism, the autonomic nervous system plays a major role in controlling bronchial musculature, bronchial vessels, and

Fig. 30-1. *Structure of selected agents useful in asthma.*

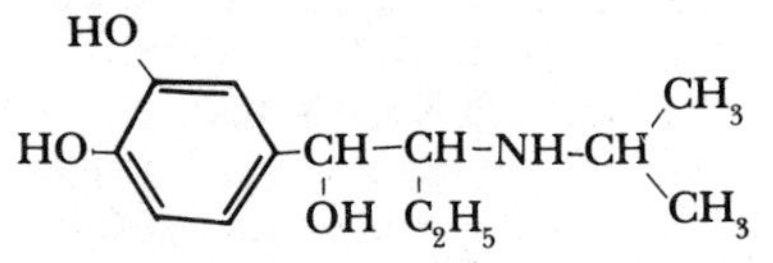

Isoetharine

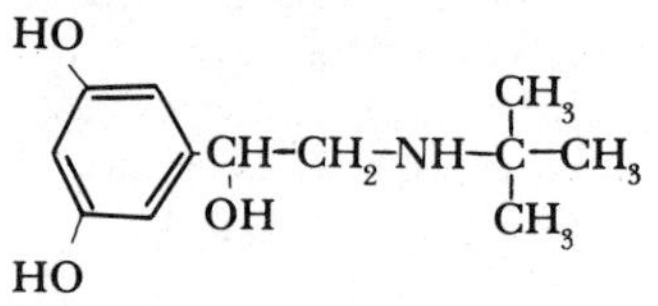

Terbutaline

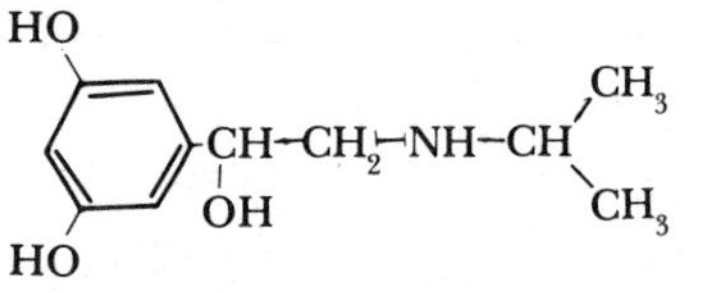

Metaproterenol

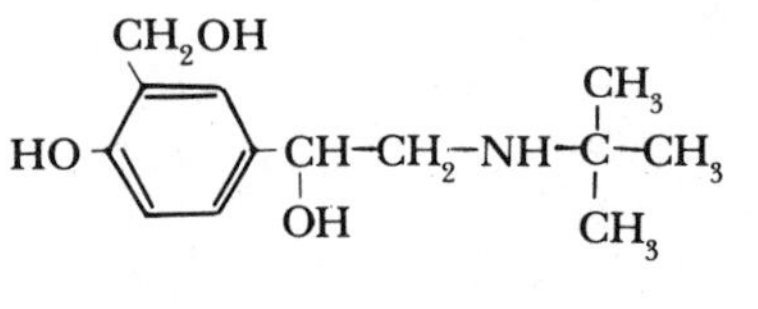

Albuterol (salbutamol)

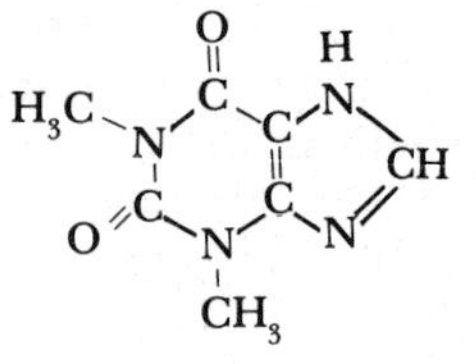

Theophylline

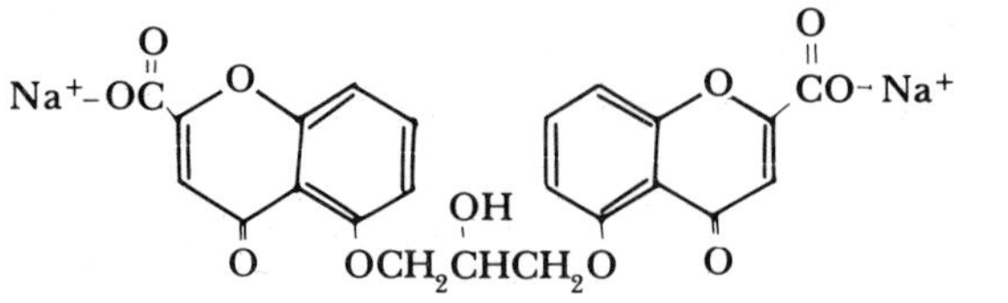

Cromolyn

bronchial gland. The stimulation of parasympathetic fibers (vagus) causes vasodilatation, bronchoconstriction, and enhanced glandular secretion. It is clearly evident that cholinomimetic agents (e.g., methacholine) are contraindicated in bronchial asthma. The stimulation of sympathetic fibers (beta$_2$ receptor sites) causes bronchial dilatation and diminished glandular secretion. Beta-adrenergic agonists (e.g., terbutaline) are extremely useful antiasthmatic agents [1].

CYCLIC AMP AND BRONCHIAL ASTHMA.

Cyclic AMP prevents bronchial smooth muscle contraction, causes bronchial relaxation, and inhibits the release of mediators. The metabolism of cyclic AMP takes place according to the following reactions:

$$\text{ATP} \xrightarrow{\text{Adenylate cyclase}} \text{cyclic AMP} \xrightarrow{\text{phosphodiesterase}} 5' \text{ AMP}$$

Agents that stimulate the activity of adenylate cyclase (beta$_2$ agonists), inhibit the activity of phosphodiesterase (aminophylline), or enhance the effects of beta$_2$ agonists on their receptor sites (corticosteroids) are extremely useful antiasthmatic agents. Conversely, substances that block the beta-adrenergic receptor sites (propranolol), stimulate the cholinergic receptor sites (cholinomimetic agents), or stimulate the alpha-adrenergic receptor sites (prostaglandin

F$_{2\alpha}$) cause bronchoconstriction. Furthermore, the muscarinic cholinergic receptor antagonists (ipratropium bromide) are potential bronchodilators [2].

BRONCHODILATORS.

These agents are sympathomimetic agents that stimulate beta receptor sites.

Epinephrine. Epinephrine may be used subcutaneously in status asthmaticus. It has a rapid onset of action of 3 to 5 minutes and short duration of action of 15 to 20 minutes.

Selective Beta$_2$ Stimulants. The selective beta$_2$-adrenergic stimulants cause bronchodilatation without cardiac acceleration. Metaproterenol and terbutaline are available in tablet form. Terbutaline is also available for subcutaneous injection. Metaproterenol and albuterol are available in metered dose inhalers (Fig. 30-1).

XANTHINES (AMINOPHYLLINE).

The main therapeutic effect of aminophylline is bronchodilatation. In addition, aminophylline causes CNS stimulation, cardiac acceleration, diuresis, and gastric secretion. Aminophylline is available in oral, rectal (pediatric), and intravenous solution to be used in status asthmaticus.

CORTICOSTEROIDS. Prednisone is available in oral form, and beclomethasone may be used as an aerosol, especially in children. The corticosteroids have the following beneficial effects:

They cause relaxation of bronchospasm.
They decrease mucus secretion.
They potentiate beta-adrenergic receptor agonist actions.
They antagonize cholinergic action.
They stabilize lysosomes.
They have antiinflammatory properties.
They inhibit antibody formation.
They antagonize histamine actions.

Since these agents may produce a large number of side effects, they should be used judiciously as adjuncts with other medications.

CROMOLYN SODIUM. Cromolyn sodium (Fig. 30-1) exerts its effects by preventing the release of the mediators. It is used as aerosol powder four times a day only as a prophylactic medication. Since cromolyn is not a bronchodilator, it is not used in status asthmaticus.

Part Three: Chronic Bronchitis

Chronic bronchitis may occur in heavy cigarette smokers and in individuals exposed chronically to high concentrations of environmental pollutants. It may cause hypersecretion of the mucus and interference with its clearance, and it may cause malfunctioning of the alveolar macrophages and increase susceptibility to bronchopulmonary infection. The treatment of bronchitis includes the following [3]:

Stopping or curtailing smoking, and eliminating the "provocative" irritants.
Antibiotic therapy. If infection is present or suspected, active or prophylactic treatment with antibiotics such as ampicillin, tetracycline, or cephalothin may be indicated.
Therapy with bronchodilators and adrenocorticoids. Adrenergic agonists, xanthine derivatives, or prednisolone may be helpful when their uses are indicated and justified.
Anticholinergic drugs including ipratropium (Atrovent). These reduce secretion in both upper and lower respiratory tract and are effective bronchodilators.

QUESTIONS ON PULMONARY PHARMACOLOGY

Select one answer that best completes the statement or answers the question.

____ 251. Antitussive preparations should be used:
  A. In productive cough.
  B. In unproductive cough.
  C. Only when hypoxia is imminent.
  D. Only when infection is imminent.

____ 252. All of the following have antitussive properties *except* which one?
  A. Morphine.
  B. Codeine.
  C. Dextromethorphan.
  D. Deserpidine.

____ 253. Which one of the following agents does not depress respiration?
  A. Methadone.
  B. Meperidine.
  C. Levorphanol.
  D. Dextromethorphan.

____ 254. Which one of the following agents is devoid of analgesic property?
  A. Levopropoxyphene.
  B. Dextropropoxyphene.
  C. Dihydromorphenone.
  D. Dihydrocodeinone.

____ 255. Which one of the following substances is not actually an expectorant?
  A. Ammonium chloride.
  B. Potassium citrate.
  C. Guaiacols.
  D. Acetylcysteine.

____ 256. Which one of the following substance(s) is (are) able to increase the concentrations of cyclic AMP in the lung?
  A. Propranolol.
  B. Methacholine.
  C. Prostaglandin $F_{2\alpha}$.
  D. A and B.
  E. None of the above.

_____ 257. Which one of the following agents when used in a therapeutic dose is expected to influence the heart the least?
  A. Propranolol.
  B. Terbutaline.
  C. Aminophylline.
  D. Atropine.

_____ 258. The use of beclomethasone in an asthmatic patient accomplishes all of the following *except* which one?
  A. It potentiates cholinergic agonists.
  B. It potentiates beta-adrenergic agonists.
  C. It stabilizes lysosomes.
  D. It antagonizes histamine action.

ANSWERS AND EXPLANATIONS ON PULMONARY PHARMACOLOGY

251. B.

252. D.

Explanation: Deserpidine is a *Rauwolfia* derivative having reserpinelike actions.

253. D.

254. A.

255. D.

256. E.

257. B.

Explanation: Beta$_2$-adrenergic stimulants such as terbutaline cause bronchodilatation without causing cardiac acceleration.

258. A.

REFERENCES

1. Austen, K. F., and Lichtenstein, L. M. *Asthma: Physiology, Immunopharmacology and Treatment.* New York: Academic, 1973.

2. Boushey, H. A., and Holtzman, M. J. Bronchodilators and Other Agents Used in the Treatment of Asthma. In B. G. Katzung (ed.), *Basic and Clinical Pharmacology.* Los Altos, Calif.: Lange, 1982. Pp. 205–213.

3. Burrows, B. Chronic Bronchitis and Emphysema. In J. B. Wyngaarden and L. H. Smith, Jr. (eds.), *Cecil's Textbook of Medicine* (6th ed.). Philadelphia: Saunders, 1982. Pp. 363–371.

4. Daniele, R. P. Asthma. In J. B. Wyngaarden and L. H. Smith, Jr. (eds.), *Cecil's Textbook of Medicine* (6th ed.). Philadelphia: Saunders, 1982. Pp. 359–363.

5. Herzog, H. *Asthma.* Basel: Karger, 1980.

6. Murray, J. F. Respiratory Diseases. In J. B. Wyngaarden and L. H. Smith, Jr. (eds.), *Cecil's Textbook of Medicine* (6th ed.). Philadelphia: Saunders, 1982. Pp. 335–339.

31. The Pharmacology of Histamine and Antihistamines

The most powerful weapon on earth is the human soul on fire.

Ferdinand Foch

Histamine is synthesized according to the following reaction:

Histidine $\xrightarrow{\text{Histidine decarboxylase}}$ histamine

Histamine may be used diagnostically to identify patients with pheochromocytoma (it increases the release of catecholamines) and to differentiate pernicious anemia (lack of acid release indicates achlorhydria). Histamine is stored mostly in mast cells. It is also found in platelets, leukocytes, and basophils, in skin, in the lung, in gastric mucosa, and to a certain extent in blood, plasma, sputum, gastric juice, blister fluid, and pus [1]. The histamine release in the brain and perhaps other sites involves exocytosis, since this K^+-induced release is a Ca^{2+}-dependent process. Histamine is released by many factors:

Histamine is involved in IgE-mediated immune responses initiating and maintaining a host of inflammatory and allergic reactions, including lysosomal enzyme release from neutrophils, lymphocyte proliferation in response to mitogens, lymphocyte-mediated cytolysis, and antibody production and secretion.

Histamine, as a normal constituent of gastric mucosa, controls both microcirculation and gastric secretion. The gastric secretagogues are acetylcholine, histamine, and gastrin. The action of acetylcholine is blocked by atropine, and the action of histamine is blocked by cimetidine, burimamide, and metiamide. No specific antagonist is available for gastrin.

Histamine is released by numerous drugs including reserpine, codeine, meperidine, hydralazine, morphine, *d*-tubocurarine, dextrans, papaverine, and compound 48/80. However, it should be emphasized that the different histamine storage sites show certain degrees of specificity. For example, the histamine in mast cells is not released following K^+-induced depolarization or by reserpine, factors that release histamine from neurons. Conversely, compound 48/80, which releases histamine from mast cells, is ineffective in releasing histamine from neurons.

Histamine is metabolized by histamine *N*-methyltransferase (HMT) to *N*-methylhistamine, which is then deaminated by monoamine oxidase type B into methylimidazole acetic acid (MIA).

ACTIONS OF HISTAMINE.
Histamine in the peripheral system causes

Capillary dilatation and increased permeability

Bronchoconstriction and contraction of gastrointestinal muscles
Stimulation of chromaffin cells, releasing catecholamines
Stimulation of sensory nerve endings, causing pain
Vasodilation, tachycardia, headache
Stimulation of exocrine secretion, causing hypersecretion of mucus in the lung
Stimulation of gastric secretion

HISTAMINE RECEPTOR SITES. The diversified actions of histamine are brought forth by interaction with different types of receptors according to the following specifications:

Histamine 1 (H_1) mediates such actions as bronchoconstriction, and contraction of smooth muscles in the gastrointestinal tract. These effects are blocked by classic antihistaminics such as pyrilamine.
Histamine 2 (H_2) mediates gastric secretion, which is blocked by cimetidine. Other effects such as vasodilatation and hypotension are mediated via both H_1 and H_2 receptors [2, 3].

H_1 RECEPTOR BLOCKING AGENTS. By examining the structure of histamine and H_1 antihistaminics, one recognizes that a substituted ethylamine moiety $(CH_2-CH_2-NH_2)$ is present. Extensive numbers of H_1 blockers have been synthesized (Fig. 31-1). They have the following derivatives:

Histamine 1 (H_1) Blockers

Ethanolamine derivatives
    Diphenhydramine (Benadryl)
    Dimenhydrinate (Dramamine)
Phenothiazine derivative
    Promethazine (Phenergan)
Ethylenediamine derivative
    Pyrilamine (Allertoc, Neo-Antergan)
Alkylamine derivative
    Chlorpheniramine (Chlor-Trimeton)
Piperazine derivatives
    Meclizine (Bonine)
    Cyclizine (Marezine)

Histamine 2 (H_2) Blockers

Cimetidine (Tagamet)
Ranitidine (Zantac)

PHARMACOLOGIC EFFECTS. The pharmacology of H_1 receptor antagonists is qualitatively similar in that they antagonize (competitive H_1 blockers) the

Fig. 31-1. *Structure of selected H_1 and H_2 blockers.*

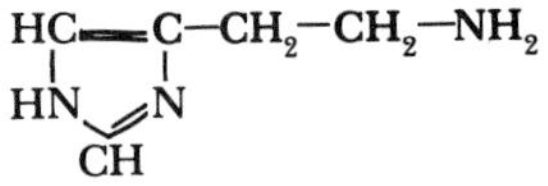

Histamine

Histamine$_1$ receptor blockers

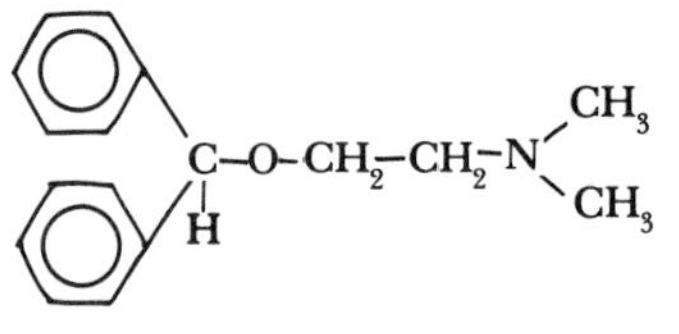

Diphenhydramine

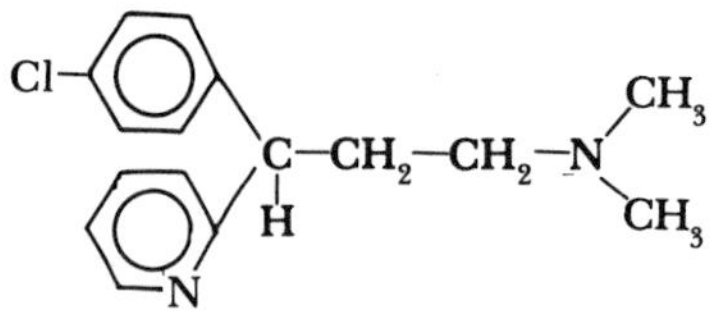

Chlorpheniramine

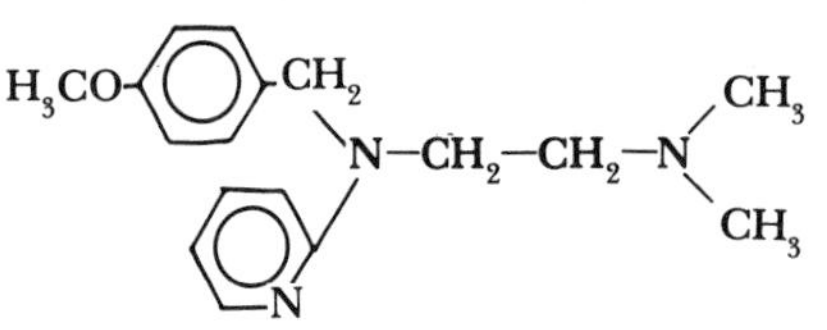

Pyrilamine

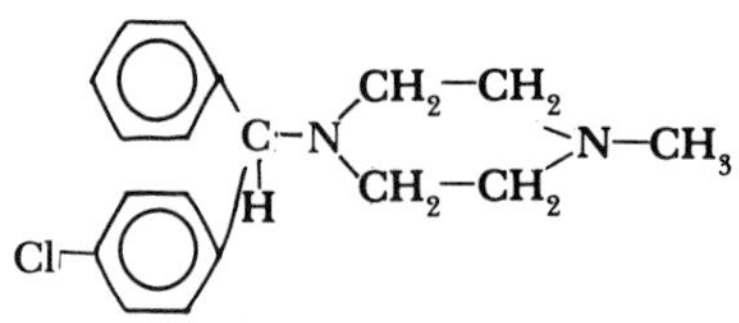

Chlorcyclizine

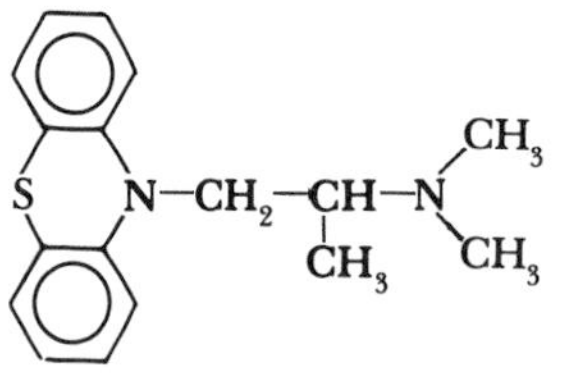

Promethazine

Histamine$_2$ receptor blocker

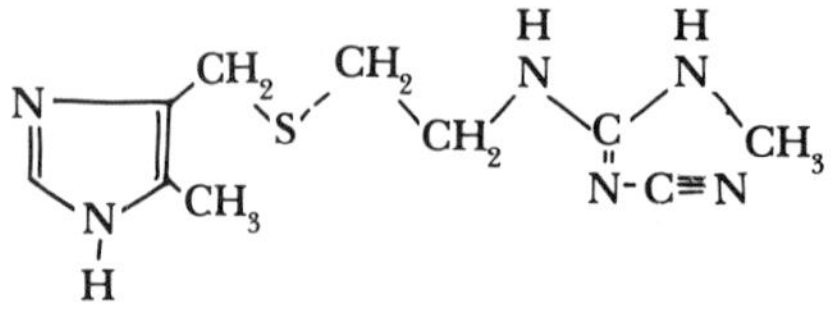

Cimetidine

histamine-mediated bronchoconstriction, vasodilatation, and enhanced capillary permeability. In addition to blocking H_1 receptors, some of these agents have anticholinergic properties. Diphenhydramine has strong atropinelike effects whereas pyrilamine has weak anticholinergic effects. Some antihistaminics such as benztropine (Cogentin) are used in parkinsonism and in neuroleptic-induced pseudoparkinsonism. Furthermore, diphenhydramine is most effective in reversing the neuroleptic-induced dystonia. The usefulness of these agents in these extrapyramidal disorders is related to their anticholinergic effects. Some antihistaminics such as cyproheptadine (Periactin) also block serotonin receptor sites. As a result they have been advocated in allergic dermatitis characterized by urticaria or pruritus. Some antihistaminics such as promethazine and diphenhydramine have local anesthetic properties. They may be used substitutively in patients who are allergic to both "amide" and "ester" types of local anesthetics. Some

phenothiazine antihistaminics such as promethazine have alpha-adrenergic blocking effects. Therefore, like phenothiazine neuroleptics, promethazine may cause orthostatic hypotension.

THERAPEUTIC USES. In addition to the specific uses discussed, the general therapeutic uses of antihistaminics include treatment of allergic reactions, motion sickness, vestibular disturbances, and nausea and vomiting of pregnancy.

SIDE EFFECTS. The most common side effect of these agents is sedation, which occurs in various degrees with all of them. For example, diphenhydramine, dimenhydrinate, and promethazine cause marked sedation. Pyrilamine causes moderate sedation whereas chlorpheniramine, meclizine, and cyclizine have mild or negligible sedative properties.

ACUTE POISONING. The acute poisoning with most antihistaminics does not cause severe CNS depression as one would expect from their sedative property but becomes manifest in mydriasis, fever, flushed face, CNS excitement, hallucination, ataxia, athetosis, and convulsions. Some of these effects, which resemble the reactions seen in atropine poisoning, may indeed be due to their anticholinergic properties. Diazepam is effective and should be used in reversing the excitement and convulsions.

HISTAMINE 2 (H₂) BLOCKING AGENTS. Cimetidine and ranitidine are selective H₂ blockers with ability to reduce the secretion of gastric acid elaborated by gastrin, histamine, pentagastrin, and to a certain extent acetylcholine. They do not alter other gastric secretions or gastric motility. These agents are effective in acid-pepsin disease and Zollinger-Ellison syndrome. The toxic manifestations of cimetidine include gynecomastia in men and galactorrhea in women, rare blood dyscrasias (granulocytopenia), and CNS manifestations such as slurred speech and disorientation, especially in elderly patients.

QUESTIONS ON THE PHARMACOLOGY OF HISTAMINE AND ANTIHISTAMINES

Select one answer that best completes the statement or answers the question.

—— 259. Agents releasing histamine include:
   A. Reserpine.
   B. Codeine.
   C. Meperidine.
   D. Hydralazine.
   E. All of the above.

—— 260. Agents releasing histamine include:
   A. d-Tubocurarine.
   B. Dextrans.
   C. Papaverine.
   D. Compound 48/80.
   E. All of the above.

—— 261. The action of histamine is characterized by all of the following *except* which one?
   A. Bronchodilatation.
   B. Vasodilatation.
   C. Tachycardia.
   D. Gastric secretion.

—— 262. Which one of the following agents possessing anticholinergic and to a certain extent antihistaminic properties is used in parkinsonism?
   A. Diphenhydramine.
   B. Promethazine.
   C. Benztropine.
   D. Chlorpheniramine.

—— 263. Which one of the following phenothiazine derivatives is devoid of neuroleptic property?
   A. Promethazine.
   B. Chlorpromazine.
   C. Thioridazine.
   D. Fluphenazine.

—— 264. Which one of the following substances blocks both histamine and serotonin receptor sites?
   A. Cyproheptadine.
   B. Cimetidine.
   C. Colistimethate sodium.

   D. Captamine HCl.

—— 265. Antihistaminic-induced toxicity is characterized by:
   A. Mydriasis.
   B. Ataxia.
   C. Convulsions.
   D. Can be treated by diazepam.
   E. All of the above.

ANSWERS AND EXPLANATIONS ON THE PHARMACOLOGY OF HISTAMINE AND ANTIHISTAMINES

259. E.
260. E.
261. A.
   Explanation: Histamine causes bronchoconstriction.
262. C.
263. A.
264. A.
265. E.
   Explanation: Diazepam is effective in reversing the excitement and convulsions.

REFERENCES

1. Douglas, W. W. Histamine and 5-Hydroxytryptamine (Serotonin) and Their Antagonists. In A. G. Gilman, L. S. Goodman, and A. Gilman (eds.), *The Pharmacological Basis of Therapeutics* (6th ed.). New York: Macmillan, 1980. Pp. 608–646.
2. Ganellin, C. R., and Parsons, M. E. (eds.), *Pharmacology of Histamine Receptors*. Bristol, England: John Wright, 1982.
3. Yellin, T. O. *Histamine Receptors*. Jamaica, N.Y.: SP Medical and Scientific Books, 1979.

VIII. The Pharmacology of Eicosanoids, Cyclic Nucleotides, and Calcium Channel Blocking Agents

32. The Pharmacology of Eicosanoids: Prostaglandins, Prostacyclin, Thromboxanes, and Leukotrienes

> I would rather discover a single causal connection than win the throne of Persia.
>
> *Democritus*

All naturally occurring prostaglandins are derived by cyclization of 20-carbon unsaturated fatty acids, such as arachidonic acid, which in turn are synthesized from the essential fatty acid, linoleic acid. The prostaglandins are named according to their ring substitutions and the number of additional side-chain double bonds, as seen in prostaglandins E_1, $F_{1\alpha}$, and $F_{2\alpha}$ (Fig. 32-1).

In addition to serving as precursor for the synthesis of prostaglandins, arachidonic acid is also a precursor for the synthesis of prostacyclin, thromboxanes, and leukotrienes according to the following scheme [6]:

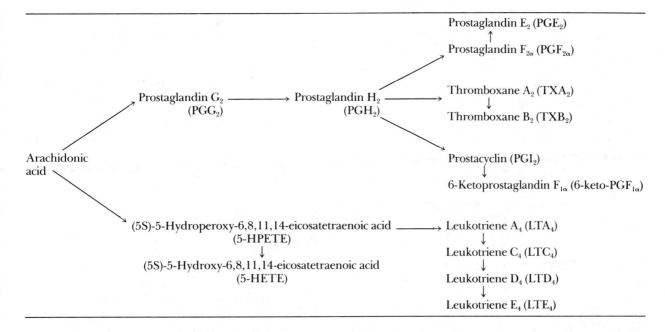

PHARMACOKINETIC PROPERTIES OF EICOSANOIDS.
Prostaglandins are inactivated rapidly ($t\frac{1}{2} < 1$ minute) in the pulmonary, hepatic, and renal vascular beds, by prostaglandin dehydrogenase, and by prostaglandin reductase. In addition, the aliphatic side chain undergoes relatively slow beta and omega oxidation. The rapid rate of metabolism and removal logically protects the cardiovascular system from smooth muscle stimulating effects of prostaglandins. Prostacyclins are also rapidly metabolized by prostaglandin dehydrogenase. Thromboxane A_2 is hydrated in the blood to thromboxane B_2. The thromboxanes are metabolized extensively, and the metabolites appear in the urine [3].

THE PHYSIOLOGY OF EICOSANOIDS.
The most important known effects of prostaglandins and other eicosanoids are contraction and relaxation of smooth muscles.

Smooth Muscles. VASCULAR SMOOTH MUSCLES. PGE_2 and PGI_2 cause arteriolar dilation in the systemic and pulmonary vascular beds. $PGF_{2\alpha}$, PGE_2, and TXB_2 constrict human umbilical cord. LTC_4 and LTD_4, which release PGE, decrease the peripheral vascular resistance. 5-HPETE and 5-HETE do not influence vascular smooth muscles.

RESPIRATORY SMOOTH MUSCLES. PGE_1, PGE_2, and PGI_2 cause bronchodilation and oppose the actions

Fig. 32-1. *Structure of selected prostaglandins and their precursor, arachidonic acid.*

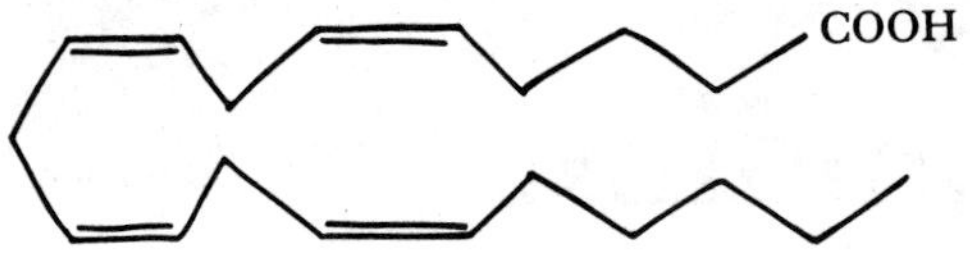

Arachidonic acid

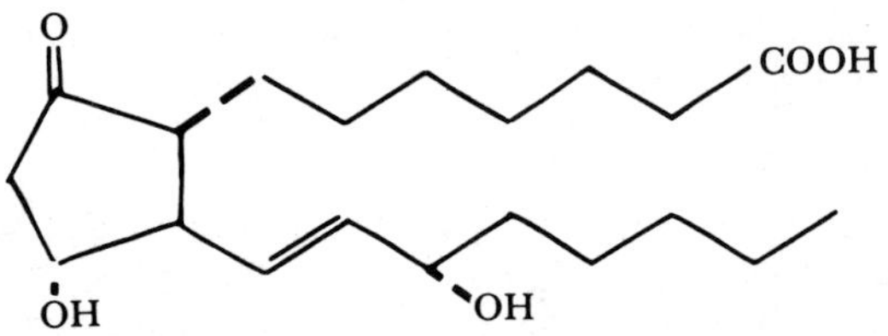

Prostaglandin E_1 (PGE$_1$)

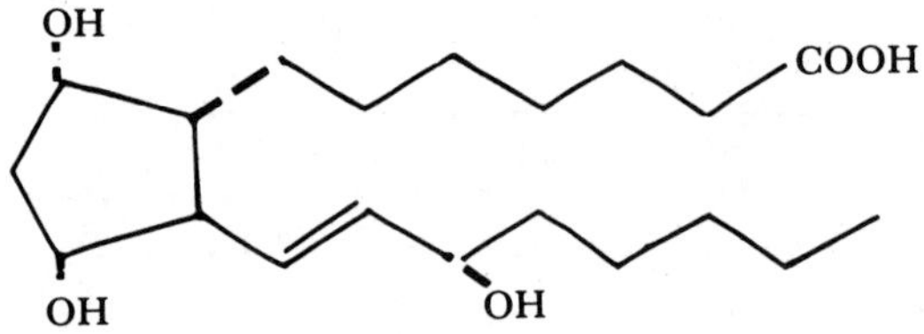

Prostaglandin $F_{1\alpha}$ (PGF$_{1\alpha}$)

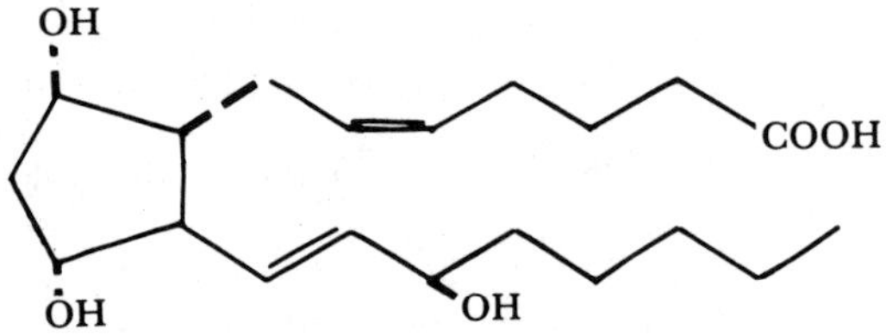

Prostaglandin $F_{2\alpha}$ (PGF$_{2\alpha}$)

of acetylcholine, histamine, and bradykinin. On the other hand, PGF$_{2\alpha}$, LTC$_4$, LTD$_4$, TXA$_2$, and HPETE are all bronchoconstricting substances possessing different potencies [1].

GASTROINTESTINAL SMOOTH MUSCLES. PGE$_2$ contracts longitudinal but relaxes circular smooth muscles whereas PGF$_{2\alpha}$ contracts both.

REPRODUCTIVE SMOOTH MUSCLES. PGE$_1$, PGE$_2$, and PGF$_{2\alpha}$ cause contraction of pregnant and nonpregnant human uterus and produce laborlike contractions. In contrast to the action of oxytocin, this effect is observed in all stages of pregnancy [1].

In general, the constricting or relaxing effects on the smooth muscles are not mediated via classic neurotransmitters such as acetylcholine, catecholamine, or histamine, since they are not altered by antihistaminic substances, by anticholinergic agents, or by either alpha- or beta-adrenergic receptor blocking agents [3].

Cardiovascular System. PGE$_2$ and PGF$_{2\alpha}$ have positive inotropic effect and in general increase cardiac output [4].

Blood. PGE$_1$ inhibits platelet aggregation whereas TXA$_2$ induces platelet aggregation. PGA$_2$, PGE$_1$, and PGE$_2$ enhance erythropoiesis by increasing the renal cortical release of erythropoietin.

Kidneys. PGE$_1$, PGE$_2$, and PGI$_2$ increase renal blood flow and produce diuresis, natriuresis, and kaliuresis. PGE$_1$ and PGE$_2$ antagonize the action of antidiuretic hormone (ADH) [2].

Endocrine System. PGE$_1$ and PGF$_{2\alpha}$ stimulate the release of ACTH. PGE$_1$ and PGE$_2$ enhance the release of growth hormone. PGF$_{2\alpha}$ increases the release of prolactin. PGE$_2$ increases the release of luteinizing hormone. PGF$_{2\alpha}$ reduces progesterone output and causes regression of corpus luteum.

Metabolic Effects. PGE$_1$ inhibits the basal and the catecholamine-stimulated lipolysis [7].

Nociception. PGE$_1$ and PGE$_2$ cause pain by sensitizing the afferent nerve endings to noxious chemical and physical stimuli.

Inflammatory and Immune Responses. Prostaglandins are involved in the genesis and manifestation of inflammation. Furthermore, prostaglandins are thought to regulate the functions of both B and T lymphocytes [5].

CNS. PGE$_1$ and PGE$_2$ cause sedation.

Pyrexia. PGE$_1$ causes fever when injected intracerebroventricularly.

THE PHARMACODYNAMICS OF EICOSANOIDS. Some, but not all, pharmacologic effects of eicosanoids are mediated via alterations in the concentration of cyclic AMP. For example, PGE$_1$ and PGE$_2$ inhibit platelet aggregation by increasing the concentration of cyclic AMP. Conversely, TXA$_2$, which induces platelet aggregation, inhibits the synthesis of cyclic AMP.

THERAPEUTIC USES OF EICOSANOIDS. Prostaglandins are mostly used as abortifacients. They may be administered (1) by vaginal suppository (dinoprostone), which contains PGE$_2$, (2) by intramuscular injection of carboprost tromethamine, which contains 15-methyl PGF$_{2\alpha}$, and (3) by intraamnionic administration of dinoprost tromethamine, which contains PGF$_{2\alpha}$. Other possible uses include ductus arteriosus (PGE_1) to maintain patency, and utilization as a vasodilator (PGE_1) in peripheral vascular diseases. Furthermore, high levels of $PGF_{2\alpha}$ may cause dysmenorrhea, since substances such as indomethacin and ibuprofen are effective in relieving its agonizing symptoms.

Additional therapeutic usefulness must await a more comprehensive understanding of the roles of eicosanoids in health and disease states.

QUESTIONS ON THE PHARMACOLOGY OF EICOSANOIDS

Select the answer that best completes the statement or answers the question.

_____ 266. All of the following statements are correct about dysmenorrhea *except* which one? It may be:
A. Associated with a high level of prostaglandin $F_{2\alpha}$.
B. Treated with indomethacin.
C. Treated with ibuprofen.
D. Treated with arachidonic acid.

_____ 267. All of the following statements are correct about the pharmacokinetics of prostaglandins *except* which one?
A. They are metabolized by pulmonary, hepatic, and renal vascular beds.
B. They are metabolized by a dehydrogenase.
C. They have a relatively long half-life of greater than 24 hours.
D. They are metabolized by reductase.

_____ 268. The bronchodilating action of prostaglandin E_1 is shared by:
A. Acetylcholine.
B. Histamine.
C. Prostaglandin E_2.
D. Bradykinin.

_____ 269. The vascular effects of prostaglandins are blocked by:
A. Diphenhydramine.
B. Atropine.
C. Phenoxybenzamine.
D. Propranolol.
E. None of the above.

_____ 270. The action of prolactin is increased by all of the following substances *except* which one?
A. Prostaglandin $F_{2\alpha}$.
B. Chlorpromazine.
C. Bromocriptine.
D. Thioridazine.

ANSWERS AND EXPLANATION ON THE PHARMACOLOGY OF EICOSANOIDS

266. D.
267. C.
268. C.
269. E.
270. C.

Explanation: Prostaglandin $F_{2\alpha}$ increases the release of prolactin. Chlorpromazine and thioridazine (neuroleptics), by blocking dopaminergic receptor sites, enhance the release and action of prolactin whereas bromocriptine, by stimulating the dopaminergic receptor sites, inhibits it. Bromocriptine is used to inhibit postpartum lactation.

REFERENCES

1. Cuthbert, M. F. *The Prostaglandins: Pharmacological and Therapeutic Advances.* Philadelphia: Lippincott, 1973.
2. Dunn, M. J., Patrono, C., and Cinotti, G. A. *Prostaglandins and the Kidney: Biochemistry, Physiology and Clinical Applications.* New York: Plenum, 1983.
3. Goldyne, M. E. Prostaglandins and Other Eicosanoids. In B. G. Katzung (ed.), *Basic and Clinical Pharmacology.* Los Altos, Calif.: Lange, 1982. Pp. 196–204.
4. Herman, A. G., et al. *Cardiovascular Pharmacology of the Prostaglandins.* New York: Raven, 1982.
5. Ramwell, P. *Prostaglandin Synthesis Inhibitors: New Clinical Applications.* New York: Liss, 1980.
6. Samuelsson, B., Paoletti, R., and Ramwell, P. W. *Advances in Prostaglandin, Thromboxane, and Leukotriene Research,* Vol. II. New York: Raven, 1983.
7. Von Euler, U. S., and Eliasson, R. *Prostaglandins.* New York: Academic, 1967.

33. The Pharmacology of the Cyclic Nucleotide System

A large number of pharmacologic substances exert their unique effects by interacting with a component of cell membrane called "receptor site." The interaction of an agonist with a receptor may result in the synthesis or release of a "mediator" or "messenger," which conveys the message and translates it into physiologic effects. Among all putative messengers, the cyclic nucleotides play grand roles in bringing forth the actions of seemingly endless groups of physiologic events and pharmacologic substances [3].

THE SYNTHESIS OF CYCLIC NUCLEOTIDES.
Cyclic AMP and cyclic GMP are synthesized and catabolized according to the reactions shown in Figure 33-1. The basal activities of adenylate cyclase and guanylate cyclase are lower than the basal activities of the cyclic nucleotide phosphodiesterases. Furthermore, they not only show dissimilar subcellular distribution but are subject to different regulatory mechanisms.

The interaction of an agonist such as epinephrine with its receptor site results in synthesis and accumulation of cyclic AMP. This activates a cyclic AMP–dependent protein kinase, which mediates the catalytic transfer of a gamma phosphate from ATP to a protein, the final substrate sponsoring the physiologic effects of the agonist that had initially interacted with the receptor site. Figure 33-2, depicting the epinephrine-mediated conversion of glycogen to glucose, is cited as one example of the concept of cyclic AMP–mediated physiologic events.

The fasting hypoglycemia may result in conversion of glycogen into glucose. This metabolic effect is triggered initially by hypoglycemically mediated release of epinephrine from adrenal medulla, which interacts with epinephrine receptor sites on the hepatocytes. The interaction activates the membrane-bound adenylate cyclase, converting ATP into cyclic AMP. The adenylate cyclase itself is thought to be regulated by a multiple component unit that shows selectivity of binding and specificity of action. In the outer component of the membrane there exists an activating receptor, which is able to interact with many substances including beta-adrenergic agonists, and an inhibitory receptor, which is able to interact with many substances including alpha-adrenergic agonists. The inner surface of membrane contains the GTP regulatory proteins that interact with both activating and inhibiting receptors on one side of the membrane

and the adenylate cyclase on the other. The collective cascading and sequential interactions of these multi-compartmental units result in the synthesis of cyclic AMP.

The intracellular receptor for cyclic AMP is a protein kinase containing two regulatory and two catalytic subunits (R_2C_2). The interaction of cyclic AMP with this protein causes dissociation of catalytic subunits (C) from regulatory dimer (R). The catalytic subunits are able to phosphorylate a variety of proteins, such as lipase to lipase phosphate, glycogen synthase to glycogen synthase phosphate, and inactive phosphorylase kinase to active phosphorylase kinase. The active phosphorylase kinase converts the inactive phosphorylase *b* to the active phosphorylase *a*, which in turn catalyzes the conversion of glycogen to glucose 1-phosphate and its sequential conversion to glucose, correcting the hypoglycemia (Fig. 33-2).

Calcium (Ca^{2+}) plays a major role in the regulation of cyclic nucleotide metabolism, and the Ca^{2+} effects show tissue specificity. In physiologic ranges, Ca^{2+} activates adenylate cyclase from brain. This Ca^{2+}-mediated activation of adenylate cyclase is thought to be mediated via binding of Ca^{2+} to calmodulin, a low-molecular-weight Ca^{2+}-binding protein homologous to skeletal muscle troponin C. In high doses, Ca^{2+} inhibits adenylate cyclase in heart as well as in the brain, perhaps by interacting with an inhibitory calcium binding site. In addition, Ca^{2+}-calmodulin-mediated events in the cytoplasm activate cyclic nucleotide phosphodiesterase (a partly cytoplasmic soluble enzyme) and reduce the concentration of cyclic AMP (Fig. 33-2). The calmodulin-sponsored and Ca^{2+}-mediated alterations in the concentrations of cyclic AMP are of paramount importance in conferring pharmacodynamic properties on numerous neuropharmacologic agents [5].

In mammalian brain, dopaminergic receptor sites are divided into two general categories: dopamine receptor 1 (D_1) and dopamine receptor 2 (D_2), with distinct affinity for pharmacologic substances. D_1 uses cyclic AMP as a second messenger; D_2 does not. Substances such as chlorpromazine and haloperidol are nonspecific in that they block both D_1 and D_2 whereas atypical neuroleptics such as sulpiride block only D_2 receptors [1]. The clinical importance of this receptor affinity for specific agonists and antagonists and the role that calmodulin may play in expressing these events are being unfolded gradually.

Neuroleptics, such as prochlorperazine (Compa-

Fig. 33-1. *Metabolism of cyclic AMP and cyclic GMP.*

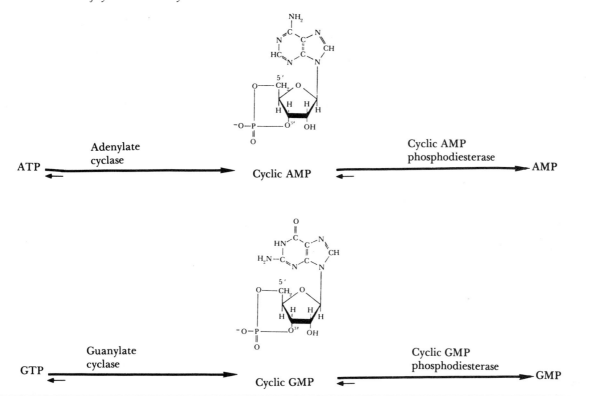

ATP $\xrightarrow{\text{Adenylate cyclase}}$ Cyclic AMP $\xrightarrow{\text{Cyclic AMP phosphodiesterase}}$ AMP

GTP $\xrightarrow{\text{Guanylate cyclase}}$ Cyclic GMP $\xrightarrow{\text{Cyclic GMP phosphodiesterase}}$ GMP

zine), used as an antiemetic agent in children, may cause acute dystonia. The incidence of dystonia is highest among children who are dehydrated or have relative hypoparathyroidism, conditions that may alter the Ca^{2+} homeostasis in the body and depress its level in the brain. Since the acute dystonia disappears rapidly after administration of diphenhydramine, an antihistaminic agent with strong anticholinergic property, an interference with action of dopaminergic receptor by prochlorperazine has been postulated. It is remarkable to note that the pediatricians had effectively treated phenothiazine-induced acute dystonia in children by administration of caffeine (a phosphodiesterase inhibitor) almost a decade before the discovery of cyclic AMP.

Agents such as chlorpromazine that block both D_1 and D_2 receptors are excellent neuroleptics but cause extrapyramidal side effects—pseudoparkinsonism, for example. Agents such as sulpiride that block only D_2 cause little or no extrapyramidal side effects. The interaction of neuroleptics with dopamine-initiated and calmodulin-fostered enhancement of cyclic AMP may play a definite role in down regulation or up regulation of dopaminergic receptors. Tardive dyskinesia, which occurs following chronic administration of neuroleptics in large doses, may be simply a biochemical expression of calmodulin-directed receptor plasticity [2].

In addition to Ca^{2+} calmodulin-dependent expression of neurotransmitter activities, numerous Ca^{2+}-dependent but calmodulin-independent events take place [5].

In order to illustrate the importance of cyclic nu-

cleotides in pharmacology further, additional selected cyclic AMP–mediated hormonal events are cited [4].

DISORDER OF ADENYLATE CYCLASE AND PSEUDOHYPOPARATHYROIDISM. Pseudohypoparathyroidism is a disorder characterized by hypocalcemia, neuromuscular irritability, tetany, and convulsions. Unlike patients with idiopathic hypoparathyroidism or patients whose parathyroids have been removed, the patients with pseudohypoparathyroidism do not respond to parathyroid hormone but do respond to vitamin D. This rare genetic disorder is caused by the absence of "coupling protein," which couples the hormone with the catalytic subunit of adenylate cyclase.

CALCITONIN. The concentration of calcitonin in the plasma increases in hypercalcemia. Calcitonin is effective in combating hypercalcemia in patients with vitamin D intoxication and hyperparathyroidism. Calcitonin does not have antiparathyroid effect and does not block the activation of adenylate cyclase by parathyroid hormone. The mechanism of action of calcitonin is not known.

ADRENOCORTICOTROPIC HORMONE (ACTH). ACTH stimulates the adrenal gland to secrete the glucocorticoids and mineralocorticoids.

Fig. 33-2. *Cyclic AMP–mediated conversion of glycogen to glucose in liver* (bottom) *and of dopamine-mediated events in the striatum* (top).

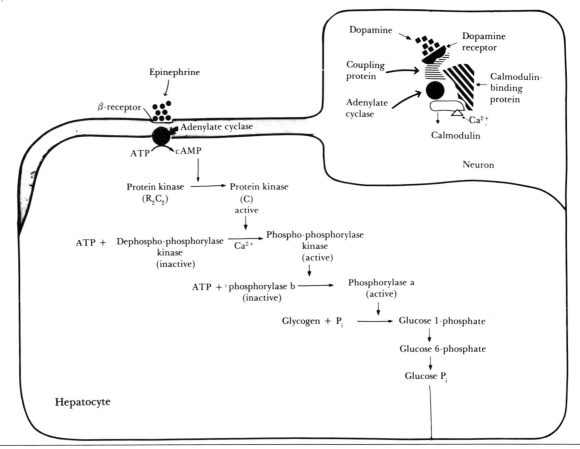

ACTH is thought to exert these effects by enhancing the concentration of cyclic AMP.

ANTIDIURETIC HORMONE (ADH). ADH activates adenylate cyclase at the basolateral membrane, increasing cyclic AMP, which in turn increases the permeability of the luminal cell surface to water.

GLUCAGON AND INSULIN. The hyperglycemic effect (antiinsulin) of epinephrine and glucagon is mediated via cyclic AMP. Insulin has been shown to inhibit the activity of adenylate cyclase and to stimulate the activity of phosphodiesterase.

GONADOTROPINS. Luteinizing hormone (LH) and follicle-stimulating hormone (FSH) are responsible for increasing testicular growth, spermatogenesis, and steroidogenesis. All these effects are mediated via cyclic nucleotides.

THE TROPIC HORMONES. Melanocyte-stimulating hormone (MSH), thyrotropin-releasing hormone (TRH), and thyroid-stimulating hormone (TSH) use cyclic AMP as a second messenger and exert their effect through this mechanism.

QUESTIONS ON THE PHARMACOLOGY OF THE CYCLIC NUCLEOTIDE SYSTEM

Select one answer that best completes the statement or answers the question.

____ 271. Which one of the following actions of histamine is mediated by elevation in the concentration of cyclic AMP?
   A. Gastric secretion.
   B. Hypertension.
   C. Bradycardia.
   D. Leukocytosis.

____ 272. Which one of the following statements best describes the actions of morphine and enkephalin on adenylate cyclase? These agents:
   A. Inhibit adenylate cyclase in toxic doses.
   B. Activate adenylate cyclase in therapeutic doses.
   C. Produce a selective and naloxone-reversible inhibition of adenylate cyclase.
   D. Produce a nonspecific and naloxone-insensitive activation of adenylate cyclase.

____ 273. The actions of which one of the following hormone(s) is (are) mediated via generation of cyclic AMP?
   A. Adrenocorticotropic hormone.
   B. Antidiuretic hormone.
   C. Gonadotropins.
   D. Thyrotropin-releasing hormone.
   E. All of the above.

____ 274. Pseudohypoparathyroidism is caused by lack of

membrane-bound:
   A. Na$^+$K$^+$ ATPase.
   B. Ca^{2+} ATPase.
   C. "Coupling protein," which couples parathyroid hormone with adenylate cyclase.
   D. Phosphodiesterase.
____ 275. Which one of the following substances does *not* increase the concentration of cyclic AMP?
   A. Insulin.
   B. Glucagon.
   C. Epinephrine.
   D. Aminophylline.
   E. Terbutaline.

ANSWERS AND EXPLANATION ON THE PHARMACOLOGY OF THE CYCLIC NUCLEOTIDE SYSTEM

271. A.
272. C.
273. E.
274. C.
275. A.
   Explanation: Insulin inhibits the activity of adenylate cyclase and stimulates the activity of phosphodiesterase.

REFERENCES

1. Cattabeni, F., et al. *Long-term Effects of Neuroleptics*. New York: Raven, 1980.
2. Costa, E. Receptor plasticity: Biochemical correlates and pharmacological significance. *Adv. Biochem. Psychopharmacol.* 24:363, 1980.
3. Greengard, P. *Cyclic Nucleotides, Phosphorylated Proteins, and Neuronal Function*. New York: Raven, 1978. Pp. 1–119.
4. Volicer, L. *Clinical Aspects of Cyclic Nucleotides*. New York: Spectrum, 1977.
5. Watterson, D. M., and Vincenzi, F. F. Calmodulin and cell functions. *Ann. N.Y. Acad. Sci.* 356:1, 1980.

34. The Pharmacology of Calcium Channel Blocking Agents

Curiosity is one of the permanent and certain characteristics of a vigorous mind.

Samuel Johnson

Numerous pharmacologic agents exert their therapeutic effects or their side effects by attenuating or blocking the physiologic actions of calcium ions. A few of these agents and their actions will be cited. In addition, limited discussion will be devoted to elaborating the pharmacology of the newly introduced calcium channel blocking agents with therapeutic usefulness in various cardiovascular diseases.

DRUGS THAT INTERFERE WITH PHYSIOLOGIC ACTIONS OF CALCIUM. Ethylenediaminetetraacetic Acid (EDTA).
EDTA, by chelating Ca^{2+} ion, is a direct anticoagulant in an in vitro system. EDTA is poorly absorbed from the gastrointestinal tract. The rapid intravenous administration of Na_2EDTA causes hypocalcemic tetany. In addition to EDTA, ethylene glycol-bis-(beta-aminoethylether)-N,N'-tetraacetic acid (EGTA), potassium fluoride, and potassium citrate are Ca^{2+}-binding agents. Fluoride poisoning causes gastrointestinal disturbances, clonic convulsions, hypotension, and respiratory and cardiac failure.

Phenytoin. Phenytoin exerts its anticonvulsant action by interfering with Ca^{2+}-facilitated norepinephrine release, which is thought to be responsible for increasing posttetanic potentiation, for creating a high-frequency train of impulses, and for spreading seizure activity from an epileptic focus to the rest of the brain. Phenytoin is also effective in digitalis-induced arrhythmias.

ANTICONVULSANT-INDUCED HYPOCALCEMIA.
Phenobarbital and phenytoin and related compounds induce the hepatic microsomal enzymes, convert the active vitamin D (D_3 and 25-OHD$_3$) to inactive metabolites, reduce the circulating level of 25-OHD$_3$, and decrease the intestinal absorption of calcium. Anticonvulsant-induced hypocalcemia and osteomalacia occur more frequently among patients with diseases involving malabsorption of vitamin D and in individuals with diminished exposure to sunlight.

Neomycin. Neomycin, a broad-spectrum antibiotic, is used sometimes in combination with erythromycin for preparation of bowel for surgery. The large (> 10 gm/day) oral administration of neomycin has caused superinfection and malabsorption syndrome for a variety of substances, including calcium.

Antipsychotics and Calmodulin. Chlorpromazine and some other phenothiazine derivatives are generalized depressants of smooth muscles, cardiac muscles, and skeletal muscles in a dose-dependent fashion. They cause orthostatic hypotension (vasodilation), negative inotropism directly (antiarrhythmic effects), muscular relaxation, and in large doses even catalepsy and paralysis (depression of gamma motor efferent mechanism). Since chlorpromazine binds to calmodulin, some of these effects are mediated via interference with calcium-mediated events.

CALCIUM CHANNEL ANTAGONISTS.
Calcium channel antagonists are divided into two broad categories: inorganic and organic compounds [3].

The inorganic compounds include cations such as Mn^{2+}, Co^{2+}, and La^{3+}. These agents are thought to exert their effect by one or a combination of the following effects:

By binding to the surface negative charges, they modify membrane excitability.
By occupying the cation coordination sites for Ca^{2+}, they interfere with channel activity.
By entering the cells, they substitute for Ca^{2+}. Since their actions are nonspecific, the inorganic Ca^{2+} channel blocking agents have no therapeutic usefulness in man-

Fig. 34-1. *Structure of selected calcium channel blocking agents used in medicine.*

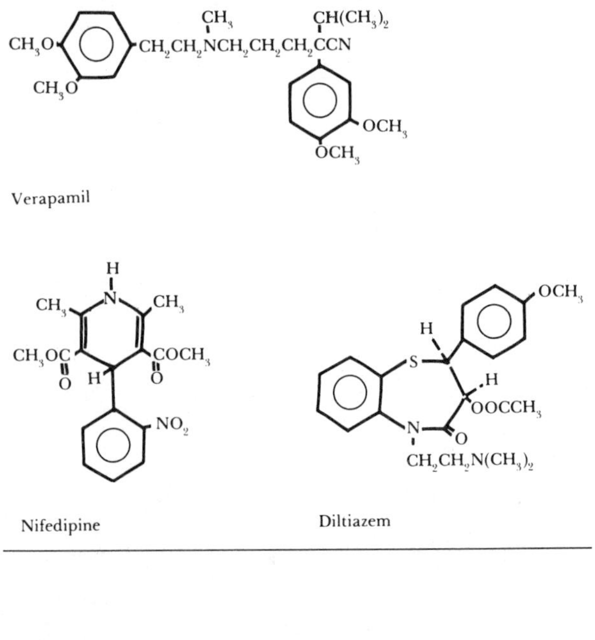

Verapamil

Nifedipine

Diltiazem

190

Fig. 34-2. *Potential-operated and receptor-operated calcium channels. (Views from F. Bronner and M. Peterlik,* Calcium and Phosphate Transport Across Biomembranes. *New York: Academic, 1980; N. Lakshminarayanaiah,* Calcium Channels in the Barnacle Muscle Membrane. *In G. B. Weiss [ed.],* New Perspectives on Calcium Antagonists. *Bethesda, Md.: American Physiological Society, 1981; D. J. Triggle,* Calcium Antagonists: Basic Chemical and Pharmacological Aspects. *In G. B. Weiss [ed.],* New Perspectives on Calcium Antagonists. *Bethesda, Md.: American Physiological Society, 1981; S. Tsuyoshi Ohnishi and M. Endo,* The Mechanism of Gated Calcium Transport Across Biological Membranes. *New York: Academic, 1981.)*

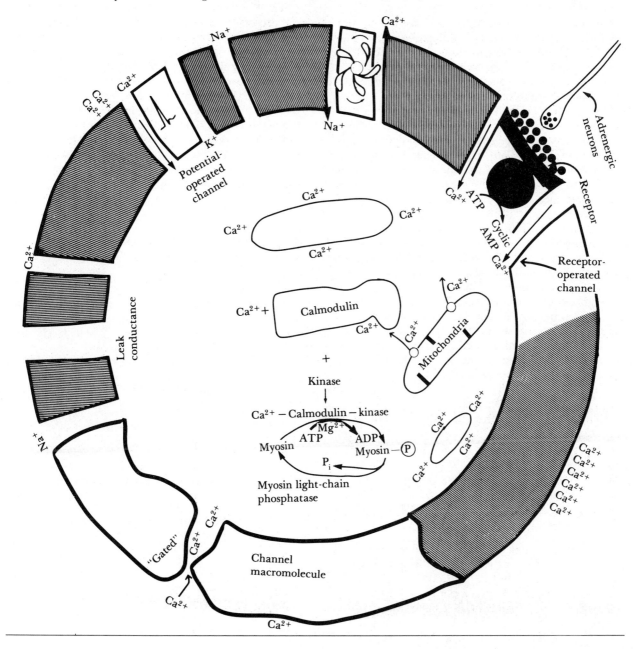

aging cardiovascular diseases. However, it is interesting that La^{3+} has analgesic property similar to that of morphine. Furthermore, the La^{3+}-induced analgesia is blocked either by naloxone or by Ca^{2+}.

The organic compounds include verapamil (Calan, Isoptin), nifedipine (Procardia), and diltiazem (Cardizem).

The organic channel blockers (Fig. 34-1) are being used increasingly in vasospastic angina, in cardiac arrhythmias, in hypertension, and in hypertrophic cardiomyopathy [2, 5, 9, 12].

ELECTRICALLY GATED Ca^{2+} CHANNELS AND RECEPTOR-RELATED Ca^{2+} CHANNELS.

Several types of Ca^{2+} channels are depicted schematically in Figure 34-2 [1, 7, 8, 11]. Channels that are always open and available for influx of Ca^{2+}, and especially sodium and potassium, are referred to as "leak conductances." Organic Ca^{2+} channel blocking agents apparently do not modify the resting membrane potential.

The influx of Ca^{2+} by high-K^+ depolarization is called a potential-operated or potential-dependent channel. The influx of Ca^{2+} by occupation of a receptor by a transmitter is called a receptor-operated or receptor-dependent channel. The receptor-operated influx of Ca^{2+} is dependent on extracellular Ca^{2+} and is additive synergistically with potential-operated influx of Ca^{2+}. Channel blocking agents (Fig. 34-1) are able to block Ca^{2+} influx mediated by these systems.

Among agonists enhancing Ca^{2+} influx, norepinephrine, prostaglandin $F_{2\alpha}$, and acetylcholine may be cited. The interaction of norepinephrine with a cardiac adrenergic receptor site may increase Ca^{2+} influx by activation of adenylate cyclase, enhancing the formation of cyclic AMP. Similarly, the interaction of prostaglandin $F_{2\alpha}$ with receptor sites in the heart (positive inotropic effect), uterus (contraction), and lung (bronchoconstriction) may involve cyclic AMP–mediated Ca^{2+} influx. Furthermore, it is interesting that La^{3+} inhibits the stimulation by prostaglandin of adenylate cyclase activity. The influx of Ca^{2+} following acetylcholine is not mediated via cyclic AMP.

Although excitation-contraction coupling and stimulus-secretion coupling are mediated via influx of Ca^{2+}, it should be recalled that many of the secretory cells do not have voltage-sensing membrane functions, and Ca^{2+} influx takes place mainly through receptor-operated channels.

A Ca^{2+} pumping ATPase has been reported in the heart, the sarcolemma, and the membrane of smooth muscle. In addition, a sodium-calcium exchange mechanism also exists, but the major role in Ca^{2+} extrusion and Ca^{2+} homeostasis depends on Ca^{2+} ATPase. The potential-operated channel is also called the "gated" calcium channel.

The molecular structure and the macromolecular components of the calcium channels have not been established [6]. Nevertheless, several isolated evidences point to the fact that not only are these channels different in cardiac muscle, skeletal muscle, and smooth muscle but also multiple calcium channels may exist in the same tissues. Furthermore, the various Ca^{2+} channel blocking agents (listed in Fig. 34-1) have both structural stereospecificity and tissue selectivity. For example, verapamil inhibits an inward Ca^{2+} current, reduces the tetrodotoxin-sensitive Na^+ current, and diminishes K^+ influx and efflux in active and quiescent states. Verapamil also inhibits the Na^{2+}-dependent uptake of neurotransmitters such as serotonin, dopamine, and norepinephrine. On the other hand, nifedipine is thought to be more selective toward blocking the Ca^{2+} channels.

Known intracellular calcium-binding proteins, among others, are troponin C, certain myosin chains, and calmodulin. Ca^{2+} binds to calmodulin to form a Ca^{2+}-calmodulin complex, which subsequently binds to a kinase forming Ca^{2+}-calmodulin-kinase that in the presence of ATP subsequently phosphorylates myosin light chain [3, 10].

The intracellular concentration of calcium (10^{-7}M) is substantially lower than its extracellular concentration (10^{-4}M). This low intracellular concentration of Ca^{2+} is accomplished by several mechanisms: (1) enhancing the efflux of Ca^{2+} by activating Ca^{2+} ATPase and Na^+-Ca^{2+} antiport mechanism, (2) uptake of cytoplasmic Ca^{2+} into the cisternae of the sarcoplasmic or endoplasmic reticulum, and (3) transporting Ca^{2+} into mitochondrial matrix (Fig. 34-2).

The Ca^{2+} channel blocking agents such as verapamil are effective in reentrant paroxysmal supraventricular tachycardias, in atrial flutter, and fibrillation. In addition, verapamil is effective in the treatment of obstructive cardiomyopathy. Nifedipine, a potent dilator of coronary arteries, is useful in angina originating from spasm of the coronary artery [4].

The application and usefulness of these drugs in medicine now should be regarded as the dawn of a new era not only in comprehension of the multiplicity of calcium actions in health and diseases but also in the introduction and application of highly specific calcium channel blocking agents.

QUESTIONS ON THE PHARMACOLOGY OF CALCIUM CHANNEL BLOCKING AGENTS

Select one answer that best completes the statement or answers the question.

____ 276. Which one of the following statements about verapamil is *not* correct?
- A. It is absorbed orally but has a low bioavailability of 10 to 20 percent.
- B. It undergoes first-pass hepatic metabolism.
- C. It has an onset of action of 2 hours following an orally administered dose.
- D. It induces protracted hypertension when given intravenously.

____ 277. The intravenous administration of verapamil in a patient receiving propranolol may lead to which one of the following events?
- A. Atrial tachycardia.
- B. Diazoxide-resistant hypertension.
- C. Hypotension, bradycardia, and AV block.
- D. None of the above.

____ 278. Which one of the following is the least desirable indication for verapamil.
- A. Atrial flutter.
- B. Atrial fibrillation.
- C. Reentrant paroxysmal supraventricular tachycardia.
- D. Digitalis toxicity.

____ 279. Nifedipine is characterized by the following actions *except* which one?
- A. It is absorbed orally.
- B. It is not metabolized and is primarily excreted by the kidneys.
- C. It is a potent vasodilator.
- D. It may be coadministered with digitalis or propranolol.

____ 280. Which one of the following drugs known to influence the actions of calcium is effective in both convulsive seizure and cardiac arrhythmias?
- A. Ethosuximide.
- B. Phenytoin.
- C. Phenobarbital.
- D. Procainamide.

ANSWERS AND EXPLANATIONS ON THE PHARMACOLOGY OF CALCIUM CHANNEL BLOCKING AGENTS

276. D.
    Explanation: Verapamil, given intravenously, causes hypotension with onset and duration of action of 5 and 15 minutes respectively.
277. C.
    Explanation: Propranolol is a cardiac depressant, and the major contraindications of verapamil are sinus node diseases, AV block, and left ventricular dysfunction.
278. D.
279. B.
280. B.

REFERENCES

1. Bronner, F., and Peterlik, M. *Calcium and Phosphate Transport Across Biomembranes*. New York: Academic, 1981.
2. Cauvin, C., Loutzenhiser, R., and Van Breemen, C. Mechanisms of calcium antagonist-induced vasodilation. *Ann. Rev. Pharmacol. Toxicol.* 23:373, 1983.
3. Cheung, W. Y. *Calcium and Cell Function*, Vols. I and II. New York: Academic, 1980.
4. Comess, K. A., and Fenster, P. E. Calcium Channel Blocking Agents. In G. A. Ewy and R. Bressler (eds.), *Cardiovascular Drugs and the Management of Heart Disease*. New York: Raven, 1982. Pp. 179–190.
5. Fleckenstein, A. Specific pharmacology of calcium in myocardium, cardiac pacemakers, and vascular smooth muscle. *Annu. Rev. Pharmacol. Toxicol.* 17:149, 1977.
6. Lakshminarayanaiah, N. Calcium Channels in the Barnacle Muscle Membrane. In G. B. Weiss (ed.), *New Perspectives on Calcium Antagonists*. Bethesda, Md.: American Physiological Society, 1981. Pp. 19–33.
7. Triggle, D. J. Calcium Antagonists: Basic Chemical and Pharmacological Aspects. In G. B. Weiss (ed.), *New Perspectives on Calcium Antagonists*. Bethesda, Md.: American Physiological Society, 1981. Pp. 1–18.
8. Tsuyoshi Ohnishi, S., and Endo, M. *The Mechanism of Gated Calcium Transport Across Biological Membranes*. New York: Academic, 1981.
9. Vanhoutte, P. M., and Leusen, I. *Vasodilatation*. New York: Raven, 1981.
10. Watterson, D. M., and Vincinzi, F. F. Calmodulin and Cell Functions. *Ann. N.Y. Acad. Sci.* 356:1, 1980.
11. Weiss, G. B. (ed.). *New Perspectives on Calcium Antagonists*. Bethesda, Md.: American Physiological Society, 1981.
12. Zelis, R., and Flaim, S. F. Calcium blocking drugs for angina pectoris. *Annu. Rev. Med.* 33:465, 1982.

IX. Chemotherapy of Microbial Diseases

35. Antimicrobial Chemotherapy

Life is no brief candle—it is a splendid torch.

George Bernard Shaw

Prior to discussion of the pharmacologic properties of individual antibiotics and chemotherapeutic agents, a few basic principles will be presented in summary form.

GENERAL PHARMACODYNAMICS OF CHEMOTHERAPEUTIC AGENTS.
Antimicrobial agents exert their effects by four different mechanisms:

1. Inhibition of cell wall synthesis—e.g., penicillins, cephalosporins, bacitracin, cycloserine, and vancomycin
2. Inhibition of function(s) of cellular membrane(s)—e.g., amphotericin B, colistin, nystatin, and polymyxin
3. Inhibition of nucleic acid synthesis (antimetabolites)—e.g., sulfonamides, trimethoprim, nalidixic acid, rifampin, and pyrimethamine
4. Inhibition of protein synthesis—e.g., chloramphenicol, erythromycins, tetracyclines, and aminoglycosides

ACTIONS AND SPECTRUM OF THE ACTIVITY.
While exerting their effects, the antimicrobial agents are able either to cause death of the cells (bactericidal—e.g., penicillin) or to inhibit microbial replication (bacteriostatic—e.g., sulfonamides). While exerting their effects, the antimicrobial agents may have either a narrow spectrum of activity or a broad spectrum of activity inhibiting both gram-positive and gram-negative bacteria (e.g., tetracyclines).

ANTIBIOTIC SYNERGISM AND ANTAGONISM.
In the eradication of infectious diseases, antibiotics are sometimes used in combinations that must be selected carefully. Not all antibiotics have synergistic effects; indeed, they may have antagonistic effects when used in an inappropriate combination. For example, penicillin, streptomycin, bacitracin, and polymyxins have synergistic effects and may be used together in certain combinations. On the other hand, chloramphenicol, tetracyclines, erythromycin, and sulfonamides are seldom used in combination. As a matter of fact, some of these agents, such as chloramphenicol, can even antagonize the bactericidal actions of penicillins or aminoglycosides.

SELECTION OF ANTIBIOTICS.
The administration of antibiotics or chemotherapeutic agents is not always necessary. They should not be used when the illness has not resulted from bacterial infection or has resulted from a bacterial infection that is in an advanced stage of resolution. Furthermore, antibiotics are ineffective in viral infections [13].

The occurrence of fever does not necessarily indicate either bacterial or viral infection. For example, fevers of unknown origin (FUO) occur in neoplasias (e.g., Hodgkin's and other lymphoma, hypernephroma, preleukemia, and atrial myxoma), in hypersensitivity diseases (e.g., systemic lupus erythematosus, Still's disease, and temporal arteritis), in granulomatous diseases (e.g., sarcoidosis), and in inherited diseases (e.g., familial Mediterranean fever, type I hyperlipidemia, and Fabry's disease—an X-linked inherited error of glycosphingolipid) [14].

When diagnosis of infection is certain and the decision has been made to use chemotherapy, four factors should be thoughtfully considered: the patient, the disease, the organism(s), and the drug(s).

The Patient. The first factor to be considered is the host's defenses and whether or not they are functional. Host defenses are controlled by (1) intact skin and mucous membranes, (2) active circulating phagocytes and effective humoral mediators, (3) active fixed phagocytes in the reticuloendothelial system, and (4) functional immune responses from T cells and B cells [1]. It should be recalled that chemotherapeutic agents control the infective organisms only to allow the host's defense mechanism to gain effective control. In an immune-deficient and compromised host, the prognosis of chemotherapy is uncertain.

The Disease. A knowledge of the type of disease produced by the pathogenic microorganism is vital to provide appropriate and effective chemical therapy. For example, in some infections of the CNS, the secretion of antidiuretic hormone (ADH) increases. In this case, inappropriate fluid therapy may cause water intoxication [13].

The Microorganisms. A detailed microbiologic analysis and assessment are necessary to provide appropriate chemotherapeutic agents. For example, penicillin G is effective in streptococcal infection but not in tuberculosis. Furthermore, the sensitivity of the organism to chemotherapy and the response of the patient to it should be known. Thus acute infections due to group A streptococci or pneumococci respond within 48 hours to treatment with penicillin G. On the other hand, in typhoid fever no noticeable alteration in temperature may be noted in 4 to 5 days after treatment with chloramphenicol [13].

The Drugs. The selection of antibiotics is mostly based on the pattern of sensitivity of the infecting organism(s). In addition, other factors such as the age of the patient, the status of the patient's liver to metabolize the drug(s), the status of the patient's kidney to excrete the drug or its metabolites, genetic disorders altering the pharmacokinetics of the drug(s), and the history of drug allergy must all be taken into serious consideration.

SINGLE DRUG OR COMBINATION ANTIBIOTICS. Antibiotics may be used in combination. The advantages of this regimen are the following:

Synergistic augmentation of therapeutic efficacy
Reduction of toxicity from drugs with dissimilar mechanisms of action
Effective treatment for mixed infection
Effective treatment for infection of unknown etiology
Prevention or delay of the emergence of bacterial resistance

The disadvantages of treatment with multiple medications are the following:

Emergence of superinfection
Occurrence of antibiotic antagonism if the wrong combination is chosen
Enhanced toxicity if the wrong combination is chosen
Increased cost

PROPHYLACTIC ANTIBIOTICS. There are certain absolute indications for prophylactic treatment with antibiotics [2]:

1. To protect the heart in rheumatic patients. Benzathine penicillin is used to prevent streptococcal throat infection in order to prevent the recurrence of rheumatic fever.
2. To protect patients with bacterial endocarditis. Penicillin is used in dental extractions of patients with rheumatic fever or congenital cardiac abnormalities.
3. To prevent tuberculosis. Isoniazid is used as a prophylactic therapy in normal subjects who have come in contact with patients with active tuberculosis.
4. To prevent gas gangrene. Large doses of penicillin are used in severe contaminated trauma and for amputation through the thigh in obliterative arterial disease.

Relative, but debatable, indications for prophylactic treatment with antibiotics are postoperative infections only if the risk of sepsis exists [2].

COMPLICATIONS OF ANTIMICROBIAL THERAPY. The complications of therapy with antibiotics are bacterial resistance to drugs, the emergence of superinfections, and the appearance of toxic reactions.

Bacterial Resistance. Microorganisms show resistance to drugs by diversified mechanisms [4]. The microorganism may produce an enzyme that destroys the drug; staphylococci produce beta-lactamase, which destroys penicillin G. The microorganism may change its permeability to the drug; tetracyclines accumulate only in susceptible bacteria, and the resistant bacteria do not transport tetracy-

clines. The microorganism may develop a metabolic pathway other than the one inhibited originally by the drug; sulfonamide-resistant bacteria can utilize preformed folic acid. The microorganism may develop a de novo target different from the one originally acted on by the drug; erythromycin-resistant organisms have an altered receptor site on the 50S subunit of the bacterial ribosomes.

The bacterial resistance may be genetic or nongenetic in character.

NONGENETIC RESISTANCE. Once the infection has been controlled by chemotherapeutic agents, a few bacteria may remain "dormant" (inactive) in the host but are not able to multiply. Furthermore, these non-multiplying bacteria are resistant to drugs. However, in the event of immunosuppression, they resume multiplying and once more show susceptibility to the action of the chemotherapeutic agents.

GENETIC RESISTANCE. In this case, a stable genetic alteration occurs in the microorganism. The change may involve either chromosomal resistance or extrachromosomal resistance. The chromosomal resistance develops following a spontaneous mutation in a locus that controls susceptibility to a given chemotherapeutic agent. The microorganism also contains extrachromosomal genetic elements called plasmids (episomes). Genetic material and plasmids are transferred by

Transduction. The plasmid DNA is transferred by a virus to another bacterium.
Transformation. The naked DNA is passed from one bacterium to another.
Conjugation. The genetic material is transferred during a mating (conjugation) process.
Translocation or transposition. An exchange of short DNA sequence occurs between two plasmids or one plasmid and a portion of bacterial chromosome within a bacterial cell [4].

Microorganisms resistant to one drug are also resistant to related drugs in the same categories or to totally unrelated drugs (cross resistance). Resistance to antibiotic and chemotherapeutic agents may be abolished or delayed by one or a combination of the following actions:

Avoiding the unnecessary use of antibiotics
Using antibiotics in full adequate indicated doses
Avoiding the topical use of antibiotics for a prolonged period of time
Whenever possible, using the narrow-spectrum antibiotics
When following a combination drug regimen, using the full dosage [2]

Emergence of Superinfections. One of the hazards of chemotherapy is the alteration in the normal microbial population ("normal flora") of upper respiratory, intestinal, and genitourinary tracts, producing new infection(s) (superinfection). These infections, which may be caused by *Proteus* strains, staphylococci, and *Pseudomonas* and *Candida* organisms, are difficult to treat and hence are potentially dangerous.

Appearance of Toxic Reactions. Either hypersensitivity reactions or direct toxicities not attributable to hypersensitivity reactions may take place. They will be discussed with individual antibiotic and chemotherapeutic agents.

Part One: Sulfonamides and Trimethoprim

Sulfonamides (Fig. 35-1) are structurally related to para-aminobenzoic acid (PABA). Substances resembling sulfonamides but devoid of antibacterial activities are some oral hypoglycemic agents (tolbutamide) and some carbonic anhydrase inhibitors (acetazolamide). The presence of a free para-amino group is essential for antibacterial action. Succinylsulfathiazole (Sulfasuxidine) and phthalylsulfathiazole (Sulfathalidine) are agents with a substituted para-amino group. These intestinal antiseptics are slowly hydrolyzed in the intestine, releasing sulfathiazole, which exerts antiseptic effects against the coliform and clostridial organisms.

ANTIBACTERIAL ACTION. As bacteriostatic agents, sulfonamides are active against both gram-positive and gram-negative bacteria, including streptococci, gram-negative bacilli, and *Chlamydia, Nocardia*, and *Actinomyces* organisms. Sulfonamides alone or with trimethoprim are the drugs of choice in urinary tract infections, nocardiosis, and toxoplasmosis. Sulfonamides are also used topically in burn therapy.

MECHANISM OF ACTION. Sulfonamides, by competing with PABA, inhibit the synthesis of folic acid that is essential for bacterial production of pu-

Fig. 35-1. *Structure of selected sulfonamides.*

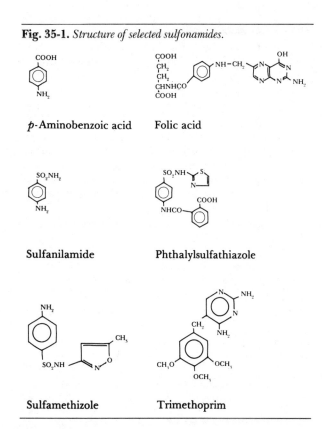

p-Aminobenzoic acid   Folic acid

Sulfanilamide   Phthalylsulfathiazole

Sulfamethizole   Trimethoprim

rines and the ultimate synthesis of nucleic acids. They also become incorporated into folic acid.

DEVELOPMENT OF RESISTANCE. The widespread use of sulfonamides against gonococci, meningococci, beta-hemolytic streptococci, and coliform organisms has resulted in the emergence of resistant strains. In general, organisms that are impermeable to sulfonamides or produce large amounts of PABA are resistant to sulfonamides. Furthermore, resistance in a previously sensitive organism may occur as a result of mutation, causing (1) overproduction of PABA or (2) alteration in folic acid–synthesizing enzymes [7].

PHARMACOKINETICS. Sulfonamides are absorbed orally, become bound to plasma proteins, are distributed widely throughout the body including the cerebrospinal fluid, and become metabolized in the liver by acetylation. The acetylated metabolites, which have no bacteriostatic activity, retain the toxic property of the parent compounds. The free sulfonamides undergo glomerular filtration and then are partially resorbed whereas the acetylated derivatives are not resorbed and are excreted readily. The urinary concentration of acetylated derivative is higher than the plasma level. The urinary solubility of the sulfonamides decreases when the pH of the urine decreases. The tendency toward crystalluria increases in acidic pH's. Conversely, the solubility of the sulfonamides increases greatly in alkaline pH's. The recently introduced sulfonamides are more soluble at the usual urinary pH. The incidence of crystalluria may be diminished by (1) enhancing fluid intake, (2) alkalinization of the urine, and (3) taking a mixture of sulfonamides. On the basis of pharmacokinetic principles, the sulfonamides may be classified in four separate categories:

1. Sulfonamides with rapid rate of absorption and elimination are sulfisoxazole (Gantrisin), sulfamethoxazole (Gantanol), sulfacytine (Renoquid), and sulfamethizole (Thiosulfil). These highly soluble, recently introduced sulfonamides have excellent antibacterial activity with a minimum or an absence of the renal toxicity of the sulfonamides of yesteryear.

2. Sulfonamides with rapid rate of absorption but slow rate of elimination, which are relatively toxic agents and no longer used in the United States, include sulfamethoxypyridazine and sulfadimethoxine.

3. Sulfonamides that are poorly absorbed are succinylsulfathiazole (Sulfasuxidine), phthalylsulfathiazole (Sulfathalidine), and sulfasalazine (Azulfidine). These agents are used as intestinal antiseptics. Sulfasalazine is used in the therapy of regional enteritis and ulcerative colitis.

4. Sulfonamides that are used topically are sulfacetamide (Sulamyd, Isopto Cetamide), which is used in ophthalmic infections, and mafenide (Sulfamylon)

and silver sulfadiazine (Silvadene), which are used in infections associated with burns.

TOXICITIES OF THE SULFONAMIDES. Many of the adverse reactions to sulfonamides are due to hypersensitivity reactions, which include dermatitis, leukopenia, hemolytic anemia, and drug fever. Stevens-Johnson syndrome is a very severe, but rare, hypersensitivity reaction that occurs only with some of the long-acting sulfonamide preparations.

Renal lesions may be due to precipitation of sulfonamide and their acetyl derivatives in the urinary tract. Renal damage may also be attributable to a direct toxic effect of sulfonamides on the kidney tubules.

Sulfonamides may cause jaundice and kernicterus in the newborn because of displacement of bilirubin from protein-binding sites. Therefore, sulfonamides should not be used in pregnancy.

TRIMETHOPRIM-SULFAMETHOXAZOLE COMBINATION: BACTRIM, SEPTRA. These combination drugs (usually five parts sulfa to one part trimethoprim) interfere with the synthesis of active folic acid in two separate reactions. Sulfonamides compete with PABA and prevent the conversion of PABA to dihydrofolic acid. Trimethoprim, by inhibiting the activity of dihydrofolic acid reductase, prevents the conversion of dihydrofolic acid into tetrahydrofolic acid, necessary for the synthesis of DNA according to the following summarized reactions:

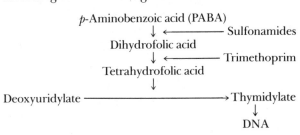

These drug combinations have the following therapeutic advantages:

They cause synergistic antibacterial effects.
They have bactericidal activity.
The emergence of bacterial resistance is decreased.
The spectrum of antibacterial activity is enhanced.
The toxicity is reduced.

Folic acid deficiency may also occur after prolonged usage of methotrexate or in patients who had preexisting folic acid deficiency. Folinic acid may be administered to overcome the folic acid deficiency–related megaloblastic anemia.

CLINICAL USES. Oral trimethoprim is used in chronic recurring urinary tract infection.

Oral trimethoprim-sulfamethoxazole is used in *Shigella* and some *Salmonella* infections, particularly

Fig. 35-2. *Structure of selected urinary tract antiseptics.*

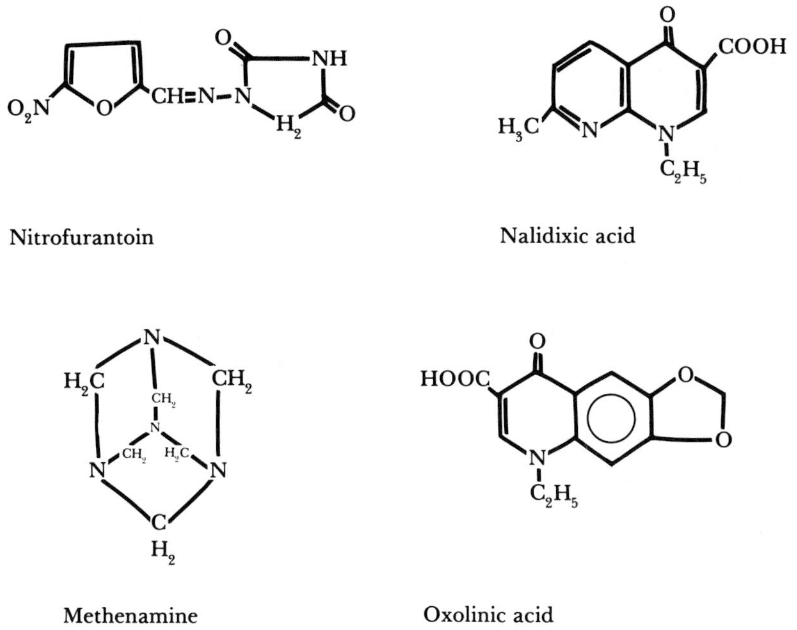

Nitrofurantoin

Nalidixic acid

Methenamine

Oxolinic acid

when they are resistant to ampicillin and chloramphenicol.

High doses of oral trimethoprim-sulfamethoxazole are used in *Pneumocystis* pneumonia. This combination, along with polymyxin, has been shown to be effective in *Serratia* or *Pseudomonas* sepsis.

Intravenous trimethoprim-sulfamethoxazole is indicated in severe *Pneumocystis carinii* pneumonia, gram-negative bacterial sepsis, and shigellosis.

Oral trimethoprim with sulfonamide has been used in leishmaniasis and toxoplasmosis and in falciparum malaria [7].

Part Two: Urinary Antiseptics

Nitrofurantoin, nalidixic acid, methenamine, and oxolinic acid are orally active urinary antiseptics (Fig. 35-2) that have no systemic antibacterial activity.

NITROFURANTOIN. Nitrofurantoin (Furadantin), which is active against many strains of *E. coli*, is bacteriostatic in nature. Most species of *Proteus, Pseudomonas, Enterobacter*, and *Klebsiella* are resistant.

NALIDIXIC ACID (NEGGRAM). Nalidixic acid, which is active against many strains of *Escherichia coli, Proteus mirabilis*, and *Klebsiella-Enterobacter*, is bactericidal in nature. It inhibits DNA synthesis.

OXOLINIC ACID (UTIBID). The antibacterial spectrum and the mechanism of action of oxolinic acid are similar to those discussed for nalidixic acid.

METHENAMINE MANDELATE (MANDELAMINE). Methenamine decomposes in solution to generate formaldehyde, which in a concentration of 20 μg per milliliter inhibits all bacteria-causing urinary tract infection. Urea-splitting microorganisms (*Proteus* species) raise the pH of the urine and hence inhibit the release of formaldehyde and the action of methenamine. On the other hand, acidification of urine enhances the antibacterial action of methenamine [9].

Part Three: Penicillins

All penicillins (Fig. 35-3) are composed of a thiazolidine ring attached to a beta-lactam. This in turn carries a free amide group (O=CNH) on which a substitution occurs and an attachment (R) is made. In the case of benzyl penicillin, the R is a benzyl group. Penicillin may be metabolized by amidase to 6-aminopenicillanic acid, which has antibacterial activity, or by penicillinase (bacterial beta-lactamase) to penicilloic acid, which is devoid of antibacterial activity but is antigenic in nature and acts as a sensitizing structure [3]. The main cause of bacterial resistance to penicillin is indeed the production of penicillinase by the microorganisms.

Penicillin is an organic acid that is commonly supplied as sodium and potassium salts. Penicillin V (Pen-Vee K, V-Cillin K) and phenethicillin (Syncillin, Maxipen) are different from penicillin G (benzyl penicillin) in that they are more acid resistant. In addition to the broad-spectrum penicillins such as ampicillin and amoxicillin, there is a newer group of "anti-Pseudomonas" penicillins effective against gram-negative bacilli that includes carbenicillin, ticarcillin, azlocillin, mezlocillin, and piperacillin. The latter two are also useful against *Klebsiella pneumoniae* and *Bacteroides fragilis*. The penicillinase-resistant penicillins are oxacillin, cloxacillin, dicloxacillin, methicillin, and nafcillin. These agents are the drugs of choice for infections caused by penicillinase-producing *Staphylococcus aureus*.

MECHANISM OF ACTION. Penicillins inhibit the formation of cell walls and hence are bactericidal in action. Penicillin exerts its effect by binding to cellular receptors now identified as transpeptidation enzymes. By binding to and inhibiting transpeptidation reactions, it interrupts the synthesis of cell wall peptidoglycan. Penicillin also removes or inactivates an inhibitor of the lytic enzymes (autolysin), resulting in lysis of microorganisms in an isotonic environment [3]. In general, penicillins are more active against gram-positive organisms.

BACTERICIDAL ACTIONS. The penicillin-susceptible organisms are non-penicillinase-producing strains of most cocci, gram-positive bacilli, and spirochetes.

Fig. 35-3. *Catabolism of penicillin by the action of amidase and penicillinase. (Modified from G. L. Mandell and M. A. Sande, Penicillins and Cephalosporins. In A. G. Gilman, L. S. Goodman, and A. Gilman [eds.],* The Pharmacological Basis of Therapeutics *[6th ed.]. New York: Macmillan, 1980.)*

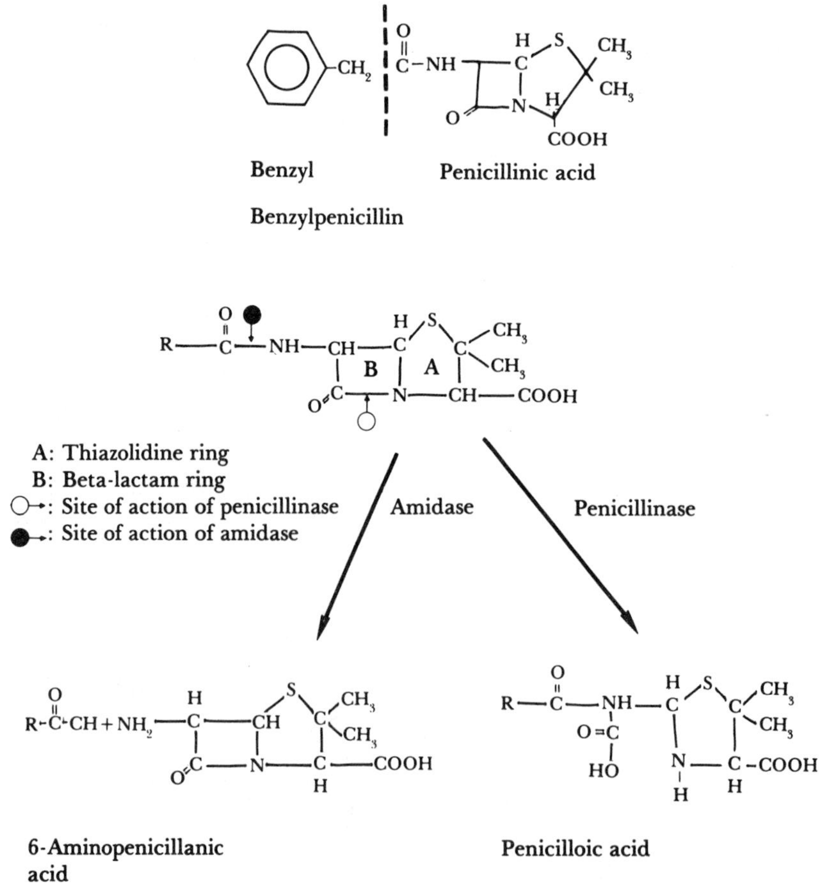

Table 35-1. *Comparative Pharmacology of Penicillin Derivatives*

	Property		
Drug	Acid Stability	Penicillinase Resistance	Spectrum of Activity
Penicillin G	No	No	Narrow spectrum
Penicillin V, phenethicillin	Yes	No	Narrow spectrum
Methicillin	No	Yes	Narrow spectrum
Dicloxacillin	Yes	Yes	Narrow spectrum
Nafcillin	No	Yes	Narrow spectrum
Amoxicillin	Yes	No	Broad spectrum
Ampicillin	Yes	No	Broad spectrum

THERAPEUTIC USES. Penicillin G may be used actively and prophylactically in the following cases:

Streptococcal infections—streptococcal pharyngitis (including scarlet fever); streptococcal pneumonia, arthritis, meningitis, and endocarditis; streptococcal otitis media and sinusitis; infectious endocarditis
Pneumococcal infections
Staphylococcal infections—generally resistant to penicillin G
Meningococcal disease
Gonococcal infections
Syphilis
Actinomycosis, anthrax, and gas gangrene

PHARMACOKINETICS. Thirty percent of an oral dose of penicillin is absorbed from the gastrointestinal tract. Penicillin G is rapidly destroyed at pH_2 of gastric secretion. Penicillin is widely distributed throughout the body and, except in meningitis, does not pass across the blood-brain barrier. Penicillin is metabolized slightly by the liver but mainly is excreted by the kidney. Probenecid blocks the active tubular secretion of penicillin and hence prolongs its action. Penicillin is readily absorbed from intramuscular sites, and long-acting repository forms such as penicillin G procaine and penicillin G benzathine are available. Table 35-1 summarizes the pharmacologic properties of several semisynthetic penicillins.

CARBENICILLINS. Carbenicillin (Geopen). This agent, which is acid labile (not active orally), is used in severe gram-negative infections caused by *Pseudomonas* and *Proteus* strains.

Carbenicillin Indanyl (Geocillin). This agent, which is acid stable (active orally), is used for urinary tract infections caused by *Proteus* and *Pseudomonas aeruginosa* strains.

Ticarcillin. This agent is a substitute for carbenicillin in the treatment of serious gram-negative infections.

BROAD-SPECTRUM PENICILLIN. Amoxicillin and ampicillin are broad-spectrum penicillins used in

Urinary tract infections
Upper respiratory tract infections
Bacterial endocarditis
Otitis media
Typhoid fever

ADVERSE REACTIONS TO PENICILLINS. Penicillins, which are the safest antibiotics, produce few direct toxic reactions. Most of the serious side effects are hypersensitivity reactions. Penicillins and their by-products, penicilloic acid and penicilloyl-polylysine, are antigenic in susceptible individuals who develop IgG antibodies to them. Furthermore, all penicillins cross-sensitize and cross-react. Allergic reactions including anaphylactic shock occur in sensitized patients following repeated administration of penicillin. Anaphylactic reactions, which are more common following parenteral administration of penicillin, may be reduced by the administration of corticosteroids.

The direct toxicity of penicillin in large doses may include phlebitis if the agent is given intravenously, injection site inflammatory reactions when given intramuscularly, degeneration of nerve if injected into a nerve, and CNS excitability if given intrathecally.

The broad-spectrum penicillins such as ampicillin and amoxicillin may cause gastrointestinal irritation. Occasionally, the overgrowth of staphylococci, *Pseudomonas* and *Proteus* organisms, or yeasts may cause enteritis. Methicillin and nafcillin may cause granulocytopenia. Methicillin has caused nephritis. Carbenicillin may cause hypokalemic alkalosis [3].

Part Four: Penicillin Substitutes

CEPHALOSPORINS. Cephalosporins (Fig. 35-4) are structurally related to penicillins. The nucleus of the cephalosporin, 7-aminocephalosporanic acid, resembles 6-aminopenicillanic acid, the nucleus of penicillin. Cephalosporins have a broad spectrum of antimicrobial activity and are effective against a variety of gram-positive and some strains of gram-negative bacteria such as *E. coli*, *Klebsiella*, and *Proteus* species. In addition, cephalosporins are effective against some strains of *Enterobacter*, *Serratia*, and *Pseudomonas*. Among gram-positive bacteria, enterococci, penicillin-resistant pneumococci, and methicillin-resistant staphylococci are also resistant to cephalosporins [3]. Furthermore, the second-generation and newer cephalosporins, such as cefamandole, cefoxitin, cefuroxime, and moxalactam (Fig. 35-4), have an even broader spectrum of activity and are more active than the first-generation and older cephalosporins such as cephalothin against gram-negative microorganisms [3, 9].

Mechanism of Action. Like penicillins, cephalosporins exert their effects by inhibiting the formation of cell walls in the bacteria. Clinical resistance among second- and third-generation cephalosporins has been reported. These agents are resistant to penicillinase.

Pharmacokinetics. Cephalexin, cefaclor, cefadroxil, and cephradine are absorbed well from the gastrointestinal tract and are given orally. Cephaloridine, cephalothin, cephapirin, cefoxitin, cefotaxime, cefamandole, and cefazolin are poorly absorbed from the gastrointestinal tract and must be given parenterally. Since cephalosporins have short half-lives, they must be administered on a frequent basis. First- and second-generation cephalosporins (but not the third generation) do not penetrate into the central nervous system readily and therefore are not effective for the treatment of meningitis. The cephalosporins are eliminated by glomerular filtration and active tubular secretion, which are blocked by probenecid. The acetylated derivatives of cephalosporins such as cephalothin and cephapirin are metabolized in the liver to inactive metabolites [3].

Clinical Use. Cephalosporins, often with aminoglycoside antibiotics, are used in suspected bacteremia from *Staphylococcus*, *Klebsiella*, coliform bacteria, *Proteus*, or *Pseudomonas*. Cephalosporins are alternatives to penicillin G for the treatment of streptococcal and pneumococcal infections. The third-generation cephalosporins are the drugs of choice in gram-negative bacillary meningitis. Cephalosporins are used on a very limited basis prior to and following some surgical procedures bearing high risks for infections.

Adverse Reactions. The adverse reactions caused by cephalosporins resemble those discussed for penicillin and include injection site complications, phlebitis

Fig. 35-4. *Structure of cephalothin and other penicillin substitutes.*

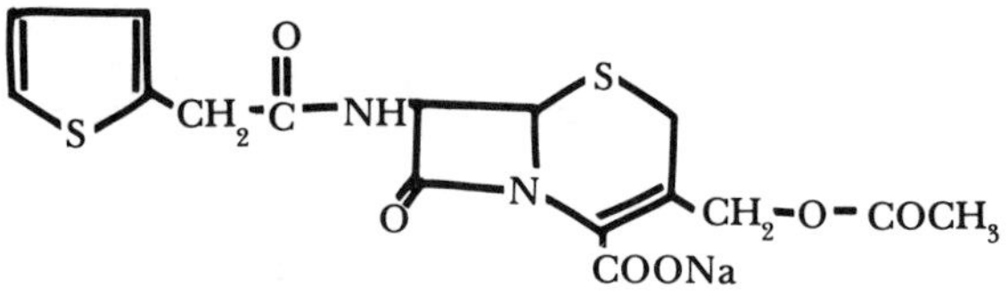

Cephalothin sodium

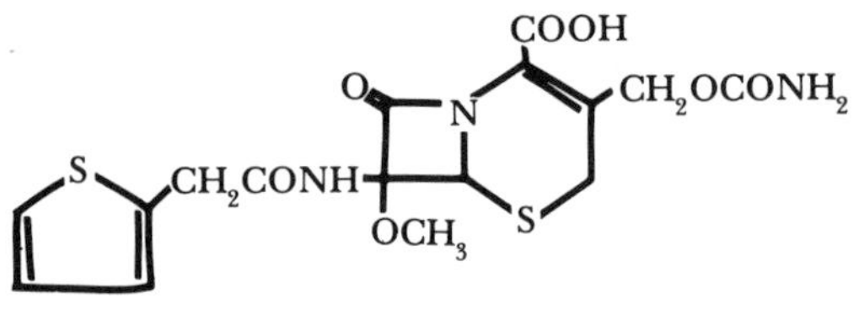

Cefoxitin

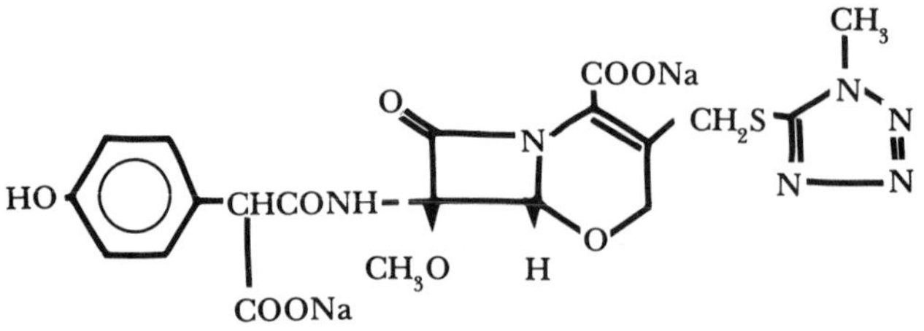

Moxalactam sodium

following intravenous administration, hypersensitivity reactions, and rare anaphylactic shock. Infrequent nephrotoxicity does occur with some cephalosporins.

ERYTHROMYCIN (ERYTHROCIN, ILOTYCIN). Antimicrobial Activity and Clinical Use. Erythromycin, as a penicillin alternative, is a medium- to broad-spectrum antibiotic. It possesses both bactericidal and bacteriostatic activity depending on the concentration of the drug being used and the microorganisms being treated. Erythromycin is effective against gram-positive organisms such as *Streptococcus pyogenes* and *S. pneumoniae*. In larger doses, erythromycin is effective against *S. epidermidis* and *S. aureus*. In addition, gram-positive bacilli such as *Clostridium perfringens*, *Corynebacterium diphtheriae*, and *Listeria monocytogenes* are susceptible to erythromycin. Erythromycin is also effective against *Mycoplasma pneumoniae* and *Legionella pneumophila*, which causes Legionnaires' disease.

Mechanism of Action. Erythromycin exerts its effect by binding to a 23S rRNA on the 50S ribosomal subunit and hence inhibiting protein synthesis. Aminoacyl translocation reactions and elongation of the peptide chain are blocked [8].

Development of Resistance. Resistance occurs from the methylation of rRNA receptors, preventing the attachment of erythromycin to 50S ribosomes.

Pharmacokinetic Properties. Since erythromycin is destroyed by gastric secretions, it is supplied as enteric-coated tablets that are absorbed well from the upper part of the small intestine. Erythromycin stearate is acid resistant. Erythromycin is largely excreted in the bile, while the urinary excretion is negligible.

Adverse Reaction. Some derivatives of erythromycin and especially erythromycin estolate cause cholestatic hepatitis.

CLINDAMYCIN (CLEOCIN). Clindamycin has a similar antibacterial spectrum and shows some cross resistance to erythromycin. It exerts its effects by binding to the 50S subunit of bacterial ribosomes and by inhibiting protein synthesis. Clindamycin is an alternative to penicillin, being effective against staphylococcal, streptococcal, and pneumococcal infections. In addition, it is effective against anaerobic infections, especially those caused by *Bacteroides*. Clindamycin, which is absorbed well orally, may cause skin rashes, diarrhea, and pseudomembranous colitis.

VANCOMYCIN (VANCOCIN). Vancomycin, a bactericidal antibiotic, exerts its effect by inhibiting cell wall synthesis in gram-positive bacteria. It is effective in methicillin-resistant organisms and as an alternative to semisynthetic penicillins or cephalosporins in severe staphylococcal infections. Furthermore, it is effective in streptococcal endocarditis infection and for the treatment of pseudomembranous colitis. Vancomycin is not absorbed well orally, and with the exception of treatment of enterocolitis, when it is given orally, it must be administered intravenously. Toxic reactions such as ototoxicity and nephrotoxicity do occur. Fever, chills, injection site complications, and phlebitis also take place.

SPECTINOMYCIN (TROBICIN). Spectinomycin binds to the 30S ribosomal subunit and inhibits protein synthesis in gram-negative bacteria. Spectinomycin is given as a single intramuscular injection for the treatment of acute uncomplicated genital and rectal gonorrhea in patients who are either allergic to penicillin or infected with penicillinase-producing microorganisms [12].

Part Five: Aminoglycoside Antibiotics

Aminoglycosides (Fig. 35-5) contain a hexose nucleus, a streptidine (in streptomycin), or deoxystreptamine (other aminoglycosides), to which amino sugars are attached by glycosidic linkages [6].

MECHANISM OF ACTION. Aminoglycosides are bactericidal and inhibit protein synthesis in susceptible microorganisms. They produce this effect (1) by interfering with the initiation complex of peptide formation, (2) by inducing misreading of the code on the mRNA template, which causes incorporation of inappropriate amino acid into peptide, and (3) by rupturing the polysomes into monosomes, which become nonfunctional [6].

MECHANISM OF RESISTANCE. Resistance to aminoglycosides may occur following one or a combination of the following mechanisms [6]:

Interference with the transport of aminoglycoside into bacterial cells
Deletion of receptors on the 30S ribosomal subunit, not allowing aminoglycosides to function
Bacterial biotransformation of aminoglycosides to inactive forms

Fig. 35-5. *Structure of streptomycin and tobramycin.*

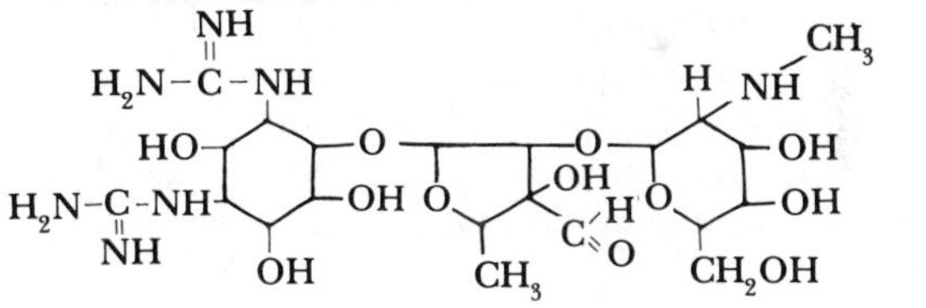

Streptomycin

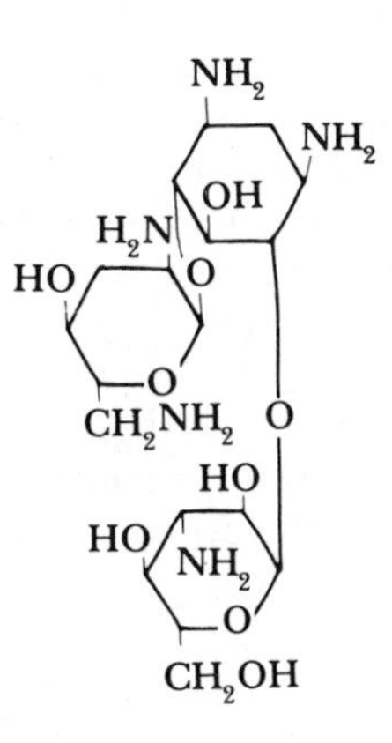

Tobramycin

In addition, since the initial transport of aminoglycosides into bacterial cells is an oxygen-dependent process, microorganisms that are able to grow under anaerobic conditions show or develop resistance.

ANTIMICROBIAL ACTIONS. Aminoglycosides are effective against aerobic gram-negative enteric bacteria, especially in bacteremia, sepsis, or endocarditis. Some aminoglycosides—gentamicin, tobramycin, kanamycin, and amikacin—are also effective against other aerobic gram-negative bacilli.

PHARMACOKINETICS. The aminoglycosides are poorly absorbed from the gastrointestinal tract. Therefore, they are administered intramuscularly. Furthermore, since they do not penetrate into the CNS, they may have to be given intrathecally or intraventricularly for meningitis. Aminoglycosides are excreted by glomerular filtration, which is greatly reduced in renal impairment, causing toxic blood levels.

TOXIC REACTIONS. The greatest toxic reactions following aminoglycoside administration are cochlear damage and vestibular impairment, causing vertigo and disturbance in maintaining postural equilibrium. Aminoglycosides given during pregnancy cause deafness in the newborn. In addition to ototoxicity, nephrotoxicity and reversible neuromuscular blockade, causing respiratory paralysis, do occur with high doses.

STREPTOMYCIN. Streptomycin is combined with isoniazid and given in nondisseminated pulmonary tuberculosis. Streptomycin is a drug of choice in plague and tularemia and, in combination with tetracyclines, in the management of brucellosis. In combination with penicillin G, it is effective in bacterial endocarditis.

GENTAMICIN (GARAMYCIN). Gentamicin is used in serious infections by gram-negative organisms. It is effective in urinary tract infections, bacteremia, meningitis, infected burns, pneumonia, osteomyelitis, and peritonitis. In combination with carbenicillin it is used in infections resulting from *P. aeruginosa*. Furthermore, gentamicin in combination with penicillin is used in bacterial endocarditis.

TOBRAMYCIN (NEBCIN). The clinical pharmacology of tobramycin resembles that of gentamicin. However, tobramycin is more effective against *P. aeruginosa*.

KANAMYCIN (KANTREX). Kanamycin is effective in the treatment of bacteremia caused by gram-negative enteric organisms. In combination with clindamycin, kanamycin is used in penetrating abdominal wounds [6].

AMIKACIN (AMIKIN). Among aminoglycosides, amikacin has the broadest antimicrobial spectrum. It is usually reserved for the treatment of serious infections resistant to other aminoglycosides.

NEOMYCIN (MYCIFRADIN, NEOBIOTIC). Neomycin is used orally for preoperative chemoprophylaxis in hepatic coma and in colonic surgery. It is also used topically in infections of the skin and mucous membranes.

Part Six: Chloramphenicol

ANTIMICROBIAL ACTIVITY. Chloramphenicol (Chloromycetin) (Fig. 35-6) has a broad spectrum of bacteriostatic activity for many bacteria and for rickettsiae. It is a drug of choice in (1) *Salmonella* infection (e.g., typhoid fever), (2) *Haemophilus influenzae* infection, meningitis, laryngotracheitis, or pneumonia not responding to ampicillin, (3) infection with *Bacteroides*, (4) meningococcal infection in patients allergic to penicillin, and (5) rickettsial infections [5].

DEVELOPMENT OF BACTERIAL RESISTANCE. The resistance to chloramphenicol results from the production by microorganisms of chloramphenicol acetyltransferase, which metabolizes the drug.

MECHANISM OF ACTION. Chloramphenicol exerts its effects (1) by binding to 50S ribosomal subunits and thus inhibiting bacterial protein synthesis, (2) by preventing peptide bond formation, and (3) by inhibiting the synthesis of mitochondrial proteins in the host.

PHARMACOKINETICS. Chloramphenicol is completely absorbed from the gastrointestinal tract and distributed widely throughout the body including the cerebrospinal fluid. Chloramphenicol is metabolized in the liver by glucuronyl transferase, and the metabolites are excreted by the kidneys. Newborn infants are not able to metabolize chloramphenicol readily.

TOXIC REACTIONS. Chloramphenicol causes dose-dependent and dose-independent hematologic reactions. Fatal aplastic anemia occurs in genetically susceptible patients taking chloramphenicol on a chronic basis. Reversible and dose-dependent disturbances of hemopoiesis, characterized by altered maturation of red blood cells, vacuolated nucleated red blood cells in the marrow, and reticulocytopenia, take place.

Gray Baby Syndrome. Newborn infants are deficient in glucuronyl transferase. When treating newborns, one should be sure that chloramphenicol dosage does not exceed 50 mg/kg/day. Large doses cause gray baby syndrome, characterized by vomiting, hypothermia, gray color, and shock.

Fig. 35-6. *Structure of tetracycline and chloramphenicol.*

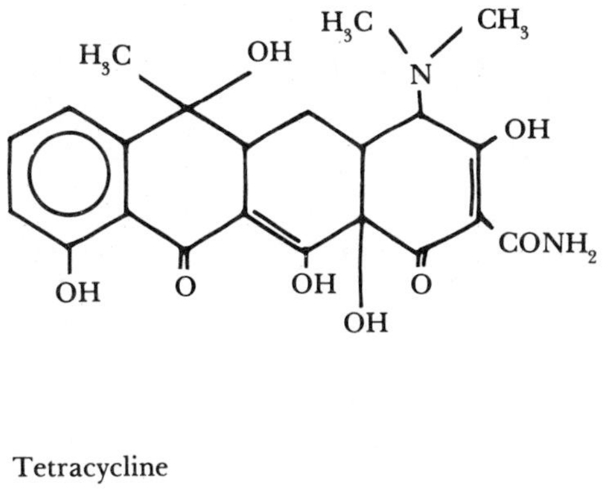

Tetracycline

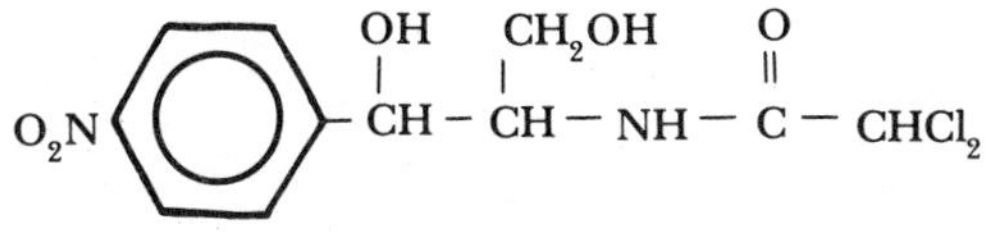

Chloramphenicol

Part Seven: Tetracyclines

The tetracyclines include the following antibiotic agents:

Tetracycline (Achromycin, Panmycin)
Chlortetracycline (Aureomycin)
Oxytetracycline (Terramycin)
Demeclocycline (Declomycin)
Doxycycline (Vibramycin)
Minocycline (Minocin, Vectrin)
Methacycline (Rondomycin)

Tetracyclines (Fig. 35-6), which are bacteriostatic in nature, have the broadest spectrum of activity, being effective against gram-positive and gram-negative bacteria, rickettsiae, mycoplasmas, amebas, and chlamydiae.

MECHANISM OF ACTION. Tetracyclines enter bacterial cells by passive diffusion and by active transport and then accumulate intracellularly. This sequence does not occur in mammalian cells. The tetracyclines bind to 30S subunits of bacterial ribosomes in a way that blocks the binding of the aminoacyl tRNA to the acceptor site on the mRNA ribosome complex [5].

DEVELOPMENT OF RESISTANCE. The resistant mutant develops resistance (1) by not transporting tetracycline, (2) by not accumulating tetracycline, and (3) by plasmid-controlled resistance transmitted by transduction or by conjugation [5].

PHARMACOKINETICS. The absorption of tetracyclines from the gastrointestinal tract is nonuniform in nature. Chlortetracycline is absorbed to the extent of 30 percent; tetracycline, oxytetracycline, and demeclocycline are absorbed to the extent of 60 to 80 percent; doxycycline and minocycline are absorbed to the extent of 90 to 100 percent. The unabsorbed tetracycline may modify the intestinal flora. The absorption of tetracyclines is impaired by divalent cations (Ca^{2+}, Mg^{2+}, Fe^{2+}), by Al^{3+}, and by extreme alkaline pH's. Tetracyclines distribute widely throughout the body fluid, pass across the placental barrier, and accumulate in the growing bones. The concentration of chlortetracycline in spinal fluid is only one-fourth that in the plasma. Minocycline, a more lipid-soluble tetracycline, reaches a high concentration in tears and saliva and is able to eradicate the meningococcal carrier state. The tetracyclines are metabolized in the liver and excreted mainly by the bile and urine. The concentrations of tetracyclines in the bile are 10 times higher than those in serum.

THERAPEUTIC USES. Tetracyclines are effective in Rocky Mountain spotted fever, murine typhus, recrudescent epidemic typhus, scrub typhus, Q fever, lymphogranuloma venereum, psittacosis, tularemia, brucellosis, gonorrhea, certain urinary tract infections, granuloma inguinale, chancroid, syphilis, and disease due to *Bacteroides* and *Clostridium* [11].

ADVERSE REACTIONS. Tetracyclines in general cause toxic and hypersensitivity reactions—gastrointestinal irritations that are disabling and may result in the discontinuation of medications. With continuous usage, tetracyclines may alter the normal flora, allowing the growth of *Pseudomonas, Proteus,* staphylococci, resistant coliforms, *Clostridium,* and *Candida* [5]. These superinfections should be recognized and treated appropriately with vancomycin and other drugs.

Liver Toxicity. Tetracyclines have caused hepatic necrosis, especially when given in large doses intravenously, in pregnant women and in patients with preexisting liver impairment.

Renal Toxicity. Outdated tetracycline preparations cause a Fanconi-like syndrome characterized by nausea, vomiting, polyuria, polydipsia, proteinuria, acidosis, glycosuria, and aminoaciduria. With the exception of doxycycline, tetracyclines do accumulate in patients with renal impairment. Tetracyclines produce nitrogen retention, especially when given with diuretics.

Photosensitivity. The systemic administration of demeclocycline causes photosensitization to ultraviolet light or sunlight.

Vestibular Reactions. Minocycline causes vertigo and dizziness.

Damage to Bone and Teeth. Tetracyclines are bound to calcium and become deposited in bone, damaging the developing bone and teeth.

Tissue Injury. Intravenous administration of tetracyclines has caused venous thrombosis [5].

Part Eight: Polypeptide Antibiotics

BACITRACIN (BACIQUENT). Bacitracin, which inhibits cell wall synthesis, is active against gram-positive bacteria. In combination with polymyxin and neomycin, it is often used in topical infections, and in open infections such as infected eczema, dermal ulcers, and surgical wounds. The parenteral administration of bacitracin may cause nephrotoxicity.

POLYMYXINS. Polymyxin B (Aerosporin) and polymyxin E, colistin (Coly-mycin), which are bactericidal, are effective in gram-negative bacterial infections, especially *Pseudomonas* infection. Polymyxins are cationic detergent peptides, possessing both lipophilic and lipophobic groups that are able to bind and subsequently damage the bacterial cell membranes. Polymyxins are not absorbed orally and must be administered parenterally for systemic infections. Reversible nephrotoxicity (proteinuria, hematuria, and cyclindruria), neurotoxicity characterized by giddiness, numbness, paresthesias, neuromuscular blockade, confusion, ataxia, and convulsions occur.

QUESTIONS ON ANTIMICROBIAL CHEMOTHERAPY

Select the answer that best completes the statement or answers the question.

____ 281. Chemotherapeutic agents that inhibit bacterial cell wall include:
   A. Penicillins.
   B. Cephalosporins.
   C. Bacitracin.
   D. Cycloserine.
   E. All of the above.

____ 282. Chemotherapeutic agents that exert their effects by inhibiting the function(s) of cell members include:
   A. Amphotericin B.
   B. Colistin.
   C. Nystatin.
   D. Polymyxin.
   E. All of the above.

____ 283. Chemotherapeutic agents that inhibit nucleic acid synthesis include:
   A. Sulfonamides.
   B. Trimethoprim.
   C. Nalidixic acid.
   D. Rifampin.
   E. All of the above.

____ 284. Chemotherapeutic agents that inhibit protein synthesis include:
   A. Chloramphenicol.
   B. Erythromycin.
   C. Tetracycline.
   D. Aminoglycosides.
   E. All of the above.

____ 285. Which one of the following drugs is mismatched with the indicated action or reaction assigned to it?
   A. Penicillin—bactericidal.
   B. Sulfonamide—bacteriostatic.
   C. Tetracycline—broad spectrum of activity.
   D. Sulfonamide—neurotoxicity.

____ 286. What is (are) the advantage(s) of using combined antibiotics?
   A. Enhanced therapeutic efficacy.
   B. Elimination of toxicity.
   C. Delaying of the emergence of bacterial resistance.
   D. A, B, and C.
   E. A and C.

____ 287. The indication(s) for prophylactic treatment with antibiotics is (are):
   A. To protect the heart in rheumatic patients.
   B. To protect patients with bacterial endocarditis.
   C. To prevent tuberculosis.
   D. A, B, and C.
   E. A and B.

____ 288. Substances that resemble sulfonamide in structure but are devoid of antibacterial activity include:
   A. Tolbutamide.
   B. Carbamazepine.
   C. Ethosuximide.
   D. Amitriptyline.

____ 289. Which one of the following agents is an intestinal antiseptic?
   A. Phthalylsulfathiazole.
   B. Nitrofurantoin.
   C. Nalidixic acid.
   D. Methenamine.

____ 290. Resistance to the bacteriostatic activity of sulfisoxazole develops by:
   A. Overproduction of para-aminobenzoic acid.
   B. Inhibition of dehydrofolate reductase.
   C. Lack of excretion of urinary folic acid.
   D. Lack of conversion of sulfisoxazole to its acetylated derivative.

____ 291. Which one of the following penicillins is not stable in acid pH?
   A. Penicillin G.
   B. Penicillin V.
   C. Dicloxacillin.
   D. Amoxicillin.

____ 292. Which one of the following penicillins is not penicillinase resistant?
   A. Methicillin.
   B. Nafcillin.
   C. Dicloxacillin.
   D. Penicillin V.

____ 293. Which one of the following penicillins has a relatively broad spectrum of antibacterial actions?
   A. Phenethicillin.
   B. Nafcillin.
   C. Amoxicillin.
   D. Penicillin G.

____ 294. Carbenicillin indanyl is characterized by which of the following actions?
   A. It is not active orally.
   B. It is used for urinary tract infection.
   C. It is effective against *Proteus*.
   D. It is destroyed by acidic pH.
   E. B and C.

____ 295. Which one of the following drugs is mismatched with the assigned toxicity?
   A. Methicillin—granulocytopenia.
   B. Cimetidine—granulocytopenia.
   C. Nafcillin—granulocytopenia.
   D. Carbenicillin—granulocytopenia.

296. Which one of the following statements is not true about erythromycin?
  A. It has a narrow spectrum of antibacterial activity.
  B. It is effective against gram-positive organisms.
  C. It binds to a 23S rRNA on the 50S ribosomal subunit and hence inhibits protein synthesis.
  D. It is mainly excreted in the bile.

297. Which one of the following statements is not true about spectinomycin?
  A. It binds to the 30S ribosomal subunit and inhibits protein synthesis.
  B. It is given intravenously daily for 10 days.
  C. It is effective in patients allergic to penicillin.
  D. It is effective against penicillinase-producing *Neisseria gonorrhoeae*.

298. Aminoglycosides exert their effects by:
  A. Interfering with the initiation complex of peptide formation.
  B. Causing misreading of the code on the mRNA template.
  C. Rupturing polysomes into monosomes.
  D. All of the above.

299. Resistance to aminoglycosides develops by:
  A. Interference with transport of aminoglycoside into bacterial cells.
  B. Deletion of receptor on the 30S ribosomal subunit, not allowing aminoglycoside to function.
  C. Bacterial transformation of aminoglycoside to inactive forms.
  D. All of the above.

300. Streptomycin has therapeutic use in:
  A. Pulmonary tuberculosis.
  B. Plague.
  C. Tularemia.
  D. Brucellosis.
  E. All of the above.

301. Chloramphenicol is characterized by all of the following actions *except* which one?
  A. It has a narrow spectrum of activity.
  B. It is a drug of choice in *Salmonella* infection.
  C. It is used in meningococcal infection in patients allergic to penicillin.
  D. Bacterial resistance results from the development of chloramphenicol acetyltransferase.

302. Polymyxin antibiotics:
  A. Are bactericidal.
  B. Are effective against gram-negative bacteria, especially the *Pseudomonas* infections.
  C. Are cationic detergents.
  D. Possess both lipophilic and lipophobic groups.
  E. All of the above.

ANSWERS ON ANTIMICROBIAL CHEMOTHERAPY

281. E.
282. E.
283. E.
284. E.
285. D.
286. E.
287. D.
288. A.
289. A.
290. A.
291. A.
292. D.
293. C.
294. E.
295. B.
296. A.
297. B.
298. D.
299. D.
300. E.
301. A.
302. E.

REFERENCES

1. Gallin, J. I. The Compromised Host. In J. B. Wyngaarden and L. H. Smith, Jr. (eds.), *Cecil's Textbook of Medicine* (6th ed.). Philadelphia: Saunders, 1982. Pp. 1395–1402.
2. Garrod, L. P. Principles and Practice of Antibacterial Chemotherapy. In G. S. Avery (ed.), *Drug Treatment: Principles and Practice of Clinical Pharmacology and Therapeutics* (2nd ed.). New York: Adis, 1980. Pp. 1122–1141.
3. Jawetz, E. Penicillins and Cephalosporins. In B. G. Katzung (ed.), *Basic and Clinical Pharmacology*. Los Altos, Calif.: Lange, 1982. Pp. 487–495.
4. Jawetz, E. Principles of Antimicrobial Drug Action. In B. G. Katzung (ed.), *Basic and Clinical Pharmacology*. Los Altos, Calif.: Lange, 1982. Pp. 481–485.
5. Jawetz, E. Chloramphenicol and Tetracyclines. In B. G. Katzung (ed.), *Basic and Clinical Pharmacology*. Los Altos, Calif.: Lange, 1982. Pp. 496–500.
6. Jawetz, E. Aminoglycosides and Polymyxins. In B. G. Katzung (ed.), *Basic and Clinical Pharmacology*. Los Altos, Calif.: Lange, 1982. Pp. 501–507.
7. Jawetz, E. Sulfonamides and Trimethoprim. In B. G. Katzung (ed.), *Basic and Clinical Pharmacology*. Los Altos, Calif.: Lange, 1982. Pp. 515–519.
8. Jawetz, E. Drugs with Specialized Functions. In B. G. Katzung (ed.), *Basic and Clinical Pharmacology*. Los Altos, Calif.: Lange, 1982. Pp. 530–537.
9. Mandell, G. L., and Sande, M. A. Sulfonamides, Trimethoprim-Sulfamethoxazole, and Urinary Tract Antiseptics. In A. G. Gilman, L. S. Goodman, and A. Gilman (eds.), *The Pharmacological Basis of Therapeutics* (6th ed.). New York: Macmillan, 1980. Pp. 1106–1125.
10. Mandell, G. L., and Sande, M. A. Penicillins and Cephalosporins. In A. G. Gilman, L. S. Goodman, and A. Gilman (eds.), *The Pharmacological Basis of Therapeutics* (6th ed.). New York: Macmillan, 1980. Pp. 1126–1161.
11. Sande, M. A., and Mandell, G. L. Tetracyclines and Chloramphenicol. In A. G. Gilman, L. S. Goodman, and A. Gilman (eds.), *The Pharmacological Basis of Therapeutics* (6th ed.). New York: Macmillan, 1980. Pp. 1181–1191.
12. Sande, M. A., and Mandell, G. L. Miscellaneous Antibacterial Agents: Antifungal and Antiviral Agents. In A. G. Gilman, L. S. Goodman, and A. Gilman (eds.), *The Pharmacological Basis of Therapeutics* (6th ed.). New York: Macmillan, 1980. Pp. 1222–1248.

13. Smith, H. *Antibiotics in Clinical Practice* (3rd ed.). Baltimore: University Park, 1977.
14. Wolff, S. M. The Febrile Patient. In J. B. Wyngaarden and L. H. Smith, Jr. (eds.), *Cecil's Textbook of Medicine* (6th ed.). Philadelphia: Saunders, 1982. Pp. 1392–1393.

X. Antiviral Agents, Immunopharmacology and Cancer Chemotherapy, and Antifungal Agents

36. Antiviral Agents

Men take their needs into consideration, never their abilities.

Napoleon Bonaparte

As ubiquitously occurring obligate intracellular parasites, viruses are able to infect humans, other animals, plants, and even bacteria by invading, confiscating, and utilizing the cellular metabolic machinery of the host. A viral infection can be inconsequential (papovaviruses, causing warts), disabling (picornaviruses, causing polio), or fatal (rhabdoviruses, causing rabies).

CLASSIFICATION OF THE VIRUSES. The viruses possess and utilize either RNA or DNA but not both nucleic acids. The following listing cites only a few examples of RNA- and DNA-containing viruses.

RNA-Containing Viruses	DNA-Containing Viruses
Rotaviruses, causing diarrhea	Adenoviruses, causing pharyngitis
Enteroviruses, causing polio	Poxviruses, causing smallpox
Paramyxoviruses, causing mumps and measles	Herpesviruses, causing herpes simplex
Orthomyxoviruses, causing influenza	
Rhabdoviruses, causing rabies	

Viruses are subclassified according to their structural features. For example, viral nucleic acid may be double stranded, as in poxviruses, or single stranded, as in rhabdoviruses. Furthermore, viruses may be enveloped (rhabdoviruses) or nonenveloped (adenoviruses).

MULTIPLICATION OF A VIRUS. The complete virus particle, known as a virion, contains an outer protein coat (capsid). Viral multiplication proceeds in steps.

Entry of a Virion and Release of Nucleic Acid. This step [1] has three parts (Fig. 36-1):

Adsorption. The virion becomes attached to a specific receptor on the surface of a susceptible cell in the host.
Penetration. The virion then enters the cells, either with fusion of its capsid with the plasma membrane or by engulfment in a phagocytic vacuole.
Eclipse phase. The capsid is removed to allow the expression of the viral genes. In the DNA virus, DNA is replicated by DNA polymerase of the host, and it may be coded by the virus and synthesized on the ribosomes of the host. The RNA viruses can replicate RNA directly from their RNA genome.

Replication of the Genome and Synthesis of Viral Proteins. During this phase the synthetic events take place:

Early mRNA synthesis (transcription)
Early protein synthesis (translation)
DNA synthesis (genome replication)
Late mRNA synthesis
Late protein synthesis

In a virus with a double-stranded DNA genome, the synthesis of mRNA and protein that occurs prior to the formation of viral DNA is called early function whereas that occurring after viral DNA synthesis is called late function [2].

Assembly and Release. After synthesis of nucleic acids and structural proteins, they are transported to the site of nucleocapsid assembly. The assembly of nucleocapsid for most DNA-containing viruses takes place in the nucleus; the assembly of nucleocapsid of RNA-containing viruses takes place in the cytoplasm [2].

Nonenveloped viruses with icosahedral symmetry are released in the extracellular fluid after disintegration of the cell by the infecting virus. On the other hand, the enveloped viruses are released through complex mechanisms involving synthesizing of viral membrane protein, binding of this protein to the inner surface of the host cell, replacing the cellular membrane protein with the viral membrane protein, and migration of the nucleocapsid toward "budding" through the modified membrane, "wrapping" themselves into a portion of the membrane in the process [2].

ANTIVIRAL DRUGS. These agents are amantadine (Symmetrel), idoxuridine (Stoxil), trifluorothymidine (Viroptic), adenine arabinoside, vidarabine (Vira-A), and acyclovir (Zovirax).

Amantadine. The antiviral activity of amantadine is restricted to the RNA viruses, especially influenza type A. It exerts its effects by preventing the penetration and uncoating of the virus. Amantadine may be used either prophylactically or therapeutically against influenza type A virus. It is absorbed well from the gastrointestinal tract and is eliminated extensively (90%) by the kidneys. In renal failure, the doses of amantadine should be reduced. Since amantadine releases catecholamine, it may cause insomnia, nervousness, dizziness, and ataxia in toxic doses.

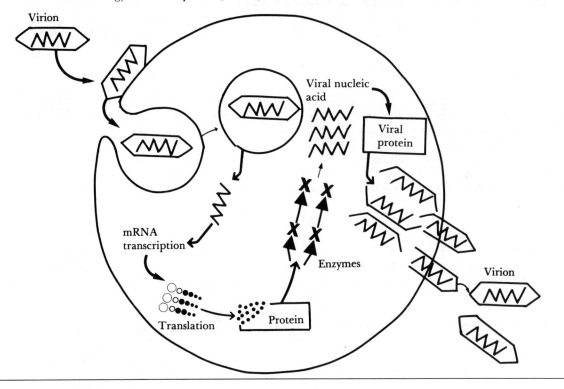

Idoxuridine (Stoxil, Dendrid, Herplex). Idoxuridine (5-iodo-2′-deoxyuridine) is a pyrimidine antimetabolite. Its antiviral activity is limited to DNA viruses, especially the herpes simplex viruses in the cornea. It is effective in herpetic keratitis, for which it is administered topically. Idoxuridine is thought to engage in its antiviral activity by becoming phosphorylated first and then becoming incorporated into viral DNA. Idoxuridine is too toxic to be given systemically since bone marrow depression and other serious complications occur.

Trifluorothymidine (Viroptic). Trifluorothymidine, a halogenated thymidine analogue, exerts its effects by becoming incorporated into the DNA of DNA-containing viruses, primarily the herpesviruses. It is used in herpes simplex keratitis.

Adenine Arabinoside, Vidarabine (Vira-A). Vidarabine (Fig. 36-2), an adenosine analogue, is phosphorylated to the triphosphate derivative and then inhibits viral DNA polymerase. It is the least toxic agent used topically in herpes simplex keratitis and systemically in herpetic encephalitis or in neonatal disseminated herpes infection. Vidarabine is rapidly metabolized to hypoxanthine arabinoside.

Acyclovir (Zovirax). Acyclovir is an analogue of guanosine or deoxyguanosine with an acyclic side chain. It exerts its effects by becoming phosphorylated and then inhibits viral DNA polymerase. Acyclovir is used topically in herpes simplex infection and in severe initial genital herpes. In addition, it is

Fig. 36-2. *Structure of selected antiviral agents.*

Acyclovir

Vidarabine

used intravenously in mucosal and cutaneous herpes simplex infection.

QUESTIONS ON ANTIVIRAL AGENTS

Select the statement that best answers the question.

_____ 303. All of the following statements apply to amantadine *except* which one?
    A. It is used in influenza type A virus.
    B. It is used in mild Parkinson's disease.
    C. It releases catecholamine.
    D. It is not effective orally since it undergoes rapid hepatic first-pass metabolism.

_____ 304. All of the following statements apply to idoxuridine *except* which one?
    A. It should be administered intravenously in bolus dosage.
    B. It is a pyrimidine antimetabolite.
    C. It is effective in herpetic keratitis.
    D. It is effective mainly against DNA viruses.

_____ 305. Vidarabine is characterized by all of the following actions *except* which one?
    A. It is metabolized to hypoxanthine arabinoside.
    B. It is used only topically.
    C. It inhibits viral DNA polymerase.
    D. It is an adenosine analogue.

ANSWERS AND EXPLANATIONS ON ANTIVIRAL AGENTS

303. D.
Explanation: Amantadine is absorbed well orally and is mainly excreted by the kidneys.

304. A.

305. B.
Explanation: Vidarabine is used topically in herpes simplex keratitis and systemically in herpetic encephalitis or in neonatal herpes infection.

REFERENCES

1. Steigman, A. J. Viral Diseases. In G. S. Avery (ed.), *Drug Treatment: Principles and Practice of Clinical Pharmacology and Therapeutics* (2nd ed.). New York: Adis, 1980. Pp. 1142–1157.
2. Vilcek, J. Fundamentals of Virus Structure and Replication. In G. J. Galasso, T. C. McRigan, and R. A. Buchanan (eds.), *Antiviral Agents and Viral Diseases of Man.* New York: Raven, 1979. Pp. 1–38.

37. Immunopharmacology and Cancer Chemotherapy

There are only three absolute virtues: objectivity, courage and a sense of responsibility.

Arthur Schnitzler

Part One: Immunopharmacology

Immunosuppressive therapy is carried out by means of corticosteroids, cytotoxic agents (alkylating agents, antimetabolites), cyclosporin A and dihydrocyclosporin C, antilymphocyte globulin and RhoGAM, lymphoid irradiation and thoracic duct drainage, and immunomodulating agents (interferons and their inducers).

THERAPEUTIC USES. Immunosuppressive agents are used in organ transplantation—liver, heart, and kidney—alone or as a combination of the available agents such as glucocorticosteroids, azathioprine, and cyclophosphamide. In addition, a combination of drug therapy and other ameliorative techniques dealing with lymphocyte depletion such as thoracic duct drainage or total lymph node irradiation may be indicated.

Immunosuppressive agents are used in autoimmune diseases. A few examples will be cited. Chronic active hepatitis not attributable to drugs, Wilson's disease, and alpha$_1$-antitrypsin deficiency have been treated with prednisone combined with azathioprine; azathioprine by itself was not effective [7]. Idiopathic thrombocytopenic purpura is treated with corticosteroids, splenectomy, and, in refractory cases, immunosuppressive agents [6]. Hemolysis due to warm-reacting autoimmune antibodies (autoimmune hemolytic anemia) involving IgG (predominantly IgG_1 and IgG_3) is initially treated with prednisone. If that is unsuccessful, splenectomy (in younger patients) or immunosuppression by azathioprine or cyclophosphamide (in older patients) is used [11].

Acute rheumatic fever is treated with antiinflammatory agents such as aspirin. Corticosteroids are reserved for patients with severe carditis who do not respond to or are unable to take salicylates [1].

Myasthenia is treated with cholinergic drugs, which have no influence on the course of the disease, or with therapeutic measures such as thymectomy, corticosteroids, or immunosuppressive agents, which are intended to induce remission of the disease itself [12].

Immunosuppressive agents are used in isoimmune disorders such as Rh hemolytic disease of the newborn.

Immunomodulating agents are being investigated for potential uses in immunodeficiency disorders, chronic infections, and neoplasm.

THE IMMUNE MECHANISM AND SUCCESS OF IMMUNOSUPPRESSIVE THERAPY. An immune response (immunity) results from the interaction of an antigen with mononuclear cells circulating in the blood and lymph. The immune response has three components [10]: (1) recognition and presentation of an antigen, (2) triggering of the effector mechanism, and (3) regulation of the response.

By phagocytosis, the body deals with foreign particles. The phagocytic cells are (1) the polymorphonuclear neutrophilic leukocytes, (2) the monocytes, and (3) the specialized macrophages such as tissue histiocytes, liver Kupffer cells, and alveolar macrophages. Other "mediator cells," such as mast cells, basophils, and platelets, release soluble mediators to enhance vascular permeability and inflammatory reactions.

Following an antigen challenge, the peripheral lymphoid system, comprised of the B cells and T cells, produces a specific immune response. Most T cells are found in the thoracic duct, the lymph nodes, and especially the thymus. Most B cells are found in bone marrow. A third population of lymphocytes exists, called null cells or L cells, which may be precursors of B or T cells. B cells, when exposed to antigens or mitogenic stimulation, will differentiate into antibody-secreting plasma cells. A subpopulation of B cells called "memory cells" is responsible for a memory humoral reaction, also called "secondary response" or "anamnestic response." Regarding the use of immunosuppressive agents, it should be recalled that it is easier to block or attenuate a primary response than to suppress an established immune response.

With the exception of $Rh_0(D)$ immune globulin, the available immunosuppressive agents are nonspecific in action.

Generalized and prolonged immunosuppression increases susceptibility to infection.

Generalized and prolonged immunosuppression increases the risk of lymphoreticular cancer.

THE CORTICOSTEROIDS. Corticosteroids such as prednisone or dexamethasone have lympholytic properties. They reduce the lymphoid contents of the lymph nodes and the spleen without influencing the myeloid or erythroid stem cells. Corticosteroids have the following pharmacologic effects related to immunosuppression [13]:

They inhibit prostaglandin E_2 and leukotriene synthesis.

They reduce the macrophage-mediated lysosomal contents.

They reduce the activity of the lymphocyte-mediated chemotactic factor and lymphotoxin.

They increase the catabolism of immunoglobulin such as IgG.

They are able to lyse helper T cells.

They interfere with the ability of reticuloendothelial macrophages to attack and destroy antibody-coated cells.

Prednisone is used in autoimmune diseases, both in organ-specific autoimmune diseases such as myasthenia gravis or idiopathic thrombocytopenic purpura and in non-organ-specific autoimmune diseases such as lupus erythematosus, rheumatoid arthritis, and periarteritis nodosa. In addition, prednisone is used in organ transplantation and is of paramount value in problems associated with organ rejection.

THE CYTOTOXIC COMPOUNDS. The Alkylating Agent Cyclophosphamide (Cytoxan). As an alkylating agent, cyclophosphamide and its active metabolites destroy the rapidly proliferating lymphocytes and hence are potent immunosuppressive agents. The metabolites devoid of alkylating properties also lack immunosuppressive property. Since the biotransformation to active metabolites takes place in the liver, inducers of microsomal enzymes do influence the therapeutic spectrum and the toxicity of the cyclophosphamide. When used in combination with prednisone and antilymphocyte globulin, cyclophosphamide prolongs the survival of organ or skin allografts. In addition, it is effective in T cell–dependent autoimmune diseases such as chronic lymphocytic thyroiditis [16].

Purine Antimetabolite Azathioprine (Imuran). When injected, azathioprine is rapidly converted to 6-mercaptopurine. The half-life of azathioprine after intravenous injection is 10 to 20 minutes, and that of 6-mercaptopurine is somewhat longer. The cytotoxic activity of these thiopurines is due to the conversion of mercaptopurine to thioinosinic acid, which in turn blocks the formation of adenylosuccinic acid and xanthylic acid. This action is thought to block the excess synthesis of inosinic acid from its precursors, glutamine and phosphoribosylpyrophosphate. Unlike cyclophosphamide, azathioprine is a potent antiinflammatory substance, reducing the number of monocytes and neutrophils at the inflammatory sites. Moreover, antibody responses are inhibited by azathioprine. Studies in humans have shown that azathioprine decreases gamma globulin and antibody levels, influencing IgG production rather than IgM. Therefore, azathioprine is an effective immunosuppressant in the early phases of immune responses. It is less effective or ineffective on the effector phase and on established reactivities [16].

Azathioprine is effective in renal transplantation, in acute glomerulonephritis, the renal component of systemic lupus erythematosus, in prednisone-resistant idiopathic thrombocytopenic purpura, and in autoimmune hemolytic anemias [14]. Depression of bone marrow is azathioprine's chief side effect.

CYCLOSPORIN A (CS-A). Cyclosporin A, a fungal metabolite, is a cyclic polypeptide consisting of 11 amino acids. It has a biologic half-life of 4 to 6 hours and displays a preferential T cell cytotoxic property in that it inhibits the factors that stimulate T lymphocyte proliferation. Cyclosporin A has been used as the sole immunosuppressant (without the use of prednisone or other drugs) for cadaveric transplants of the kidney, pancreas, and liver [14]. Cyclosporin A has caused reversible hepatic toxicity and nephrotoxicity.

Another fungal metabolite, dihydrocyclosporin C, is even more selective than cyclosporin A. It suppresses T lymphocyte production with only marginal effects on the antibody response [16].

THE ANTILYMPHOCYTE GLOBULIN. The antilymphocyte globulin (ALG) is obtained by immunization of horses with human lymphoid cells or with fetal thymus. The antilymphocyte antibody destroys T cells and impairs delayed hypersensitivity and cellular immunity without altering humoral antibody formation. The pattern of immunosuppression obtained with ALG is identical to that which occurs following thoracic duct drainage, depleting small lymphocytes [14].

$Rh_0(D)$ IMMUNE GLOBULIN. $Rh_0(D)$ immune globulin (RhoGAM) is a solution of human IgG globulin containing antibodies against the $Rh_0(D)$ antigen of the red blood cells. It is administered to a mother after the birth of her Rh-negative baby as a prophylactic measure to prevent erythroblastosis fetalis (hemolytic disease of the newborn) in infants born in succeeding pregnancies. Treatment with RhoGAM may also be indicated in Rh-negative mothers who have had ectopic pregnancies, miscarriages, or abortions in which the blood type of the fetus is unknown [14].

IMMUNOMODULATING AGENTS. In addition to its antiviral actions, interferon has antiproliferative action and modifies the functions of macrophages and natural killer cells. Thymosin, a protein synthesized by the epithelioid component of the thymus, may be potentially valuable in Di George's syndrome and other T cell–deficiency states. Levamisole increases T cell–mediated immunity and may be of value in immunodeficiency associated with Hodgkin's disease [14].

Part Two: Cancer Chemotherapy

Management of cancer includes treatment with alkylating agents (nitrogen mustards, alkyl sulfonates), antimetabolites (methotrexate, purine analogues), natural products (vinca alkaloids, antibiotics), miscellaneous compounds (hydroxyurea, procarbazine, cisplatin), hormones (estrogens, corticosteroids), and radioactive isotopes.

CAUSES OF CANCERS. Most neoplastic diseases occur from constitutional tendency or enhanced genetic susceptibility states combined with multiple exposures to "initiators" and "promoters." Among the known accelerating factors are (1) tobacco smoking (cancers of the lung, larynx, mouth, pharynx, esophagus, bladder, pancreas, and kidneys), (2) alcohol consumption (liver cancer in cirrhotic patients), (3) solar radiation (squamous- and basal-cell carcinomas), (4) ionization radiation (osteosarcoma following radium 224, leukemia with phosphorus 32), (5) occupational hazards (people manufacturing mustard gas and vinyl chloride), (6) environmental pollution (polycyclic hydrocarbons), (7) medications (synthetic estrogens), (8) infectious agents (the Epstein-Barr virus in nasopharyngeal cancer and Burkitt's lymphoma), and (9) nutrition (high dietary fat in colonic cancer), which have all been implicated as causes of cancer [4].

THE RAVAGES OF CANCER. Cancer produces (1) anorexia and cachexia, causing malnutrition and metabolic alterations, (2) hematologic complications, causing anemia and erythrocytosis, and (3) renal manifestations, causing the deterioration of kidney function, such as obstruction of the ureters, hyperuricemia, and hypercalcemia, and nephrotic syndrome, such as the development of membranous glomerulopathy [15].

Cancers create symptoms by elaborating humoral or hormonal substances such as ACTH and proACTH, lipotropin, chorionic gonadotropin, vasopressin, somatomedins, hypoglycemia-producing factors, parathyroid hormone, an osteoclast-activating factor, prostaglandins, erythropoietin, a hypophosphatemia-producing factor, calcitonin, a growth hormone, prolactin, gastrin, secretin, glucagon, a corticotropin-releasing hormone, somatostatin, and neurophysins [8].

Cancers, whether metastasizing or not, produce dysfunction of the central nervous system involving (1) the brain and cranial nerves (dementia, bulbar encephalitis, subacute cerebellar degeneration, optic neuritis, and retinal degeneration), (2) the spinal cord (gray matter myelopathy, including autonomic insufficiency, and subacute necrotic myelopathy), (3) peripheral nerves and roots (subacute sensory neuropathy, sensorimotor peripheral neuropathy, acute polyneuropathy, Guillain-Barré type, and autonomic neuropathy), and (4) neuromuscular junction and muscle (polymyositis and dermatomyositis, myasthenia syndrome, myasthenia gravis, and neuromyotonia). In addition to these disorders, metabolic encephalopathy ensues following the destruction of vital organs, producing hepatic coma (liver), pulmonary encephalopathy (lung), uremia (kidney), and hypercalcemia (bone). Furthermore, the elaboration of hormonal substances by tumors and competition between a tumor and the brain for essential nutrients cause numerous other disabling and disheartening symptoms [9].

CANCERS PRODUCING CUTANEOUS LESIONS. Some examples are lymphangiosarcoma, which produces Stewart-Treves syndrome, cancer of the urinary tract, which causes Bowen's disease, and breast cancer, which causes Paget's disease [5].

PRINCIPLES OF CANCER THERAPY. Malignant neoplastic diseases may be treated by surgery, radiation therapy, immunotherapy, or chemotherapy. The extent of a malignant disease (staging) should be ascertained for effective therapeutic intervention [3].

Surgery. Surgery is effective for localized tumors but ineffective for metastasized or disseminated tumors. The treatment regimen often combines surgery with radiotherapy or chemotherapy. For example, soft tissue sarcomas are initially treated by (1) local excision, (2) high-dose local radiation, and (3) adjuvant chemotherapy with doxorubicin, cyclophosphamide, or methotrexate [3].

Radiation Therapy. Radiation therapy, an effective alternative to surgery, is used in the locoregional (but not widely disseminated) treatment of a malignancy. The rapidly dividing malignant cells are especially sensitive to radiation therapy. Radiation therapy brings about its beneficial effects by the formation of ion pairs or reactive oxygen metabolites such as superoxide, H_2O_2, or hydroxyl radicals with the ability to cause breaks in DNA, which if not repaired will cause cell death. Radiosensitizers are agents that enhance the effect of radiation whereas radioprotectors are designed to protect normal cells. Metronidazole and bromodeoxyuridine are radiosensitizers [3].

Immunotherapy. Since tumor growth is associated with the progressive impairment of immunologic competence, the enhancement of cell-mediated immunity is a therapeutic goal. Cell-mediated immunity may be augmented by nonspecific stimulants such as levamisole, lymphokines, and interferon, which stimulate the antitumor activity of natural killer cells. Cell-mediated immunity may be invoked by specific stimulants such as vaccines composed of killed or inactivated tumor cells or tumor cell fragments. The full range of usefulness of immunotherapy remains to be realized [3].

Chemotherapy. Chemotherapeutic agents are effective in disseminated cancer. Prior to the discussion of the specific pharmacokinetics and pharmacodynamics of each class of antineoplastic agents, several fundamental concepts and therapeutic objectives are presented.

1. Since a single cell is capable of multiplying rapidly and eventually killing the host, one of the therapeutic objectives is to eradicate the last neoplastic cell.

2. Unlike normal cells, cancerous cells continue to multiply ceaselessly, and unless arrested they will kill the host. In the early phase the cancerous cells grow exponentially. However, as the tumor grows in mass, the time needed to double the number of cells also increases. The kinetics of cell multiplication may be said to follow a gompertzian growth curve. The tumor growth may be divided into three phases: (a) the subclinical phase, in which 1.0×10^4 cells are present, (b) the clinical phase, in which 1.0×10^8 cells (1 cm^3 nodule) are present, and (c) the fatal phase, in which the number of cancerous cells equals or exceeds 1.0×10^{12}.

Most human cells evolve from a single clone of malignant cells. As a tumor grows, significant mutation takes place, producing cells of diversified morphologic and biochemical characteristics. During the subclinical phase, the rapidly growing cell population is uniform in character and is highly sensitive to drug treatment; hence the necessity of early diagnosis and treatment. During the clinical phase, the nondividing (refractory to chemotherapy) and slowly growing cells are nonuniform in character and less sensitive to drug treatment [3], thus necessitating multiple drug treatment.

3. Cell destruction with antineoplastic agents follows a first-order kinetics, indicating that the drugs kill a constant fraction of cells and not a constant number of cells. This concept is depicted mathematically in the following tabulation:

No. of Treatments	% Killed	No. of Tumor Cells Killed Each Treatment	No. of Surviving Tumor Cells
Start	—	—	1,000,000
1	90	900,000	100,000
2	90	90,000	10,000
3	90	9,000	1,000
4	90	900	100
5	90	90	10
6	90	9	1

4. Cytotoxic drugs are not specific in function. They arrest not only cancerous cells but also normal cells, especially those of the rapidly proliferating tissues such as bone marrow, lymphoid system tissue, oral and gastrointestinal epithelium, skin and hair follicles, and germinal epithelium of the gonads. Consequently, the therapeutic regimen requires high-dose intermittent schedules and not low-dose continuous treatment. Succeeding doses are given as soon as the host has recovered from the previous treatment [2].

5. Antineoplastic agents may be teratogenic, carcinogenic, and immunosuppressant.

6. Antineoplastic agents exert their lethal effects on different phases of cell cycles and are cell cycle specific or cell cycle nonspecific (Table 37-1).

ALKYLATING AGENTS. These agents exert their antineoplastic actions by generating highly reactive carbonium ion intermediates that form covalent linkage with various nucleophilic compounds on both proteins and DNA. The 7 position of the purine base guanine is particularly susceptible to alkylation, resulting in miscoding, depurination, or ring cleavage. Bifunctional alkylating agents are able to cross-link two nucleic acid molecules or one protein and one nucleic acid molecule. These agents, although most active therapeutically, are notorious for their tendency to cause carcinogenesis and mutagenesis. Alkylating agents that are cell cycle phase nonspecific are most cytotoxic to rapidly proliferating tissues.

Nitrogen Mustards. The activity of nitrogen mustards depends on the presence of bis(2-chlorethyl grouping) $N {<} {{CH_2 - CH_2Cl} \atop {CH_2 - CH_2Cl}}$, which is present in mechlorethamine (Mustargen). Mechlorethamine is used in Hodgkin's disease and other lymphomas, usually in combination with other drugs, e.g., MOPP therapy (mechlorethamine, vincristine, procarbazine, and prednisone). It may cause bone marrow depression.

Chlorambucil (Leukeran). Chlorambucil is the least toxic nitrogen mustard, used as a drug of choice in chronic lymphocytic leukemia (CLL). It is absorbed orally, is slow in its onset of action, and may cause bone marrow depression.

Cyclophosphamide (Cytoxan, Endoxan). Cyclophosphamide is used in Hodgkin's disease, in lymphosarcoma and other lymphomas, as a secondary drug in acute leukemia, and in combination with doxorubicin in breast cancer. Also effective in breast cancer is the combination cyclophosphamide, methotrexate, fluorouracil, and prednisone (CMFP). In addition, cyclophosphamide is an immunosuppressive agent. Its toxic side effects include alopecia, bone marrow depression, nausea and vomiting, and hemorrhagic cystitis.

Alkyl Sulfonates. Busulfan (Myleran) is metabolized to an alkylating agent. Since it produces selective myelosuppression, it is used in chronic myelocytic leukemia (CML). It causes pronounced hyperuricemia from the catabolism of purine.

Nitrosoureas. Carmustine (BCNU), lomustine (CCNU), and semustine (methyl-CCNU) generate alkyl carbonium ions and isocyanate molecules and hence are able to interact with DNA and other macromolecules. These agents, which are lipid soluble, do cross the blood-brain barrier and therefore are ef-

Table 37-1. *Nature of the Cell Cycle*

	G1	S	G2	M
Duration in hours	18–40	16–20	2–10	0.1–1
Function	RNA and protein synthesis	DNA synthesis	RNA and protein synthesis	Mitosis
Selected examples of drugs causing lethal effects	Chlorambucil Dacarbazine 5-Fluorouracil 5-Fluorouridine Hydroxyurea Melphalan Methotrexate (early) Mitomycin C Thiotepa Vinblastine (late)	Asparaginase 5-Azacitidine Cytarabine Dacarbazine Daunorubicin Doxorubicin (adriamycin) 5-Fluorouracil 5-Fluorouridine Hydroxyurea Methotrexate Vinblastine Vincristine	Bleomycin 5-Fluorouracil 5-Fluorouridine Mitomycin C	Actinomycin D Bleomycin Chlorambucil Doxorubicin 5-Fluorouracil Lomustine Mechlorethamine Melphalan Mitomycin C Thiotepa Vinblastine

fective in treating brain tumors. They are bone marrow depressants.

Triazenes. Dacarbazine (DTIC-Dome) is metabolized to an active alkylating substance. It is used in malignant melanoma and causes myelosuppression.

ANTIMETABOLITES.

Antimetabolites are structural analogues of naturally occurring compounds, functioning as fraudulent substances for vital biochemical reactions.

Folic Acid Analogues. Methotrexate (Amethopterin) is a folic acid antagonist that binds to dihydrofolate reductase, interfering with the synthesis of the active cofactor tetrahydrofolic acid (FH$_4$), which is necessary for the synthesis of thymidylate, purine nucleotides, and the amino acids serine and methionine. Methotrexate is used in the following types of cancer [2]:

Acute lymphoid leukemia. During the initial phase, vincristine and prednisone are used. Methotrexate and mercaptopurine are used for maintenance therapy. Methotrexate is also given intrathecally with or without radiotherapy to prevent meningeal leukemia.
Diffuse histiocytic lymphoma. Cyclophosphamide, vincristine, methotrexate, and cytarabine (COMA).
Mycosis fungoides. Methotrexate.
Squamous-cell carcinoma, large-cell anaplastic carcinoma, and adenocarcinoma. Doxorubicin or cyclophosphamide, or methotrexate.
Head and neck squamous-cell carcinoma. Cisplatin and bleomycin, or methotrexate.
Choriocarcinoma. Methotrexate.

DEVELOPMENT OF RESISTANCE TO METHOTREXATE. Tumor cells acquire resistance to methotrexate by several mechanisms [3]:

Deletion of a high-affinity, carrier-mediated transport system for reduced folates

Increase in the concentration of dihydrofolate reductase
Biochemically altered reductase with reduced affinity to bind methotrexate

In order to overcome the resistance, higher doses of methotrexate are administered.

LEUCOVORIN RESCUE THERAPY. The effects of methotrexate may be reversed by the administration of leucovorin, the reduced folate. This leucovorin "rescue" prevents or reduces the toxicity of methotrexate, expressed as mouth lesions (stomatitis), gastrointestinal epithelium irritation (diarrhea), leukopenia, and thrombocytopenia.

Pyrimidine Analogues. Fluorouracil (5-FU) and fluorodeoxyuridine (floxuridine, FUdR) inhibit pyrimidine nucleotide biosynthesis and interfere with the synthesis and actions of nucleic acids. In order to exert its effect, fluorouracil must be first converted to nucleotide derivatives such as 5-fluorodeoxyuridylate (5-FdUMP). Similarly, FUdR is converted to FdUMP according to the following summarized reactions:

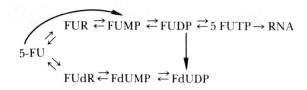

FdUMP inhibits thymidylate synthetase, inhibiting the essential formation of dTMP, one of the four precursors of DNA [3]. In addition, 5-FU is sequentially converted to 5-FUTP, which becomes incorporated into RNA, inhibiting its processing and functions. Fluorouracil is used in the following types of cancer [2]:

Breast carcinoma. Cyclophosphamide, methotrexate, fluorouracil, prednisone (CMF ± P). The alternative drugs are doxorubicin and cyclophosphamide.

Colonic carcinoma. Fluorouracil.

Gastric adenocarcinoma. Fluorouracil, doxorubicin, mitomycin (FAM), or fluorouracil and semustine.

Hepatocellular carcinoma. Fluorouracil or fluorouracil and lomustine.

Pancreatic adenocarcinoma. Fluorouracil.

DEVELOPMENT OF RESISTANCE TO 5-FLUOROURACIL (5-FU). Resistance to 5-FU occurs through one or a combination of the following mechanisms [3].

Deletion of uridine kinase
Deletion of nucleoside phosphorylase
Deletion of orotic acid phosphoribosyltransferase
Decreased thymidylate kinase

Since 5-fluorouracil is metabolized rapidly in the liver, it is used usually intravenously and not orally. 5-Fluorouracil causes myelosuppression and mucositis.

CYTOSINE ARABINOSIDE (CYTARABINE, CYTOSAR, ARA-C). Cytosine arabinoside is an analogue of deoxycytidine, differing only in the substitution of sugar arabinose for deoxyribose. It becomes converted to ara-CTP, inhibiting DNA polymerase according to the following summarized reactions:

$$\text{Ara-C} \xrightarrow{\text{Deoxycytidine kinase}} \text{ara-CMP} \xrightarrow{\text{dCMP kinase}} \text{ara-CDP}$$

$$\text{Ara-CDP} \xrightarrow{\text{NDP kinase}} \text{ara-CTP}$$

$$\text{Deoxynucleotides} \xrightarrow[\text{DNA polymerase}]{} \text{DNA}$$

Cytosine arabinoside is used in acute granulocytic leukemia [2]. Doxorubicin, or daunorubicin and cytarabine, or cytarabine and thioguanine, or cytarabine, vincristine, and prednisone are the agents employed.

Resistance to cytosine arabinoside may relate to the following:

Deletion of deoxycytidine kinase
Increased intracellular pool of dCTP, a nucleotide that competes with ara-CTP
Increased cytidine deaminase, converting ara-C to inactive ara-U

The toxic effects of cytosine arabinoside are myelosuppression and injury to gastrointestinal epithelium, causing nausea, vomiting, and diarrhea.

Purine Antimetabolites. 6-Mercaptopurine (6-MP) and 6-thioguanine (6-TG) are analogues of the purines hypoxanthine and guanine, which must be activated by nucleotide formation.

$$\text{6-MP + phosphoribosylpyrophosphate (PRPP)} \xrightarrow[]{\substack{\text{Hypoxanthine-guanine} \\ \text{phosphoribosyl} \\ \text{transferase}}} \text{6-ThioIMP}$$

$$\text{6-TG + PRPP} \xrightarrow{} \text{6-ThioGMP}$$

ThioIMP and ThioGMP are feedback inhibitors of phosphoribosylpyrophosphate amidotransferase, which is the first and rate-limiting step in the synthesis of purine. In addition, these analogues inhibit de novo biosynthesis of purine and block the conversion of inosinic acid to adenylic acid or to guanylic acid. The triphosphate nucleotides are incorporated into DNA, producing delayed toxicity after several cell divisions [3].

6-Mercaptopurine is used in acute lymphoid leukemia. Maintenance therapy uses methotrexate and 6-mercaptopurine. Mercaptopurine is absorbed well from the gastrointestinal tract. It is metabolized by (1) methylation of the sulfhydryl group and subsequent oxidation and (2) conversion to 6-thiouric acid by the aid of xanthine oxidase, which is inhibited by allopurinol. Mercaptopurine may cause hyperuricemia. Its chief toxic effects are hepatic damage and bone marrow depression.

Thioguanine is used in acute granulocytic leukemia, usually in combination with cytosine arabinoside and daunorubicin.

NATURAL PRODUCTS. Vinca Alkaloids (Vinblastine, Vincristine, and Vindesine). These agents, which bind to tubulin, block mitosis with metaphase arrest. Vinca alkaloids are used in the following types of cancer [2].:

Acute lymphoid leukemia. In the induction phase vincristine is used with prednisone.

Acute myelomonocytic or monocytic leukemia. Cytarabine, vincristine, and prednisone.

Hodgkin's disease. Mechlorethamine, vincristine, procarbazine, and prednisone (MOPP).

Nodular lymphoma. Cyclophosphamide, vincristine, and prednisone (CVP).

Diffuse histiocytic lymphoma. Cyclophosphamide, doxorubicin, vincristine, and prednisone (CHOP), or bleomycin, doxorubicin, cyclophosphamide, vincristine, and prednisone (BACOP), or cyclophosphamide, vincristine, methotrexate, and cytarabine (COMA).

Wilms's tumor. Dactinomycin and vincristine.

Ewing's sarcoma. Cyclophosphamide, or dactinomycin, or vincristine.

Embryonal rhabdomyosarcoma. Cyclophosphamide, or dactinomycin, or vincristine.

Bronchogenic carcinoma. Doxorubicin, cyclophosphamide, and vincristine.

The toxicity of vinblastine is manifested mainly in bone marrow depression; of vincristine, in paresthesias, neuritic pain, muscle weakness, and visual disturbances. Both vinblastine and vincristine may also cause alopecia.

ANTIBIOTICS. Dactinomycin, Actinomycin D (Cosmegen). The antibiotics that bind to DNA are cell-cycle phase nonspecific. Dactinomycin binds to double-stranded DNA and prevents RNA synthesis by inhibiting DNA-dependent RNA polymerase. It is administered intravenously in (1) pediatric solid tumors such as Wilms's tumor and rhabdomyosarcoma and (2) gestational choriocarcinoma. Dactinomycin causes skin reactions, gastrointestinal injury, and delayed bone marrow depression.

Mithramycin (Mithracin). The mechanism of action of mithramycin is similar to that of dactinomycin. It is used in advanced disseminated tumors of the testis and in hypercalcemia associated with cancer. Mithramycin may cause gastrointestinal injury, bone marrow depression, hepatic and renal damage, and hemorrhagic tendency.

Daunorubicin (Daunomycin, Cerubidine), Doxorubicin (Adriamycin). These agents exert their effects by binding to and causing intercalation of the DNA molecule, resulting in inhibition of DNA template function, and by causing DNA chain scission and chromosomal damage. Daunorubicin is useful in acute lymphocytic and acute granulocytic leukemia. Adriamycin is useful in solid tumors such as sarcoma, metastatic breast cancer, and thyroid cancer. These agents cause stomatitis, alopecia, myelosuppression, and cardiac abnormalities ranging from arrhythmias to cardiomyopathy.

Bleomycin (Blenoxane). Bleomycin produces its effects by chain scission and fragmentation of DNA. With the exception of skin and lungs, most tissues are able to inactivate bleomycin enzymatically. Bleomycin is used in squamous-cell carcinoma of the head, neck, and esophagus, in combination with other drugs in testicular carcinoma, and in Hodgkin's disease and other lymphomas. Bleomycin causes stomatitis, ulceration, hyperpigmentation, and erythema. In addition, it produces pulmonary fibrosis.

MISCELLANEOUS ANTINEOPLASTIC AGENTS. Asparaginase (Elspar).
Normal cells are able to synthesize asparagine whereas neoplastic tissues must obtain it from external sources. Asparaginase, by metabolizing asparagine, deprives the neoplastic tissues of asparagine, leading to the inhibition of protein and nucleic acid synthesis. The resistant tumors are thought to possess higher than ordinary amounts of asparagine synthetase. Asparaginase, which is prepared from *E. coli*, is used in the induction of remission of acute lymphocytic leukemia. Asparaginase causes malaise, anorexia, chills, fever, and hypersensitivity reactions. In general, it is not as toxic as other antineoplastic agents to bone marrow or other rapidly growing tissues.

Hydroxyurea. Hydroxyurea inhibits DNA synthesis by inhibiting the formation of ribonucleoside diphosphate reductase, which catalyzes the reduction of ribonucleotides to deoxyribonucleotides. Hydroxyurea is used in chronic granulocytic leukemia unresponsive to busulfan. In addition, it is used in acute lymphoblastic leukemia. Hydroxyurea may cause bone marrow depression.

Cisplatin (Platinol). Cisplatin binds to intracellular DNA, causing interstrand and intrastrand cross-linking. It is a cell-cycle phase nonspecific agent. Ineffective orally, it is used in testicular, bladder, and head and neck cancers. It causes nephrotoxicity, ototoxicity, and gastrointestinal injury.

Procarbazine (Matulane). This agent inhibits DNA, RNA, and protein synthesis by unknown mechanism(s). It is effective in Hodgkin's disease in combination with mechlorethamine, vincristine, and prednisone (MOPP). Procarbazine causes neurotoxicity, bone marrow depression, and gastrointestinal injury.

QUESTIONS ON IMMUNOPHARMACOLOGY AND CANCER CHEMOTHERAPY

Select the answer that best completes the statement or answers the question.

_____ 306. In organ transplantation one may use:
  A. Glucocorticoids.
  B. Azathioprine.
  C. Lymph irradiation.
  D. All have been shown to be effective.

_____ 307. Immunosuppressive agents such as prednisone and azathioprine have been shown to be effective in all the following cases *except* which one?
  A. Chronic active hepatitis.
  B. Wilson's disease.
  C. Megaloblastic anemia.
  D. Thrombocytopenic purpura.

_____ 308. Myasthenia gravis may be treated by:
  A. Thymectomy.
  B. Immunosuppressive agents.
  C. Corticosteroids.
  D. Cholinesterase inhibitors.
  E. All of the above.

_____ 309. Immunosuppressive agents:
  A. Show nonspecificity of actions.
  B. May increase susceptibility to infections.
  C. May increase the risk of lymphoreticular cancer.
  D. All of the above.

_____ 310. The immunosuppressive action of prednisone:
  A. Reduces the lymphocyte-mediated chemotactic factor and lymphotoxin.
  B. Increases the catabolism of immunoglobulin such as IgG.
  C. Lyses the helper T cells.
  D. All of the above.

_____ 311. The metabolite of azathioprine is:
  A. 6-Mercaptopurine.
  B. Merodicein.
  C. Triclocarban.
  D. Cloflucarban.

_____ 312. The chief side effect of azathioprine is:
  A. Alopecia.
  B. Hypertrichosis.
  C. Bone marrow suppression.
  D. Nephrotoxicity.

_____ 313. Azathioprine is therapeutically useful in:
  A. Acute glomerulonephritis.
  B. The renal component of systemic lupus erythematosus.
  C. Prednisone-resistant thrombocytopenic purpura.
  D. Autoimmune hemolytic anemia.
  E. All of the above.

_____ 314. Radiation therapy:
  A. Forms ion pairs or reactive oxygen metabolites that cause breaks in DNA.

B. Is useful in locoregional but not disseminated malignancy.
C. Is more effective against rapidly dividing cells.
D. All of the above.

___ 315. Metronidazole is:
A. A radiosensitizer.
B. Effective in amebiasis.
C. Used for helminthic infections.
D. All of the above.

___ 316. Cell-mediated immunity may be stimulated nonspecifically by:
A. Levamisole.
B. Lymphokines.
C. Interferon.
D. All of the above.

___ 317. Cell-mediated immunity may be stimulated specifically by:
A. Vaccines.
B. Tumor cell fragment.
C. Both A and B.
D. Neither A nor B.

___ 318. The reason(s) cancer should be diagnosed and treated early deal(s) with the fact that during the clinical phase:
A. The cells are uniform in nature.
B. The cells are rapidly growing.
C. The cells are sensitive to chemotherapy.
D. All of the above.
E. None of the above.

___ 319. Alkylating agents:
A. Produce reactive carbonium ion intermediates that form covalent linkages with proteins and DNA.
B. Cause miscoding, depurination, or ring cleavage of macromolecules.
C. Are cytotoxic to rapidly proliferating cells.
D. All of the above.

___ 320. Chlorambucil:
A. Is a drug of choice in chronic lymphocytic leukemia.
B. Causes bone marrow depression.
C. Both A and B.
D. Neither A nor B.

___ 321. The toxicity of cyclophosphamide is manifested in all of the following *except* which one?
A. Hemeralopia.
B. Alopecia.
C. Bone marrow depression.
D. Hemorrhagic cystitis.

___ 322. Allopurinol:
A. Inhibits the synthesis of uric acid.
B. Is a xanthine oxidase inhibitor.
C. May be used with busulfan.
D. None of the above.
E. A, B, and C.

___ 323. One reason nitrosoureas are effective in brain tumors is that:
A. They are lipid-soluble substances.
B. They chelate carbonium ions.
C. They chelate isocyanate molecule.
D. They inhibit the generation of carbonium ions.

___ 324. Methotrexate:
A. Inhibits the synthesis of ·tetrahydrofolic acid.
B. Interferes with the synthesis of purine nucleotides.

C. Is used in acute lymphoid leukemia.
D. All of the above.

___ 325. Resistance to methotrexate develops by which of the following mechanisms?
A. Deletion of a high-affinity carrier-mediated transport system for reduced folates.
B. Increases in the concentrations of dihydrofolate reductase.
C. Both A and B.
D. Neither A nor B.

___ 326. Leucovorin reduces the methotrexate-induced:
A. Stomatitis.
B. Diarrhea.
C. Thrombocytopenia.
D. All of the above.

___ 327. Resistance to 5-fluorouracil occurs by deletion of:
A. Uridine kinase.
B. Nucleoside phosphorylase.
C. Orotic acid phosphoribosyl transferase.
D. All of the above.

___ 328. 5-Fluorouracil is used intravenously because it is:
A. Metabolized rapidly in the liver.
B. Not absorbed orally.
C. A potent irritant to gastric mucosa.
D. A gastric secretagogue.

___ 329. Vinca alkaloids:
A. Bind to tubulin.
B. Block mitosis with metaphase arrest.
C. Are useful in acute lymphoid leukemia.
D. All of the above.

___ 330. Vincristine causes:
A. Alopecia.
B. Visual disturbances.
C. Neuritic pain.
D. Paresthesia.
E. All of the above.

ANSWERS AND EXPLANATIONS ON IMMUNOPHARMACOLOGY AND CANCER CHEMOTHERAPY

306. D.
307. C.
308. E.
309. D.
310. D.
311. A.
312. C.
313. E.
314. D.
315. D.
Explanation: Radiosensitizers are agents that enhance the effects of radiation.
316. D.
Explanation: These agents stimulate the antitumor activity of natural killer cells.
317. C.
318. D.
319. D.
320. C.
321. A.
322. E.
Explanation: Busulfan causes pronounced hyperuricemia resulting from catabolism of purine. Allopurinol, which reduces the synthesis of uric acid, is used to overcome these side effects.

323. A.
    Explanation: Nitrosoureas cross the blood-brain barrier.
324. D.
325. C.
326. D.
327. D.
328. A.
329. D.
330. E.

REFERENCES

1. Bisno, A. L. Rheumatic Fever. In J. B. Wyngaarden and L. H. Smith, Jr. (eds.), *Cecil's Textbook of Medicine* (6th ed.). Philadelphia: Saunders, 1982. Pp. 1450–1457.

2. Carter, S. K., and Mathe, G. Malignant Diseases. In G. S. Avery (ed.), *Drug Treatment: Principles and Practice of Clinical Pharmacology and Therapeutics* (2nd ed.). New York: Adis, 1980. Pp. 953–1009.

3. Chabner, B. A. Principles of Cancer Therapy. In J. B. Wyngaarden and L. H. Smith, Jr. (eds.), *Cecil's Textbook of Medicine* (6th ed.). Philadelphia: Saunders, 1982. Pp. 1032–1046.

4. Fraumeni, J. F. Epidemiology of Cancer. In J. B. Wyngaarden and L. H. Smith, Jr. (eds.), *Cecil's Textbook of Medicine* (6th ed.). Philadelphia: Saunders, 1982. Pp. 1047–1051.

5. Johnson, M. L. Cutaneous Manifestation of Internal Malignancy. In J. B. Wyngaarden and L. H. Smith, Jr. (eds.), *Cecil's Textbook of Medicine* (6th ed.). Philadelphia: Saunders, 1982. Pp. 1029–1032.

6. Marcus, A. J. Hemorrhagic Disorders: Abnormalities of Platelet and Vascular Function. In J. B. Wyngaarden and L. H. Smith, Jr. (eds.), *Cecil's Textbook of Medicine* (6th ed.). Philadelphia: Saunders, 1982. Pp. 979–992.

7. Ockner, R. K. Chronic Hepatitis. In J. B. Wyngaarden and L. H. Smith, Jr. (eds.), *Cecil's Textbook of Medicine* (6th ed.). Philadelphia: Saunders, 1982. Pp. 789–792.

8. Odell, W. O. Endocrine Manifestations of Tumors: Ectopic Hormone Production. In J. B. Wyngaarden and L. H. Smith, Jr. (eds.), *Cecil's Textbook of Medicine* (6th ed.). Philadelphia: Saunders, 1982. Pp. 1022–1026.

9. Posner, J. B. Nonmetastatic Effects of Cancer on the Nervous System. In J. B. Wyngaarden and L. H. Smith, Jr. (eds.), *Cecil's Textbook of Medicine* (6th ed.). Philadelphia: Saunders, 1982. Pp. 1026–1029.

10. Rola-Pleszczynski, M. Anatomy of the Immune Response. In P. Sirois and M. Rola-Pleszczynski (eds.), *Immunopharmacology*. New York: Elsevier North-Holland, 1982. Pp. 1–13.

11. Rosse, W. F. Hemolysis Due to Acquired Abnormalities of Erythrocytes or Their Circulation. In J. B. Wyngaarden and L. H. Smith, Jr. (eds.), *Cecil's Textbook of Medicine* (6th ed.). Philadelphia: Saunders, 1982. Pp. 869–877.

12. Rowland, L. P. Diseases of Muscle and Neuromuscular Junction. In J. B. Wyngaarden and L. H. Smith, Jr. (eds.), *Cecil's Textbook of Medicine* (6th ed.). Philadelphia: Saunders, 1982. Pp. 2166–2185.

13. Rumjanek, V. M., Hanson, J. M., and Morley, J. Lymphokines and Monokines. In P. Sirois and M. Rola-Pleszczynski (eds.), *Immunopharmacology*. New York: Elsevier North-Holland, 1982. Pp. 267–285.

14. Salmon, S. E. Drugs and the Immune System. In B. G. Katzung (ed.), *Basic and Clinical Pharmacology*. Los Altos, Calif.: Lange, 1982. Pp. 665–681.

15. Schein, P. S. Biologic Effects of Tumors. In J. B. Wyngaarden and L. H. Smith, Jr. (eds.), *Cecil's Textbook of Medicine* (6th ed.). Philadelphia: Saunders, 1982. Pp. 1022–1026.

16. Spreafico, F., Tagliabue, A., and Vecchi, A. Chemical Immunodepressants. In P. Sirois and M. Rola-Pleszczynski (eds.), *Immunopharmacology*. New York: Elsevier North-Holland, 1982. Pp. 315–348.

38. Antifungal Agents

A teacher affects eternity, no one can tell where his influence stops.

Henry Adams

Mycoses, or fungal diseases, may be endemic, occurring in a specific geographic area (e.g., coccidioidomycosis, in the western United States), and may be located in a particular system (e.g., histoplasmosis, in the lung). Mycoses may be opportunistic, occurring in depressed cell-mediated immunity, in disease states (mucormycosis, in diabetes mellitus), and in drug-induced immunosuppression (candidiasis).

FUNGAL DISEASES. The fungal diseases are histoplasmosis, coccidioidomycosis, blastomycosis, paracoccidioidomycosis, cryptococcosis, sporotrichosis, candidiasis, aspergillosis, and mucormycosis.

Histoplasmosis. Histoplasmosis, the most common endemic respiratory mycosis, is caused by *Histoplasma capsulatum*. Although mostly innocuous, it may produce symptoms ranging from flulike manifestations to chest pain, dyspnea, pericarditis, and cyanosis. Acute respiratory infection may be treated with a brief course of corticosteroid therapy. Progressive cavitary histoplasmosis may be treated with amphotericin B for several months [1].

Coccidioidomycosis. Coccidioidomycosis is a noncontagious and self-limited respiratory mycosis caused by *Coccidioides immitis*. The primary coccidioidomycosis seldom requires treatment unless the affected patient is undergoing immunosuppressive therapy. Coccidioidomycosis may become disseminated, involving skin, subcutaneous tissue, and joints. Other manifestations are osteomyelitis, meningitis, thyroiditis, tenosynovitis, and prostatitis. Amphotericin B must be used. However, the treatment is uncertain and unpredictable [1].

Blastomycosis (Gilchrist's disease). Blastomycosis is a noncontagious subacute or chronic endemic mycosis caused by *Blastomyces dermatitidis*, involving the lungs, skin, bones, and genitourinary system in the male and often disseminating to other tissues. Amphotericin B is helpful [1].

Paracoccidioidomycosis. Paracoccidioidomycosis is a noncontagious respiratory mycosis caused by *Paracoccidioides brasiliensis*. It may be acute and self-limited, or it may produce progressive pulmonary disease characterized by cavitation, infiltration, nodules, tumorlike masses, fibrosis, and calcification. It may become disseminated to other tissues. The treatment includes sulfonamides (sulfadiazine) and amphotericin B [1].

Cryptococcosis. Cryptococcosis is a noncontagious respiratory mycosis caused by *Cryptococcus neoformans* and *C. bacillispora*. They colonize the lung, causing acute or chronic pulmonary infection, disseminating to other tissues and causing meningitis, hydrocephalus, hepatic necrosis, pyelonephritis, and adrenal insufficiency. The treatment includes amphotericin B and flucytosine [1].

Sporotrichosis. Sporotrichosis is a subacute or chronic contagious mycosis of the skin and regional lymphatics caused by *Sporothrix schenckii*. It may disseminate to joints (knees, ankles, and wrists) and bones (tibia). The treatment of choice for lymphocutaneous sporotrichosis is a saturated solution of potassium iodide. Disseminated sporotrichosis is treated with amphotericin B [1].

Candidiasis. Candidiasis is a local or systemic mycosis caused by opportunistic species of *Candida*, mostly by *Candida albicans* but to a certain extent by *C. tropicalis*, *C. parapsilosis*, *C. stellatoidea*, *C. krusei*, *C. parakrusei*, *C. pseudotropicalis*, and *C. guilliermondi*. The introduction of antibiotics, myelotoxic agents, immunosuppressive agents, and corticosteroids has enhanced these opportunistic fungal infections. Systemic candidiasis commonly involves the skin (hematogenous *Candida* infection), the eyes (*Candida* endophthalmitis), and the kidneys (*Candida* pyelonephritis). *C. albicans* endocarditis occurs following prolonged intravenous therapy [1]. Mucocutaneous infections are treated with

Clotrimazole (Lotrimin, Mycelex) in 1% cream or solution.
Miconazole nitrate (Micatin, Monistat 7)
Miconazole (Monistat 7) 2% in cream or lotion
Haloprogin (Halotex) 1% cream or solution
Amphotericin B (Fungizone) 3% solution
Nystatin (Mycostatin)

Chronic mucocutaneous candidiasis responds to amphotericin B or ketoconazole (Nizoral). Systemic candidiasis should be treated by correcting the offending factor and by amphotericin B. *C. albicans* endocarditis requires valve replacement, and endophthalmitis responds poorly to amphotericin B and flucytosine.

Aspergillosis. Aspergillosis is caused most commonly by *Aspergillus fumigatus*, *A. flavus*, *A. niger*, *A. nidulans*, *A. terreus*, *A. sydowi*, *A. clavatus*, and *A. glaucus*. The fungus invades the previously damaged lung, causing aspergillar bronchitis (aspergilloma), and the bronchial tree (bronchopulmonary aspergil-

Table 38-1. *Summary Pharmacology of Antifungal Agents*

Antifungal Agent	Properties
Nystatin (Mycostatin)	Poorly absorbed from the gastrointestinal tract; is both fungistatic and fungicidal without having any effect on bacteria, viruses, or protozoa; exerts its effect by binding to the sterol moiety and hence damaging the membrane; used primarily topically to treat candidal infection of skin and mucous membrane (paronychia, vaginitis, and stomatitis), and so causes no major toxicities
Ketoconazole (Nizoral)	Active orally; has a broad-spectrum antifungal activity against numerous pathogenic fungi; mechanism of antifungal effect similar to that of nystatin; has caused phlebitis, thrombocytopenia, and pronounced pruritus
Miconazole (Monistat IV)	Available for topical application as well as parenteral administration in the treatment of systemic candidiasis and cryptococcosis
Clotrimazole (Lotrimin)	Used topically
Econazole nitrate (Spectazole)	Used topically
Flucytosine (Ancobon)	A fluorinated pyrimidine, is related to fluorouracil; absorbed orally and distributed widely in the body including the cerebrospinal fluid; having a narrow spectrum of antifungal activity, is used primarily in combination with amphotericin B for disseminated cryptococcal and candidal infections
Hydroxystilbamidine isethionate	Active against both fungal and protozoal infections; causes both renal and hepatic toxicities, and so has been largely replaced by amphotericin B
Griseofulvin (Fulvicin, Grisactin)	Fungistatic for various species of dermatophytes including *Microsporum, Epidermophyton,* and *Trichophyton,* causing diseases of skin, hair, and nails; exerts its effect by inhibiting fungal mitosis

losis), being especially severe in immunocompromised hosts [1]. The treatment of choice is amphotericin B.

Mucormycosis. Mucormycosis (phycomycosis, zygomycosis) is an opportunistic mycosis that produces rhinocerebral disease in patients with diabetic ketoacidosis, pulmonary disease in immunosuppressed patients, and local or disseminated disease in patients with open wounds or burns [1]. Amphotericin B is the only effective drug.

ANTIFUNGAL DRUGS. Amphotericin B (Fungizone) and nystatin (Mycostatin) are polyene antibiotics.

Ketoconazole (Nizoral), miconazole (Monistat IV), clotrimazole (Lotrimin), and econazole nitrate (Spectazole) are imidazole derivatives.

Flucytosine (Ancobon) (Fig. 38-1) is a uracil antimetabolite.

Hydroxystilbamidine isethionate is an aromatic diamidine.

Griseofulvin (Fulvicin, Grisactin) (Fig. 38-1) is another fungistatic antibiotic.

AMPHOTERICIN B (FUNGIZONE). Amphotericin B, which is ineffective against bacteria, rickettsiae,

Fig. 38-1. *Structure of selected antifungal agents.*

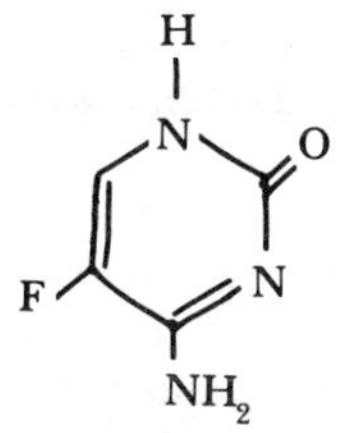

Flucytosine

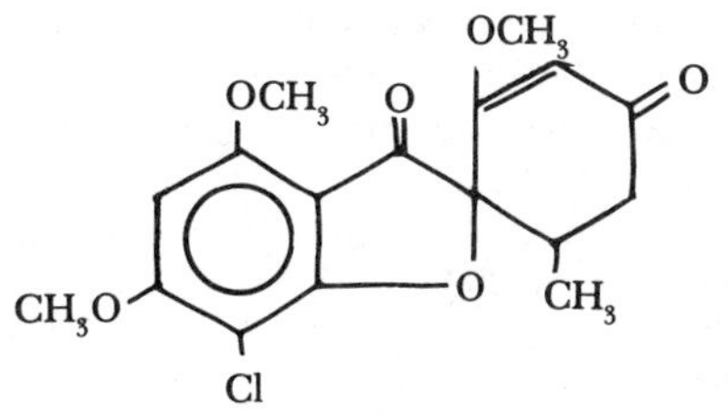

Griseofulvin

or viruses, is either fungicidal or fungistatic in nature, depending on the concentration of the drug used or the sensitivity of the fungus treated. Numerous pathogenic yeast (*C. neoformans*), pathogenic yeastlike (*Monilia*), demorphic (*Blastomyces*), filamentous (*Cladosporium*), and other fungi are highly sensitive to amphotericin B. Furthermore, the antifungal activities of amphotericin B are enhanced by flucytosine, minocycline, or rifampin, agents devoid of antifungal activity by themselves.

Pharmacodynamics. Amphotericin B exerts its antifungal effects by binding to the sterol moiety of the membrane and damaging its structural and functional integrity.

Pharmacokinetics and Proper Usage. Amphotericin B is available as a sterile lyophilized powder. Since it is insoluble in water, it is marketed with sodium deoxycholate to be dispersed in sterile water and 5% dextrose. The polyene antibiotics, amphotericin B, nystatin, and candicidin, are all poorly absorbed from the gastrointestinal tract. In the plasma, amphotericin B becomes bound to lipoproteins, including cholesterol. It is extensively metabolized, and the inactive metabolite(s) is (are) slowly excreted in the urine.

Amphotericin B is the only polyene antibiotic given parenterally. When the intravenous route of administration is contemplated, amphotericin B is dispersed fresh, as discussed, and infused slowly. The rapid administration of amphotericin B, which causes cardiac toxicity, should be avoided. Heparin (1,000 U) is often added to the infusion suspension to reduce the chance of thrombophlebitis. Amphotericin B also causes normocytic normochromic anemia, leukopenia, and thrombocytopenia.

During infusion of amphotericin B there is a rise in the patient's temperature, which may or may not be accompanied by hypotension and delirium. Often hydrocortisone sodium succinate is added to the infusion bottle during the initial but not the succeeding alternate-day treatment with amphotericin B.

Amphotericin B is a nephrotoxic substance in most patients, often causing permanent reduction of glomerular filtration rate. Hypokalemia may also occur, requiring the oral administration of potassium chloride.

Amphotericin B has been used intrathecally in patients with coccidioidal meningitis and with cryptococcal meningitis. The risks associated with this route of administration are headache, paresthesias, nerve palsies, and visual impairment.

In coccidioidal arthritis, amphotericin B may be injected intraarticularly.

The pharmacology of other antifungal agents is summarized in Table 38-1.

QUESTIONS ON ANTIFUNGAL AGENTS

Select one answer that best completes the statement or answers the question.

_____ 331. Histoplasmosis:
A. May produce flulike symptoms.
B. Is a common respiratory mycosis.
C. May be treated with amphotericin B.
D. May be treated with corticosteroids.
E. All of the above.

_____ 332. Paracoccidioidomycosis is characterized by all of the following items *except* which one?
A. It is a noncontagious respiratory mycosis.
B. It may be treated with penicillin.
C. It may be treated with sulfadiazine.
D. It may be treated with amphotericin B.

_____ 333. Cryptococcosis is characterized by all of the following items *except* which one?
A. It is a nondisseminating mycosis.
B. It is a respiratory mycosis.
C. It may be treated with amphotericin B.
D. It may be treated with flucytosine.

_____ 334. The treatment of choice for lymphocutaneous sporotrichosis is:
A. Calcium gluconate.
B. Potassium iodide.
C. Sulfadiazine.
D. Penicillin G.

_____ 335. Which of the following items or agents enhances the opportunistic nature of candidiasis?
A. Prolonged intravenous therapy.
B. Immunosuppressive agents.
C. Corticosteroids.
D. All of the above.

_____ 336. The antifungal activity of amphotericin B is enhanced by all the following agents *except* which one?
A. Chloramphenicol.
B. Flucytosine.
C. Minocycline.
D. Rifampin.

_____ 337. Amphotericin B is characterized by all of the following properties *except* which one?
A. It damages fungal membrane by binding to sterol moiety.
B. In the plasma it may be bound to cholesterol.
C. It is excreted unchanged.
D. It may be given parenterally.

ANSWERS AND EXPLANATIONS ON ANTIFUNGAL AGENTS

331. E.
332. B.
333. A.
   Explanation: Cryptococcosis disseminates to other tissues, causing meningitis, hydrocephalus, hepatic necrosis, pyelonephritis, and adrenal insufficiency.
334. B.
335. D.
336. A.
337. C.
   Explanation: Amphotericin B, the only polyene antibiotic given parenterally, is extensively metabolized in the liver. The metabolites are slowly excreted by the kidneys.

REFERENCE

1. Drutz, D. J. The Mycoses. In J. B. Wyngaarden and L. H. Smith, Jr. (eds.), *Cecil's Textbook of Medicine* (6th ed.). Philadelphia: Saunders, 1982. Pp. 1697–1713.

XI. Chemotherapy of Tuberculosis and Parasitic Diseases

39. The Pharmacology of Mycobacterial, Protozoal, and Helminthic Diseases

The price of greatness is responsibility.

Winston Churchill

Part One: Mycobacterial Diseases

TUBERCULOSIS. Tuberculosis is a necrotizing bacterial infection affecting mainly the lungs but also, to a limited extent, the kidneys, bones, lymph nodes, and meninges [17]. The treatment of tuberculosis is subdivided into chemoprophylaxis and active treatment. The drug of choice for chemoprophylaxis is isoniazid (300 mg/day for 1 year). In active tuberculosis, the primary drugs in initial treatment are isoniazid, rifampin, streptomycin, ethambutol, and pyrazinamide. The secondary drugs are para-aminosalicylic acid, ethionamide, viomycin, kanamycin, capreomycin, and cycloserine. The use of a drug combination depends on the stage of the disease.

During the initial phase, isoniazid is always used with one other drug [3]: isoniazid and rifampin, or isoniazid and streptomycin, or isoniazid and ethambutol. In advanced or cavitary pulmonary tuberculosis, often three drugs are used: isoniazid, rifampin, and streptomycin, or isoniazid, rifampin, and ethambutol.

The pharmacologic properties of the drugs most often used are summarized in Table 39-1.

Not all mycobacterial infections are caused by *Mycobacterium tuberculosis* or *M. leprae*. These "atypical mycobacteria" require treatment with secondary medications as well as other chemotherapeutic agents. For example, *M. marinum* causes skin granulomas, and effective drugs are rifampin and minocycline. *M. fortuitum* causes skin ulcers, and the indicated medications are ethambutol, cycloserine, and rifampin in combination with amikacin.

LEPROSY (HANSEN'S DISEASE). Leprosy is a chronic granulomatous disease, attacking superficial tissues such as the skin, nasal mucosa, and peripheral nerves [16]. It takes the form of lepromatous leprosy or tuberculoid leprosy. The sulfones, which are derivatives of 4,4'-diaminodiphenylsulfone, are bacteriostatic. Dapsone (DDS) and sulfoxone sodium are the most useful and effective agents available. They should be given in low doses initially, then increased gradually until a full dose of 300 to 400 mg per week is reached. During this period of dose adjustment, the patient must be monitored carefully. With adequate precaution and appropriate doses, sulfones may be used safely for years. Nevertheless, side effects such as anorexia, nervousness, insomnia, blurred vision, paresthesia, and peripheral neuropathy do occur. Hemolysis is common, especially in patients with glucose 6-phosphate dehydrogenase deficiency. A fatal exacerbation of lepromatous leprosy and an infectious mononucleosislike syndrome rarely occur. Clofazimine (Lamprene) may be effective in patients who are resistant to the sulfones, and exacerbation of leprosy is reduced dramatically. Red discoloration of the skin and eosinophilic enteritis have occurred following use of clofazimine [3].

Table 39-1. *Selected Pharmacologic Properties of Drugs Most Often Used in Tuberculosis*

Drug	Properties
Isoniazid	Bactericidal for growing tubercle bacilli; is absorbed orally and metabolized by acetylation; a structural analogue of pyridoxine, may cause pyridoxine deficiency, peripheral neuritis, and, in toxic doses, pyridoxine-responsive convulsions; mechanism of action not known
Streptomycin	Given intramuscularly; exerts its effects only on extracellular tubercle bacilli; when combined with other drugs, delays the emergence of streptomycin-resistant mutants; is ototoxic and may cause deafness
Rifampin	Absorbed from gastrointestinal tract and excreted mainly into bile; binds to DNA-dependent RNA polymerase and inhibits RNA synthesis; in higher than therapeutic doses, may cause flulike syndrome and thrombocytopenia
Ethambutol	Suppresses growth of isoniazid- and streptomycin-resistant tubercle bacilli; most important but not commonly occurring side effects are optic neuritis, decreased visual acuity, and inability to perceive the color green

Part Two: Protozoal Diseases

AMEBIASIS. Amebiasis is an infection of the large intestine produced by *Entamoeba histolytica*, causing mild diarrhea to fulminant dysentery. The treatment is directed toward (1) the asymptomatic passer of cysts, (2) acute amebic dysentery, and (3) amebic hepatitis and abscess [11].

Treatment of the Asymptomatic Carrier. The effective drugs are an 8-hydroxyquinoline derivative, such as iodoquinol (drug of first choice) and diloxanide furoate (alternative drug) [14].

Treatment of Acute Amebic Dysentery. Dehydroemetine is given for 5 days for rapid relief of symptoms, after which the patient is switched to metronidazole. When the response to metronidazole is not satisfactory, dehydroemetine plus tetracycline or dehydroemetine plus paromomycin is given concurrently with metronidazole.

Treatment of Amebic Hepatitis and Abscess. Metronidazole is the drug of first choice. Dehydroemetine and chloroquine are alternative drugs.

MALARIA. The causative organisms are protozoa of the genus *Plasmodium*. Four species are known to infect the human being only: *P. falciparum, P. vivax, P. malariae*, and *P. ovale* [4].

The major antimalarial agents are 4-aminoquinoline derivative (e.g., chloroquine), 8-aminoquinoline derivative (e.g., primaquine), folic acid antagonist (e.g., pyrimethamine), and alkaloid (e.g., quinine). They may be classified according to their effectiveness in interfering with various stages of parasitization. An agent such as primaquine destroys the schizonts in the liver soon after infection has taken place [13].

Blood Schizonticides. Agents such as quinine, quinacrine, amodiaquine, and chloroquine suppress the symptoms of malaria by destroying the schizonts and merozoites in the erythrocytes.

Gametocides. Agents such as primaquine, by destroying gametocytes in the blood, prevent infection by *Anopheles* mosquitoes.

Sporonticides. Agents such as chloroguanide and pyrimethamine help to eradicate the disease by preventing sporogony and multiplication of the aforementioned parasites.

Secondary Tissue Schizonticides. Primaquine destroys exoerythrocytic tissue schizonts such as those developing in the liver.

Selected pharmacologic properties of the antimalarial agents most often used are listed in Table 39-2. Other pharmacologic agents sometimes used in combination with antimalarial agents include:

Table 39-2. *Pharmacologic Properties of Antimalarial Agents*

Antimalarial Drugs	Properties
Chloroquine (Aralen); amodiaquine (Camoquin) is an alternative drug for chloroquine	Destroys schizonts in erythrocytes by interfering with synthesis of DNA; phosphate salts are active orally; hydrochloride salt reserved for intravenous uses; accumulates in normal and parasitized erythrocytes; overdosage has caused reversible corneal damage and permanent retinal damage; in toxic doses, will cause visual disturbances, hyperexcitability, convulsion, and heart block; an antimalarial of choice in all cases except with chloroquine-resistant *P. falciparum*; has a certain degree of effectiveness in amebiasis and late stages of rheumatoid arthritis
Primaquine	Attacks plasmodia in exoerythrocytic stages; is effective for preventing relapse and for prophylaxis when leaving an infested area; may cause hemolytic anemia especially in patients who are deficient in glucose 6-phosphate dehydrogenase
Quinine	A naturally occurring alkaloid obtained from cinchona bark with a mechanism of action similar to that of chloroquine; very useful in treating chloroquine-resistant *P. falciparum*; in toxic doses, may cause "cinchonism" characterized by tinnitus, headache, nausea, and visual disturbances
Pyrimethamine (Daraprim)	A folic acid antagonist (antifol) with pharmacologic actions similar to those of chloroguanide, methotrexate, or trimethoprim; may be used in combination with sulfadoxine for suppression and with sulfadiazine for treatment of chloroquine-resistant *P. falciparum*

Sulfonamides. Sulfadoxine or sulfadiazine is used with pyrimethamine.

Sulfones. Dapsone (DDS) is used in place of or in addition to sulfonamides and pyrimethamine.

Acridines. Quinacrine (Atabrine) has action similar to that of chloroquine.

Biguanides. Chloroguanide (proguanil, Paludrine) has suppressive as well as prophylactic actions.

LEISHMANIASIS. Leishmaniasis is produced by protozoa of the genus *Leishmania* and is transmitted by the bites of sandflies. Four separate species are generally known [5]: *L. donovani* is the cause of kala-azar. *L. tropica* is the cause of oriental sore. *L. mexicana* is the cause of forest yaws. *L. brasiliensis* is the cause of espundia.

Agents effective in leishmaniasis are pentavalent antimonials, pentamidine, amphotericin B (Fungizone), cycloguanil embonate (cycloguanil pamoate), dehydroemetine resinate (Mebadin), and metronidazole (Flagyl).

TRYPANOSOMIASIS. Trypanosomiasis is produced by protozoans of the genus *Trypanosoma*, which cause Gambian or mid-African sleeping sickness (*T. gambiense*), Rhodesian or East African sleeping sickness (*T. rhodesiense*), and Chagas's disease in Central and South American (*T. cruzi*) [6].

Agents effective in trypanosomiasis are the aromatic diamidines (pentamidine, stilbamidine, propamidine):

Pentamidine is a drug of choice for prevention and early treatment of *T. gambiense* infections. It cannot reach the CNS.

Malarsoprol is a drug of choice for *T. gambiense* infections refractory to pentamidine or for late meningoencephalitic stages of infection. It reaches the CNS.

Nifurtimox (Lampit) is a drug of choice for acute Chagas's disease.

Suramin (Naphuride) is effective only in African sleeping sickness.

TOXOPLASMOSIS. Toxoplasmosis is caused by *Toxoplasma gondii*, an intracellular parasite causing, in humans, acquired toxoplasmosis (asymptomatic) and congenital toxoplasmosis (symptomatic). The congenitally infected infants with toxoplasmosis may show rash, fever, hepatomegaly, splenomegaly, chorioretinitis (retinochoroiditis), and convulsions [2].

Pyrimethamine, in combination with sulfadiazine, is the treatment of first choice in *T. gondii* infection. Corticosteroid is added to the therapeutic regimen in patients with severe chorioretinitis.

Part Three: Helminthic Diseases

TRICHINOSIS. Trichinosis is caused by the intestinal nematode *Trichinella spiralis*. The most striking lesions are in the skeletal muscles, causing myositis and basophilic granular degeneration of the muscle fibers.

The first drug of choice is thiabendazole (50 mg/kg/day for 5–7 days), and an alternative drug is mebendazole. Thiabendazole, which is often given with corticosteroids, is not effective against larvae. Within 48 hours the muscular pain and tenderness will be obtuned [1].

Infection by Other Intestinal Nematodes. HOOKWORM. Hookworm is either *Ancylostoma duodenale* or *Necator americanus*. The major clinical manifestations of hookworm disease are chronic intestinal blood loss and iron-deficiency anemia. Therapy includes anthelmintics and correction of anemia. The drug of first choice in hookworm infection is pyrantel pamoate or mebendazole. An alternative regimen may include thiabendazole or tetrachlorethylene [10].

STRONGYLOIDIASIS (DWARF THREADWORM). Dwarf threadworm infection (strongyloidiasis) is an intestinal infection caused by *Strongyloides stercoralis*. The drug of choice is thiabendazole.

ASCARIASIS (COMMON ROUNDWORM). Ascariasis, caused by *Ascaris lumbricoides*, is characterized by an early pulmonary phase followed by a prolonged intestinal phase. In ascariasis, the first drug of choice is pyrantel pamoate or mebendazole; piperazine serves as an alternative drug.

ENTEROBIASIS (PINWORM, SEATWORM). Enterobiasis is an intestinal infection caused by *Enterobius vermicularis* and is characterized by perianal pruritus. The first drug of choice is pyrantel pamoate or mebendazole, and alternative medications are piperazine or pyrvinium pamoate.

TRICHURIASIS (WHIPWORM). Trichuriasis is an intestinal infection in humans caused by *Trichuris trichiura* and is characterized by invasion of colonic mucosa by the adult *Trichuris* nematode. The drug of choice is mebendazole.

FILARIASIS. Filariasis, caused by *Wuchereria bancrofti* or *Brugia malayi*, is characterized by nonspecific reactions and symptoms ranging from inflammation to scarring. The treatment includes diethylcarbamazine, which is a curative as well as a suppressive agent. It is given in dosage of 2 mg per kilogram three times a day for 3 to 4 weeks. The dying parasites may cause allergic reactions, which may be alleviated with antihistaminics or corticosteroids. In addition to diethylcarbamazine, the organic antimonials and arsenicals are effective in filariasis [7].

SCHISTOSOMIASIS. Schistosomiasis is caused by three closely related species of digenetic trematodes

Table 39-3. *Summary Pharmacology of Anthelmintics*

Anthelmintics	Properties
Pyrantel pamoate (Antiminth)	Poorly absorbed from gastrointestinal tract and most of it (80%) eliminated in feces; a drug of choice in ascariasis and enterobiasis; a depolarizing neuromuscular blocking agent causing spastic paralysis of hookworm, pinworm, and roundworm infestation
Mebendazole (Vermox)	Exerts its broad-spectrum anthelmintic property by inhibiting glucose uptake irreversibly and is therefore effective against ascariasis, capillariasis, enterobiasis, and trichuriasis
Pyrvinium pamoate (Vanquin, Povan)	Not absorbed from gastrointestinal tract; thought to exert its effects by inhibiting oxygen uptake and hence inhibiting respiration in nematodes
Piperazine citrate (Antepar)	Absorbed from gastrointestinal tract; since lethal doses cause convulsive seizures, should not be used in patients with epilepsy; exerts its anthelmintic effects by causing flaccid paralysis of muscle, resulting in expulsion of the worm
Thiabendazole (Mintezol)	Absorbed rapidly from gastrointestinal tract; metabolized by hydroxylation and conjugation with glucuronic acid; commonly occurring side effects are anorexia, nausea, and dizziness; should be used with caution in patients with decreased hepatic function; mechanism of action not known, but it inhibits fumarate reductase selectively and prevents embryonic development of *Ascaris* eggs in vitro
Niclosamide (Yomesan)	Not absorbed from gastrointestinal tract; safest effective drug in cestode infections; inhibits anaerobic metabolism and glucose uptake in *Taenia solium*, against which it is highly effective; since lethal doses in adult worm do not destroy the ova, purgation 1–2 hours after niclosamide is essential or risk of cysticercosis is imminent
Metrifonate (Bilarcil)	An organophosphorus inhibiting cholinesterase in *Schistosoma haematobium*; since plasma cholinesterase in host is similarly inhibited, depolarizing neuromuscular blocking agents, other cholinesterase inhibitors, and agents metabolized by plasma cholinesterase should not be concomitantly administered with metrifonate
Praziquantel (Biltricide)	Absorbed orally; effective against all schistosomes; exerts its effects by dislodging the worm in the intestine and subjecting the tegument to proteolysis; also effective against cestodes
Oxamniquine (Vansil)	Absorbed following oral administration; very effective only in *Schistosoma mansoni* infection; following treatment, *S. mansoni* flukes shift from mesenteric veins to liver where they are destroyed; male *S. mansoni* organism more susceptible to this killing effect than female, which will not be able to produce eggs
Niridazole (Ambilhar)	Possesses both schistosomicidal and amebicidal properties; has antiinflammatory properties and is a potent inhibitor of cell-mediated responses; exerts its effects by destroying vitellogenic gland and egg production in female and spermatogenesis in male *Schistosoma haematobium* fluke, against which it is highly effective; is extensively metabolized in liver, and numerous toxicities reported for niridazole do occur especially in patients with impairment of liver function; causes hemolytic anemia in patients with glucose 6-phosphate dehydrogenase deficiency; should be used cautiously in diseases involving the CNS, such as epilepsy

(blood flukes), affecting colon, urinary bladder, liver, lungs, and central nervous system. The three species and the treatments of choice are summarized here [8]:

Schistosoma haematobium (genitourinary schistosomiasis, endemic hematuria) is best treated with praziquantel; metrifonate is used as an alternative drug.
Schistosoma mansoni (intestinal bilharziasis, schistosomal dysentery) is best treated with oxamniquine; praziquantel is used as an alternative drug.
Schistosoma japonicum (eastern schistosomiasis, katayama disease) is best treated with praziquantel; niridazole is used as an alternative drug.

TAPEWORMS. Taeniasis.
Taenia saginata (beef tapeworm) is a hermaphroditic cestode that inhabits the intestinal tract of humans. The disease, usually asymptomatic, may produce epigastric discomfort, diarrhea, weight loss, and irritability [9]. The drug of first choice is niclosamide or praziquantel, and the alternative drug is paromomycin.

Taenia solium (pork tapeworm) causes a clinical picture similar to that of infection by beef tapeworm. The pharmacologic treatment is identical.

Diphyllobothriasis.
Diphyllobothrium latum (fish tapeworm) causes either no symptoms or mild abdominal discomfort. The treatment of fish tapeworm includes the use of niclosamide or praziquantel and paromomycin as first and second drug choice respectively.

Hymenolepiasis.
Caused by *Hymenolepis nana* (dwarf tapeworm), hymenolepiasis is characterized by the presence of many adult worms in the intestine, producing epigastric pain and diarrhea. The drug of first choice is either niclosamide or praziquantel, and the alternative drug is paromomycin.

The pharmacology of most often used anthelminthics is summarized in Table 39-3.

QUESTIONS ON THE PHARMACOLOGY OF MYCOBACTERIAL, PROTOZOAL, AND HELMINTHIC DISEASES

Select one answer that best completes the statement or answers the question.

_____ 338. In advanced cavitary tuberculosis the indicated therapy(s) is (are):
  A. Isoniazid.
  B. Streptomycin.
  C. Rifampin.
  D. All of the above in combination.

_____ 339. Treatment of leprosy includes use of:
  A. Dapsone.
  B. Sulfoxone.
  C. Both A and B.
  D. Neither A nor B.

_____ 340. Treatment of acute amebic dysentery includes:
  A. Dehydroemetine.
  B. Metronidazole.
  C. Both A and B.
  D. Neither A nor B.

_____ 341. Which of the following drug(s) is (are) folic acid antagonist(s)?
  A. Pyrimethamine.
  B. Methotrexate.
  C. Neither A nor B.
  D. Both A and B.

_____ 342. Rifampin is characterized by the following *except* which one?
  A. It binds to DNA-dependent RNA polymerase.
  B. It is used in amebiasis.
  C. It may cause flulike symptoms.
  D. It is absorbed orally.

_____ 343. Primaquine is characterized by the following *except* which one?
  A. It attacks plasmodia in exoerythrocytic stages.
  B. It is effective for malarial prophylaxis.
  C. It may cause hemolytic anemia in susceptible patients.
  D. It may cause polycythemia vera.

_____ 344. Thiabendazole is characterized by the following actions *except* which one?
  A. It must be given parenterally.
  B. It is metabolized by hydroxylation.
  C. It should be cautiously given in a patient with liver impairment.
  D. It is thought to exert its effects by inhibiting fumarate reductase.

_____ 345. Niridazole is characterized by the following actions *except* which one?
  A. It has antiinflammatory properties.
  B. It has schistosomicidal and amebicidal properties.
  C. It causes hemolytic anemia.
  D. It is a drug of choice in an epilepsy patient with schistosomial infection.

ANSWERS AND EXPLANATION ON THE PHARMACOLOGY OF MYCOBACTERIAL, PROTOZOAL, AND HELMINTHIC DISEASES

338. D.
339. C.
340. C.
341. D.
342. B.
343. D.
344. A.
345. D.
Explanation. Niridazole is contraindicated in epilepsy, neurosis, and psychosis.

REFERENCES

1. Bennett, I. L., Jr., and Petersdorf, R. G. Trichinosis. In M. M. Wintrobe et al. (eds.), *Harrison's Principles of Internal Medicine* (6th ed.). New York: McGraw-Hill, 1970. Pp. 1046–1048.
2. Feldman, H. A. Toxoplasmosis. In M. M. Wintrobe et al. (eds.), *Harrison's Principles of Internal Medicine* (6th ed.). New York: McGraw-Hill, 1970. Pp. 1040–1042.
3. Mandell, G. L., and Sande, M. A. Drugs Used in the Chemotherapy of Tuberculosis and Leprosy. In A. G. Gilman, L. S. Goodman, and A. Gilman (eds.), *The Pharmacological Basis of Therapeutics* (6th ed.). New York: Macmillan, 1980. Pp. 1200–1221.

4. Plorde, J. J., and Bennett, I. L., Jr. Malaria. In M. M. Wintrobe et al. (eds.), *Harrison's Principles of Internal Medicine* (6th ed.). New York: McGraw-Hill, 1970. Pp. 1030–1034.

5. Plorde, J. J., and Bennett, I. L., Jr. Leishmaniasis. In M. M. Wintrobe et al. (eds.), *Harrison's Principles of Internal Medicine* (6th ed.). New York: McGraw-Hill, 1970. Pp. 1034–1037.

6. Plorde, J. J., and Bennett, I. L., Jr. Trypanosomiasis. In M. M. Wintrobe et al. (eds.), *Harrison's Principles of Internal Medicine* (6th ed.). New York: McGraw-Hill, 1970. Pp. 1037–1040.

7. Plorde, J. J., and Bennett, I. L., Jr. Filariasis. In M. M. Wintrobe et al. (eds.), *Harrison's Principles of Internal Medicine* (6th ed.). New York: McGraw-Hill, 1970. Pp. 1055–1057.

8. Plorde, J. J., and Bennett, I, L., Jr. Schistosomiasis. In M. M. Wintrobe et al. (eds.), *Harrison's Principles of Internal Medicine* (6th ed.). New York: McGraw-Hill, 1970. Pp. 1057–1061.

9. Plorde, J. J., and Bennett, I. L., Jr. Cestodes and Tapeworms. In M. M. Wintrobe et al. (eds.), *Harrison's Principles of Internal Medicine* (6th ed.). New York: McGraw-Hill, 1970. Pp. 1063–1067.

10. Plorde, J. J., Bennett, I. L., Jr., and Petersdorf, R. G. Other Intestinal Nematodes. In M. M. Wintrobe et al. (eds.), *Harrison's Principles of Internal Medicine* (6th ed.). New York: McGraw-Hill, 1970. Pp. 1048–1055.

11. Plorde, J. J., Feldman, H. A., and Bennett, I. L., Jr. Amebiasis. In M. M. Wintrobe et al. (eds.), *Harrison's Principles of Internal Medicine* (6th ed.). New York: McGraw-Hill, 1970. Pp. 1026–1030.

12. Rollo, I. M. Drugs Used in the Chemotherapy of Helminthiasis. In A. G. Gilman, L. S. Goodman, and A. Gilman (eds.), *The Pharmacological Basis of Therapeutics* (6th ed.). New York: Macmillan, 1980. Pp. 1013–1037.

13. Rollo, I. M. Drugs Used in the Chemotherapy of Malaria. In A. G. Gilman, L. S. Goodman, and A. Gilman (eds.), *The Pharmacological Basis of Therapeutics* (6th ed.). New York: Macmillan, 1980. Pp. 1038–1060.

14. Rollo, I. M. Drugs Used in the Chemotherapy of Amebiasis. In A. G. Gilman, L. S. Goodman, and A. Gilman (eds.), *The Pharmacological Basis of Therapeutics* (6th ed.). New York: Macmillan, 1980. Pp. 1061–1069.

15. Rollo, I. M. Drugs Used in the Treatment of Protozoal Infections. In A. G. Gilman, L. S. Goodman, and A. Gilman (eds.), *The Pharmacological Basis of Therapeutics* (6th ed.). New York: Macmillan, 1980. Pp. 1070–1079.

16. Shepard, C. C. Leprosy (Hansen's Disease). In M. M. Wintrobe et al. (eds.), *Harrison's Principles of Internal Medicine* (6th ed.). New York: McGraw-Hill, 1970. Pp. 880–883.

17. Stead, W. W. Tuberculosis. In M. M. Wintrobe et al. (eds.), *Harrison's Principles of Internal Medicine* (6th ed.). New York: McGraw-Hill, 1970. Pp. 865–880.

XII. Poisons and Antidotes

40. Principles of Toxicology

Love truth but pardon error.
Voltaire

In the exploration and description of the pharmacodynamics of various therapeutic agents, it has been emphasized repeatedly that drugs seldom exert their beneficial effects without also causing side effects. The latter can be reduced, minimized, and sometimes avoided altogether by a caring and knowledgable physician. Furthermore, it has been noted that in terms of the dose-related effects of drugs the sciences of pharmacology and toxicology rest on different ends of a therapeutic spectrum since all lifesaving therapeutic compounds can have disastrously toxic and lethal effects when used erroneously and injudiciously. The distance between a "safe" and an "unsafe" therapeutic regimen is narrow and may be traversed easily. The inevitability of this therapeutic dilemma indeed lends credence to the statement, "There are really no safe biologically active drugs. There are only safe physicians."

The modern science of toxicology is a broad-based and multidisciplinary area of investigation, which gathers, assimilates, and applies information from the seemingly diversified fields of pathology, biochemistry, pharmacology, and nutrition. It involves all aspects of our lives, from growing and preparing foods (insecticides, pesticides, food additives, food substitutes) to cleaning and protecting our environment and its resources (industrial pollution and wastes contaminating the air, the soil, the rivers, the lakes, and the oceans). Toxicology may range from the inherent poisoning associated with the unpleasant task of eliminating an unwanted pest from one's own home (insecticides, rodenticides, and fumigants) to an allergic reaction that may occur when a seemingly innocuous and very desirable substance such as a perfume is used on a chronic basis (dermatotoxicity in the cosmetic industry). Toxicology may involve an acute and episodic poisoning following a one-time ingestion of a food substance (mushroom poisoning) or the most complicated and vexing diagnostic problems in pathology (forensic toxicology). Toxicology may range from the rarely occurring neurotoxicity (paresthesias, ataxia, and ascending paralysis) caused by shellfish to the mutagenic and carcinogenic effects of radiation injury (radiotherapeutics as well as problems associated with nuclear warfare). Toxicology may involve the accidental but frequent poisoning in children (aspirin and iron poisoning) or the rarely encountered but fatal kuru (laughing sickness of cannibalistic people). A detailed description of these and other overwhelmingly important parameters in toxicology falls outside the scope of a section devoted to principles of toxicology. Nevertheless, recognition of these important areas and their numerous subdivisions prompts us to take appropriate steps to reduce and to avoid the numerous tragedies that substances

such as tetrachlorodibenzo-*p*-dioxin (TCDD, Dioxin) and similar agents have caused and continue to cause [1, 4, 5, 7, 8, 10, 11]. TCDD, a contaminant of herbicide, has a LD 50 of 0.5 µg/kg, is a potent carcinogen, and is thought to be the most toxic chemical synthesized.

ORGAN-SPECIFIC AND GENERALIZED TOXICITY. Synthetic compounds used in agriculture, industry, and medicine may produce generalized toxicity, or their toxic effects may be organ specific. A few examples are cited in Table 40-1. However, it should be reemphasized that drugs in general are capable of causing multiple toxicities. For example, chlorpromazine causes dystonia, parkinsonism, and tardive dyskinesia (brain); hyperglycemia, lactation, and amenorrhea (endocrine); pigment retinopathy (eye); solar sensitivity (skin); maculopapular, urticarial, and pruritic rash (hypersensitivity); agranulocytosis and thrombocytopenia (blood); hypotension and tachycardia (cardiovascular); constipation (gastrointestinal); and hypothermia (interference with the hypothalamic temperature-regulating mechanisms).

ACUTE AND CHRONIC TOXICITY. Drugs and toxicants often produce two distinct responses and effects when used acutely or on a chronic basis. For example, when used acutely, ethyl alcohol produces inebriation at a blood alcohol concentration of > 0.15 percent. The chronic use of alcohol in malnourished individuals has been shown to cause far more deleterious effects:

Neuropathy, characterized by dysesthesias, paralysis, and trophic skin changes
Myopathy, characterized by rhabdomyolysis, muscle pain and cramp, elevated serum creatine, phosphokinase, and myoglobinuria
Wernicke-Korsakoff syndrome, caused by thiamine deficiency and characterized by confusion, ataxia, and ocular abnormalities (nystagmus, lateral rectus palsy)
Cerebellar degeneration (degeneration of cerebellar cortex, especially the Purkinje cells, causing ataxia and truncal instability)
Amblyopia (decreased visual acuity and color perception)
Marchiafava-Bignami disease, resulting from central demyelination of the corpus collosum (also seen in chronic cyanide intoxication, causing progressive dementia)
Central pontine myelinolysis, characterized by progressive bulbar weakness and quadriparesis [3]

The differentiation between acute and chronic toxicities described for alcohol may not always be so obvious and self-evident for countless groups of sub-

Table 40-1. *Manifestation of Drug Toxicity in Specific Organs*

Organ	Drug	Effect
Brain	Trifluoperazine	Tardive and persistent dyskinesia
Eye	Chloroquine	Keratopathy and posterior pole degeneration
	Trimethadione	Hemeralopia
	Trifluoperazine	Pigment retinopathy
Ear	Kanamycin	Deafness
Lung	Busulfan	Pulmonary arteriolitis and radiation pneumonitis
	Bleomycin	Pneumonitis
Heart	Antibiotics	Septicemia and endocarditis (indirect effect)
Blood	Chloramphenicol	Thrombocytopenia
Liver	Thioridazine	Cholestatic jaundice
Gastrointestinal tract	Corticosteroids	Gastric ulceration
Kidney	Phenacetin	Interstitial nephritis and papillary necrosis
Endocrine glands	Diazoxide	Hyperglycemia due to inhibition of insulin release
Bone and teeth	Tetracyclines	Discoloration of growing teeth, enamel hypoplasia
Skin	Phenylbutazone	Erythema multiforme
	Mephenytoin	Stevens-Johnson syndrome
Hair follicles	Phenytoin	Hypertrichosis

stances ingested chronically throughout the world. As an example, chemical substances used as food additives (calcium phosphate, calcium carbonate), food substitutes (artificial sweeteners), and food preservatives (benzoic acid) are absolutely safe and innocuous when used in the amount incorporated in the foods. Nevertheless, debates about the safety of these agents used on a chronic basis and often for a lifetime are never ending. Furthermore, the unanswered questions emerging from these debates have created new enterprising industries that offer the public "100% natural" foods devoid of any "unnatural substances."

RAPID AND DELAYED TOXICITY. Pharmacologic agents may manifest their toxicities rapidly or with a considerable delay of months or even years. For example, chlorpromazine produces immediate, slow, and delayed toxicities.

Immediate Toxicity. Chlorpromazine, when used as an antiemetic in children, may cause acute dystonia characterized by intermittent or sustained muscular spasms and abnormal postures of the eyes, face, and throat accompanied by respiratory stridor and cyanosis.

Slow Toxicity. Chlorpromazine may cause pseudoparkinsonism in schizophrenic patients, characterized by tremor, rigidity, akinesia, and postural abnormality. These symptoms occur mostly within 1 to 3 months after the initiation of therapy.

Delayed Toxicity. Chlorpromazine may cause tardive dyskinesia, characterized by "persistent dyskinesia" or buccolinguomasticatory syndrome. As the term implies, tardive dyskinesia always occurs late, usually after 6 months of therapy and mostly after 2 to 3 years of continuous therapy.

Diethylstilbestrol, when given to a pregnant woman, causes occasional immediate nausea and vomiting. The slow toxicity may include fluid retention and uterine bleeding. The delayed toxicities, which appear many years later in female offspring when they reach puberty, are vaginal adenosis and clear-cell vaginal adenocarcinoma.

REVERSIBLE AND IRREVERSIBLE TOXICITY. The toxic manifestations of drugs and toxicants are generally reversible but not always. For example, thioridazine and chlorpromazine may cause cholestatic hepatitis and allergic dermatitis (hypersensitivity reactions), ejaculation disorders (interference with the autonomic nervous system), galactorrhea and gynecomastia (interference with dopamine-mediated inhibition of prolactin secretion), and agranulocytosis (nonimmunologically mediated toxic reaction due to inhibition of DNA synthesis). All these toxic reactions are reversible with dose reduction or the discontinuation of medication. On the other hand, thioridazine and chlorpromazine may cause solar sensitivity and pigment retinopathy, which are not reversible. Phenytoin causes ataxia and nystagmus, which are reversible, and hypertrichosis, which is not. The chronic inhalation of manganese dust causes bronchitis, nasopharyngitis, pneumonia, dermatitis, hypotension, and impaired hepatic and renal function, which are all reversible, and parkinsonism (damage to and disappearance of neurons in the globus pallidus), which is not reversible.

AGE-RELATED TOXICITY. Prenatal Pharmacology. Unless absolutely essential, all drugs including antiemetic agents should be avoided during pregnancy.

Drugs may cause abortion. Aminopterin, mercaptopurine, azathioprine, and cyclophosphamide have caused abortion.

Drugs may cause congenital abnormalities and defects. Aminopterin, methotrexate, oral contraceptives, and phenytoin (fetal hydantoin syndrome) have caused craniofacial and limb abnormalities, as well as slow physical and mental development.

Drugs may cause metabolic abnormalities. High doses of vitamin C cause withdrawal scurvy, and high doses of vitamin B_6 cause pyridoxine dependency.

Drugs may cause neonatal addiction. Chronic use of morphine, methadone, and heroin causes addiction in the fetus.

Drugs may cause organ malfunction. Testosterone causes clitoral hypertrophy. Lithium causes cardiovascular abnormalities.

Drugs may cause sensory defect. Streptomycin causes deafness.

Drugs may cause endocrine abnormalities. Oral antidiabetic agent has caused hypoglycemia, thiouracil and iodides have caused goiter, and corticosteroids have caused Cushing-like syndrome.

Drugs may cause myasthenia. Physostigmine and pyridostigmine have caused neonatal myasthenia.

Paranatal Pharmacology. Most lipid-soluble substances or agents with molecular weight under 1,000 may pass across the placental barrier. For example, reserpine may cause nasal congestion, anorexia, and paralytic ileus; morphine and barbiturates cause respiratory depression; diazepam and magnesium sulfate cause muscular weakness; anticoagulants and synthetic vitamin K cause hemorrhage; and a narcotic antagonist such as naloxone (Narcan) precipitates a withdrawal syndrome in an addicted infant.

Neonatal Pharmacology. The neonatal pharmacokinetic parameters differ vastly from those of an adult. A pediatric patient should not be regarded as a miniature adult, and drug dosages should not be calculated on body weight only. For example, the extent of surface area, intestinal mucosal area, and pulmonary alveolar area is greater than for the adult. The volume of distribution is different, especially in premature infants, and may change daily. The activity of drug-metabolizing enzymes is not fully developed. The rates of glomerular filtration and tubular secretion are reduced. The chloramphenicol-induced gray baby syndrome is an example of the subnormal level of glucuronyl transferase in the newborn with reduced ability to conjugate chloramphenicol with glucuronic acid.

Pharmacology of Nursing Infants. Many drugs are excreted in milk. The amount of a drug appearing in the milk depends on many factors. The higher the maternal plasma concentration of a drug, the more drug is likely to appear in the milk. Atropine poisoning has occurred in nursing infants whose mothers ingested larger than therapeutic doses of atropine. Nonionized and nonprotein-bound drugs are excreted more rapidly, while ionized drugs are excreted slowly. The longer a drug stays in maternal plasma (diminished metabolism or excretion), the more it will be excreted in the milk. Since the pH of milk is more acidic (6.7) than that of plasma, basic drugs accumulate in the milk to a higher extent than do acidic drugs, so when drugs are used in therapeutically recommended amounts, in the majority of cases the concentrations of drugs in milk and in an infant's plasma are lower than in the maternal plasma, causing no interference with breast feeding. However, toxicity has occurred, and the injudicious use of drugs should be avoided. For example, heavy smokers who intend to breast-feed should perhaps expect gastrointestinal, cardiovascular, and CNS disturbances (anorexia, vomiting, diarrhea, tachycardia, restlessness, and irritability) in their infants. Furthermore, lactating mothers on chronic medications such as anticonvulsants, neuroleptics, or anxiolytic agents should perhaps refrain from breast-feeding their infants [9]. The developing brain is far more susceptible to toxicity than is the developed one. For example, the methylmercury-contaminated fish ingested by lactating Japanese mothers have caused neurologic deficits in their infants (Minamata disease).

Mercury has also been implicated in the etiology of acrodynia (pink disease) when mercury-containing teething powder was used. Methylmercury in fungicides has caused toxicity in children in Iraq. The methylmercury toxicity is characterized by phalangeal erythema, muscular weakness, ataxia, hyperirritability, sensory impairment, visual disturbances, involuntary movement, and sometimes unconsciousness.

Fetal Alcohol Syndrome. Alcohol and its metabolite acetaldehyde are important teratogens and have been implicated in the etiology of fetal alcohol syndrome. This is characterized by facial abnormalities (midface hyperplasia), microencephaly, growth deficiency, and mental retardation. The syndrome occurs early in pregnancy after the consumption of large amounts of alcohol, which should be totally abstained from during pregnancy.

Geriatric Pharmacology. Statistical data have firmly established four isolated but interrelated facts about the aged population:

1. Longevity is increasing.
2. The aged population of the world is expanding.
3. The aged population may have multiple diseases and may be taking multiple medications.
4. The potential of drug-drug interactions and adverse drug reactions is very high among aged citizens.

The appreciation and application of concepts involved in geriatric pharmacology not only may reduce potential drug-related toxicities but also may enhance the quality of life for the aged person. As described for pediatric patients, the pharmacokinetic parameters are also varied in the aged. Since plasma albumin decreases with aging, the binding of drugs to plasma protein diminishes. Furthermore, since total body fat increases with aging, the storage of lipid-soluble substances (silent sites) is varied. As the total water in the body decreases, the volumes of distribution of drugs are altered. The metabolism of some drugs is reduced, and their half-lives are increased. Because the glomerular filtration rate and the tubular excretion rate are diminished by aging, the excretion of most drugs and their metabolites is substandard. Consequently, it is obvious that the very old patient behaves pharmacokinetically like the very young one. Unfortunately, unlike pediatric patients, elderly patients may have several diseases including cardiovascular disorders and may be taking several agents, especially those with narrow margins of safety (e.g., digitalis glycosides, and tricyclic antidepressants). It is imperative, therefore, that these pharmacokinetic principles be taken into consideration in order to avoid undue toxicities [6].

DIAGNOSIS AND MANAGEMENT OF ACUTE POISONING. The following sections present the clinical manifestations and treatments of acute poisoning with selected agricultural, industrial, and biologic agents.

Part One: Agricultural Poisons

POLYCYCLIC CHLORINATED INSECTICIDES. These agents include chlordane, heptachlor, dieldrin, and aldrin.

The clinical manifestations of poisoning are hyperexcitability, ataxia, tremors, and convulsions [2]. Treatment consists in emesis, the administration of activated charcoal followed by gastric lavage, and anticonvulsants (diazepam).

CHOLINESTERASE INHIBITORS USED AS INSECTICIDES. The cholinesterase inhibitors are divided into organophosphorus compounds, such as parathion, malathion, and tetraethylpyrophosphate (TEPP), and the carbamates, such as naphthyl-N-methylcarbamate (carbaryl, Sevin).

The clinical manifestations of acute and severe poisoning from organophosphorus insecticides include cholinergic crisis resulting from stimulation of muscarinic cholinergic receptors (bronchoconstriction, salivation, sweating, lacrimation, bradycardia, hypotension, and urinary and fecal incontinence), from stimulation of nicotinic cholinergic receptors (muscular fasciculation), and from CNS effects (with initial restlessness, tremors, ataxia, and convulsions, followed by CNS depression and respiratory and circulatory depression) [2]. The treatment of cholinergic crisis from organophosphorus compounds includes the administration of a cholinesterase reactivator such as pralidoxime (2-PAM) in the presence of atropine. Antidoting with 2-PAM is not necessary with poisoning from carbaryl, a reversible cholinesterase inhibitor.

HERBICIDES. The herbicides include paraquat (methyl viologen) and diquat. Paraquat may be absorbed topically. These herbicides are inactivated by contact with soil. Smoking marijuana contaminated with them causes delayed fibrosis of the lung. The ingestion of paraquat causes gastrointestinal upset, respiratory distress, hemoptysis, ulceration of pharynx, and cyanosis. Diquat, in addition to producing gastrointestinal and pulmonary distress and cardiac arrhythmias, may cause oliguria and progressive renal failure. The treatment, which must occur early, includes the administration of activated charcoal followed by lavage with 1% bentonite solution, hydrocortisone, furosemide, and hemodialysis [2].

Part Two: Industrial Poisons

THE ALCOHOLS AND GLYCOL. Ethyl Alcohol. This agent is metabolized mainly by alcohol dehydrogenase and exhibits zero-order kinetics (10 mg/hour). No known antidote is available. Disulfiram (Antabuse) inhibits aldehyde dehydrogenase and should never be used in combination with ethyl alcohol.

Methyl Alcohol. This agent is metabolized primarily by alcohol dehydrogenase to formaldehyde, then formic acid, causing blindness and acidosis. Ethyl alcohol, when given intravenously, competes with methyl alcohol, allowing it to be excreted unchanged by the kidneys.

Ethylene Glycol. This agent causes inebriation resembling ethyl alcohol inebriation, followed by vomiting, cyanosis, hypotension, tachycardia, tachypnea, pulmonary edema, acidosis, anuria (calcium oxalate crystals), convulsions, and unconsciousness. Death results from respiratory failure or irreversible brain damage. Ethyl alcohol may be used to antidote ethylene glycol. Following this life-supporting step, additional supportive treatment should be provided by correcting acidosis, pulmonary edema, anuria, and hypoglycemia [2].

Isopropyl Alcohol. The symptoms of isopropyl alcohol poisoning are similar to those produced by ethyl alcohol, but a more marked depression of the central nervous system may occur. Other symptoms include persistent nausea, vomiting, hematemesis, abdominal pain, dehydration, depressed respiration, and oliguria. Emergency treatment consists in artificial respiration and hemodialysis. Additional supportive therapy includes correcting electrolyte imbalance, maintaining blood pressure, correcting oliguria, and preventing renal failure [2].

THE HALOGENATED HYDROCARBONS. Carbon Tetrachloride. Carbon tetrachloride decomposes to phosgene and hydrochloric acid. In general, carbon tetrachloride occasions injuries to all organs but especially the kidneys (marked edema and fatty degeneration of the tubules) and the liver (centrilobular necrosis and fatty degeneration). The toxic manifestations include oliguria, jaundice, and coma. Carbon tetrachloride oliguria is followed by a prolonged period of diuresis. The complete return of hepatic and renal functions is possible but occurs slowly. The treatment of poisoning is basic supportive treatment. Sympathomimetic agents should not be given in hypotension since cardiac arrhythmia may ensue [2].

Trichloroethylene. Trichloroethylene causes CNS depression and unconsciousness. Respiration and circulation should be supported. Recovery is prompt without causing any residual injuries.

PETROLEUM AND SOLVENT DISTILLATES. The extensive inhalation or ingestion of petroleum products (kerosene, gasoline) causes nausea, vomiting, and pulmonary irritation (coughing, hemoptysis, and CNS and respiratory depression). Treatment includes early administration of activated charcoal and gastric lavage, artificial respiration, and any other therapy to minimize pulmonary injury.

AROMATIC HYDROCARBONS. The aromatic hydrocarbons include benzene, xylene, and toluene. Chronic exposure to benzene and toluene causes anemia. Ingestion of these agents causes gastrointestinal symptoms, dizziness, headache, ataxia, delirium, cardiac irregularities, paralysis, and convulsions. Treatment consists in controlling convulsions by diazepam, providing supportive therapy, and monitoring the hematopoietic elements [2].

CORROSIVES. The corrosives include both acidic and basic substances such as chlorine and hydrochloric acid. The clinical manifestations are burning pain in the mouth, pharynx, and abdomen, severe hypotension, asphyxia, perforation of the esophagus or stomach, peritonitis, and, after recovery, strictures of the esophagus or stomach. The corrosives should be diluted with water or milk. Gastric lavage, emesis, and chemical antidotes (acid for base and base for acid) are absolutely contraindicated. Circulation should be sustained by transfusion of 5% glucose in saline, and nutrition should be supplied by administering carbohydrate intravenously [2].

METAL POISONING. Lead Toxicity. Lead binds and inactivates sulfhydryl groups in various biologic systems. Chronic toxicity is characterized by lead colic (paroxysmal abdominal pain), lead palsy (muscle weakness, fatigue, peripheral neuritis, and wrist drop), and lead encephalopathy (ataxia, insomnia, delirium, tonic-clonic convulsions, coma, and death).

Lead, which is best absorbed from the lung (dust or vapor), becomes initially bound to erythrocytes, then redistributes to soft tissues, and finally is deposited slowly in the bones. Lead is excreted very slowly. The laboratory evidence for lead poisoning includes basophilic stippling of erythrocytes, porphyrinuria, and the inhibition of delta-aminolevulinic acid dehydratase. The treatment of toxicity includes calcium disodium edetate (Calcium Disodium Versenate) and D-penicillamine (Cuprimine). Although D-penicillamine is not as active as dimercaprol, it is more active orally and hence useful in the long-term de-leading of patients for several months [2].

Mercury Toxicity. Mercury binds with sulfhydryl groups of enzymes and other proteins. The toxic manifestations are corrosive, the inorganic mercurials causing local tissue damage followed by systemic toxicity at the sites of excretion of mercury—the kidneys, salivary glands, and colon. The organic mercurials (alkyl mercury) cause concentric constriction of the visual field, ataxia, tremors, dysarthria, paresthesias, loss of sight and hearing, and intellectual deterioration. The treatment of choice includes dimercaprol (BAL) or penicillamine (Cuprimine).

Arsenic Toxicity. Arsenic exerts its toxicity by binding to sulfhydryl groups of enzymes and tissue proteins, causing hemolysis. In addition, organic arsenicals are carcinogenic in character. The early signs of toxicity include diarrhea, thickening of the skin on the palms and soles, edema, and hyperpigmentation of the neck, eyelids, axillae, and nipples. Other signs include weakness, anorexia, nausea, salivation, dermatitis, jaundice, cirrhosis, loss of hair and nails, encephalopathy, and blood dyscrasias. The treatment of choice includes dimercaprol (BAL).

Chelating Agents in Metal Poisoning. Among heavy-metal chelators, the following have been used extensively. **Penicillamine** chelates copper, mercury, lead, and iron. It is effective and is useful for the removal of copper in Wilson's disease. **Deferoxamine** chelates iron. **Dimercaprol** (BAL) is effective in the treatment of poisoning by mercury, arsenic, and gold. It should not be used in poisoning by cadmium, iron, and selenium. BAL is metabolized in the liver. High concentrations of BAL inhibit cellular respiration [2].

Calcium Disodium EDTA. This agent is not metabolized and is not active orally. It is administered by intravenous drip. The adverse effects of EDTA include renal damage, hypersensitivity reactions, and transient bone marrow depression.

Part Three: The Asphyxiants

CARBON MONOXIDE. Carbon monoxide (CO) causes tissue anoxia by combining with hemoglobin (antimetabolite of oxygen) to form carboxyhemoglobin, which is incapable of carrying oxygen. The affinity of hemoglobin for CO is 200 times higher than that for oxygen. At approximately 60 percent saturation of hemoglobin with CO, convulsions, coma, and respiratory failure take place. Treatment includes giving 100% O_2 and artificial respiration for 1 to 2 hours and maintaining body temperature and blood pressure. The cerebral edema that may occur should be treated by giving mannitol and prednisone. The convulsions may be effectively treated with diazepam.

CYANIDE. Cyanide inactivates cytochrome oxidase by combining with ferric ion atoms in the heme proteins. Death occurs suddenly, terminating in convulsive seizures. Treatment includes the production of methemoglobin so that it may compete with cytochrome oxidase for cyanide ions. This goal may be accomplished by intravenous administration of sodium nitrite, or, if that is not available, by any nitrite that can be given by inhalation. The cyanide should be detoxified by causing its reaction with thiosulfate to form the much less toxic thiocyanate [2].

QUESTIONS ON PRINCIPLES OF TOXICOLOGY

Select the answer that best completes the statement or answers the question.

____ 346. Drugs known to cause abortion are:
   A. Aminopterin.
   B. Mercaptopurine.
   C. Azathioprine.
   D. All of the above.

____ 347. Diethylstilbestrol-induced vaginal adenocarcinoma is an example of:
   A. Delayed irreversible toxicity.
   B. Hypersensitivity reaction.
   C. Dose-dependent toxicity.
   D. Idiosyncratic reaction.

____ 348. All of the following drugs have been properly matched with their toxicity *except* which one?
   A. High-dose ascorbic acid in a pregnant woman—withdrawal scurvy in the newborn.
   B. High-dose pyridoxine in a pregnant woman—pyridoxine dependency in the newborn.
   C. Streptomycin—deafness.
   D. Lithium—hypertrichosis.

____ 349. Mercury toxicity is characterized by:
   A. Muscular weakness.
   B. Ataxia.
   C. Sensory impairment.
   D. Phalangeal erythema.
   E. All of the above.

350. Which one of the following statements about fetal alcohol syndrome is not correct?
A. It is characterized by midface hyperplasia.
B. It may be due to ethyl alcohol or acetaldehyde.
C. It is reversible.
D. It occurs early in pregnant women who consume alcohol in excess.

351. In geriatric patients, one should note that:
A. Plasma albumin level decreases.
B. Total body fat increases.
C. Total body water decreases.
D. Glomerular filtration rate decreases.
E. All of the above.

352. The toxicity of polycyclic chlorinated insecticides may be managed by:
A. Diazepam.
B. Ethosuximide.
C. Chlorthiazide.
D. Chlorpromazine.

353. The treatment of choice for irreversible cholinesterase inhibitor includes:
A. Pralidoxime (2-PAM).
B. Atropine sulfate.
C. Both A and B together.
D. Neither A nor B.

354. Which one of the following statements does not apply to paraquat poisoning?
A. It is not absorbed topically.
B. It is inactivated by soil.
C. Its ingestion causes hemoptysis.
D. Treatment may include the use of furosemide.

355. Ethyl alcohol:
A. Is metabolized by zero-order kinetics.
B. May be used in methyl alcohol poisoning.
C. Both A and B.
D. Neither A nor B.

356. Which of the following statements is correct about disulfiram (Antabuse)?
A. It inhibits the metabolism of ethyl alcohol.
B. It should never be used simultaneously with ethyl alcohol.
C. Both A and B.
D. Neither A nor B.

357. The toxic manifestation of methyl alcohol poisoning includes:
A. Blindness.
B. Acidosis.
C. Both A and B.
D. Neither A nor B.

358. Which one of the following poisons is improperly matched with the indicated treatment or antidote?
A. Cyanide poisoning—calcium gluconate.
B. Arsenic poisoning—dimercaprol.
C. Lead poisoning—calcium disodium edetate.
D. Iron poisoning—deferoxamine.

359. Death from poisoning by ethylene glycol results from:
A. Respiratory failure.
B. Hypotension.
C. Anuria.
D. Acidosis.

360. Poisoning from isopropyl alcohol resembles closely poisoning from which one of the following?
A. Methyl alcohol.
B. Ethyl alcohol.
C. Ethylene glycol.
D. Kerosene.

361. Carbon tetrachloride decomposes to:
A. Carbonic acid.
B. Hydrochloric acid.
C. Phosgene.
D. B and C.
E. None of the above.

362. The chronic toxicity of benzene includes:
A. Gastrointestinal symptoms.
B. Ataxia.
C. Respiratory alkalosis.
D. Anemia.

363. Which of the following is (are) contraindication(s) in poisoning from hydrochloric acid?
A. Gastric lavage.
B. Emesis.
C. Neutralization of HCl with NaOH.
D. Transfusion of 5% glucose in saline.
E. A, B, and C.

364. Lead poisoning may be treated with all of the following *except* which one?
A. Calcium disodium edetate.
B. D-Penicillamine.
C. Dimercaprol.
D. Deferoxamine.

365. Inorganic and organic arsenicals are characterized by:
A. Binding with sulfhydryl groups of enzymes.
B. Being carcinogenic.
C. Causing hyperpigmentation of skin including nipples.
D. Causing alopecia.
E. All of the above.

ANSWERS AND EXPLANATIONS ON PRINCIPLES OF TOXICOLOGY

346. D.
347. A.
348. D.
349. E.
350. C.
351. E.
352. A.
   Explanation: Polycyclic chlorinated insecticides such as chlordane may cause hyperexcitability and convulsions, which are reversed by diazepam.
353. C.
354. A.
355. C.
   Explanation: In methanol poisoning, ethyl alcohol is administered intravenously. The alcohol dehydrogenase shows a preference for ethyl alcohol as a substrate, allowing methyl alcohol to be excreted unchanged.
356. C.
357. C.
358. A.
359. A.
360. B.
361. D.
362. D.
363. E.
364. D.
365. E.

REFERENCES

1. Casarett, L. J., and Doull, J. *Toxicology: The Basic Science of Poisons*. New York: Macmillan, 1975.
2. Dreisbach, R. H. *Handbook of Poisoning* (11th ed.). Los Altos, Calif.: Lange, 1983.
3. Haller, R. G. Alcoholism and Neurologic Disorders. In R. N. Rosenberg (ed.), *Neurology*. New York: Grune & Stratton, 1980. Pp. 569–588.
4. Hayes, A. W. *Principles and Methods of Toxicology*. New York: Raven, 1982.
5. Marzulli, F. N., and Maibach, H. I. *Dermato-toxicology and Pharmacology. Advances in Modern Toxicology*, Vol. 4. New York: Wiley, 1977.
6. O'Malley, K., Judge, T. G., and Crooks, J. Geriatric Pharmacology and Therapeutics. In G. S. Avery (ed.), *Drug Treatment: Principles and Practice of Clinical Pharmacology* (2nd ed.). New York: Adis, 1980. Pp. 158–181.
7. Polson, C. J., and Tattersall, R. N. *Clinical Toxicology*. Philadelphia: Lippincott, 1969.
8. Roizin, L., Shiraki, H., and Grecvic, N. *Neurotoxicity*, Vol. 1. New York: Raven, 1977.
9. Shirkey, H. C. Pediatric Clinical Pharmacology and Therapeutics. In G. S. Avery (ed.), *Drug Treatment: Principles and Practice of Clinical Pharmacology* (2nd ed.). New York: Adis, 1980. Pp. 97–157.
10. Simpson, L. L. *Neuropoisons: Their Pathophysiological Actions*. Vol. 1, *Poisons of Animal Origin*. New York: Plenum, 1981.
11. Thienes, C. H., and Haley, T. J. *Clinical Toxicology* (5th ed.). Philadelphia: Lea & Febiger, 1972.

Index

Index

Serotonin receptor, amitriptyline and, 71
Serotonin uptake, antidepressant block of, 71
Silent sites, 12
Silver sulfadiazine (Silvadene), 200
Site of action, definition of, 23
Sleep disorders, 68
Somatic nervous system, 35
Specificity
  chemical and structural, 24
  stereoisomeric, 24
Spectinomycin (Trobicin), 205
  bioavailability, 6
Spermatogenesis, gossypol and, 164
Spironolactone (Aldactone), 115. See also Aldosterone
Sporonticides, 234
Sporotrichosis, potassium iodide in, 228
Steroid receptor, 12–13
Steroids
  anabolic, 164
  androgenic, 164
Stevens-Johnson syndrome, 200. See also Anticonvulsants
Streptokinase (Streptase), 131
Streptomycin, 205, 206
  in tuberculosis, 233
Stress, 67
Striatal dopamine deficiency syndrome, 49
Strongyloidiasis, thiabendazole in, 237
Structure-activity relationship, 23
Succinimide derivatives, 56
Succinylcholine chloride (Anectine, Quelicin, SuxCert, Sucostrin), 93
  adverse reactions to, 94
  metabolism of, 16, 94
  uses, 94
Succinylsulfathiazole (Sulfasuxidine), 200
Sulfacetamide (Sulamyd, Isopto Cetamide), 200
Sulfacytine (Renoquid), 200
Sulfadiazine, pyramethamine and, 235
Sulfadimethoxine, 200
Sulfamethizole (Thiosulfil), 199, 200
Sulfamethoxazole (Gantanol), 200
Sulfamethoxypyridazine, 200
Sulfasalazine (Azulfidine), 200
Sulfinpyrazone (Anturane), 85
  platelet aggregation and, 83
Sulfisoxazole (Gantrisin), 200
Sulfonamides, 199–200
  antibacterial action of, 199
  as antimalarial agents, 235
  as diuretics, 113–114
  mechanism of action of, 199–200
  pharmacokinetics of, 200
  resistance to, 200
  toxicities of, 200
Sulfones
  as antimalarial agents, 235
  leprosy treatment with, 233
Sulfonylurea derivatives, 142–143

Sulfoxone sodium, 233
Sulindac (Clinoril), 84
Sulpiride
  as antidepressant, 72
  as neuroleptic, 64
  structure of, 61
Suramin (Naphuride), in African sleeping sickness, 235
Surface area, drug absorption and, 9

Tachyphylaxis, 24
  definition of, 29–30
Taeniasis
  niclosamide, 237
  praziquantel, 237
Tamoxifen (Nolvadex), antiestrogens, 161
Tapeworms (Taeniasis), 237
Tardive dyskinesia, neuroleptic-induced, 24, 63, 242
  treatment of, 63
Terbutaline (Brethine), 44
  as bronchodilator, 174
  premature labor and, 156
  structure of, 174
Testicular feminization, 24
Testosterone, 144, 164
  mechanism of action of, 160
Testosterone-receptor complex, 12–13
Tetracaine (Pontocaine)
  as spinal anesthetic, 89
Tetrachlorethylene, 237
Tetracycline (Achromycin, Panmycin), 207, 208
Tetracyclines, 208
  absorption of, 10, 30
  administration of, 9
  adverse reactions to, 208
  mechanism of action of, 208
  pharmacokinetics of, 208
  resistance to, 208
  therapeutic uses of, 208
Tetraethylammonium, autonomic ganglion blockade by, 36
Theophylline
  phosphodiesterase inhibition by, 25, 174, 186–187
  structure of, 174
Therapeutic index, 15, 16
Thiabendazole (Mintezol), 237
  properties of, 236
  for trichinosis, 235
Thiazide diuretics, 113–114
  as antihypertensive, 119, 123
  insulin release inhibition and, 142
Thiethylperazine (Torecan), as antiemetic, 167
6-Thioguanine (6-TG), 224
Thiopental (Pentothal)
  as anesthetic, 87, 97
  in carotid endarterectomy, 88
  CNS and, 91
  onset of action of, 10
  rate of distribution of, 12
  tissue localization of, 11
Thioridazine (Mellaril)
  anticholinergic effects of, 62

Thioridazine (Mellaril)—Continued
  gastrointestinal effects of, 62
  neuroleptic properties, 61, 62
  structure of, 61
  toxic effects of, 242
Thiothixene, 64
Thromboxanes, metabolism of, 183
Thrombus formation inhibitors, 128
  heparin and, 129
Thymosin
  in Di George's syndrome, 220
  in T-cell–deficiency states, 220
Thyroglobulin (Proloid), 151
Thyroid hormone deficiency, 150, 152
Thyroid hormones, 149–153
  antagonists, 151–152
  diseases associated with, 149–150, 152
  physiologic effects of, 150–151
  synthesis of, 149, 150
Thyroid preparations, 151
Thyroid-stimulating hormone (TSH), 149
  cyclic AMP and, 188
Thyrotoxic crisis, 152
Thyrotoxicosis, 149
  treatment of, 152
Thyrotropin-releasing hormone (TRH), 149
  cyclic AMP and, 188
Thyroxine (T$_4$)
  in Hashimoto's thyroiditis, 152
  as lipid-lowering agent (Choloxin), 136
  synthesis of, 149, 150
Ticarcillin, 202, 203
Tienilic acid (Ticrynafen), 115
Timolol, 45
Tissue localization of drugs, 11
Tobramycin (Nebcin)
  actions of, 205
  structure of, 205
  uses of, 206
Tocainide, 109, 111
Tolazamide (Tolinase), 26, 142
Tolbutamide (Orinase), 142
Tolerance, definition of, 29
Tolmetin (Tolectin), 84
Toxicity, 241–244
  acute and chronic, 241–242
  age-related, 242–244
    geriatric, 243–244
    neonatal, 243
    nursing infants, 243
    paranatal, 243
    prenatal, 242–243
  metabolite formation, 18
  organ-specific and generalized, 241, 242
  rapid and delayed, 242
  reversible and irreversible, 242
  therapeutic index and, 16
Toxicology, 241
Toxoplasmosis, 199, 235
Tranquilizers, major. See Neuroleptics
Transderm-Nitro, 126
Transport mechanisms, 7, 8